AF541235

GLOBAL HEALTH CARE SYSTEMS AND MANAGEMENT

Contemporary Trends

GLOBAL HEALTH CARE SYSTEMS AND MANAGEMENT

Contemporary Trends

DR. R. KUMAR
MBBS, MS, (Ophthal.) Ex. PGI
Author of Books on Health Care, Hospitals, Women Empowerment, NGOs, Social Sciences, Health, Fiction, Biography, etc.
Columnist on Health Education, Medical Tourism and Management.

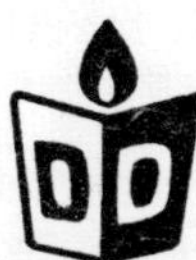

DEEP & DEEP PUBLICATIONS PVT. LTD.
F-159, Rajouri Garden, New Delhi-110027

GLOBAL HEALTH CARE SYSTEMS AND MANAGEMENT

ISBN 978-81-8450-322-7

Typeset by S.S. COMPOSERS
3190, Mohindra Park, Shakur Basti, Delhi-110034.

Printed in India at MAYUR ENTERPRISES
WZ Plot No. 3, Gujjar Market, Tihar Village, New Delhi-110018.

Published by DEEP & DEEP PUBLICATIONS PVT. LTD.
F-159, Rajouri Garden, New Delhi-110027.
Phones: 25435369, 25440916
E-mail: ddpbooks@yahoo.co.in • ddpubs@gmail.com
Showroom:
2/13, Ansari Road, Daryaganj, New Delhi-110002 • Telefax: 23245122

Contents

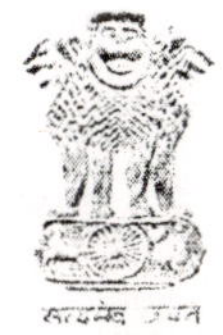

डॉ विश्व मोहन कटोच
एम डी, एफ एन ए एससी, एफ ए एम एस, एफ ए एससी, एफ एन ए
सचिव, भारत सरकार
(स्वास्थ्य अनुसंधान विभाग)
स्वास्थ्य एवं परिवार कल्याण मंत्रालय एवं
महानिदेशक, आई सी एम आर
Dr. Vishwa Mohan Katoch
MD, FNASc, FAMS, FASc, FNA
Secretary to the Government of India
(Department of Health Research)
Ministry of Health & Family Welfare &
Director-General, ICMR

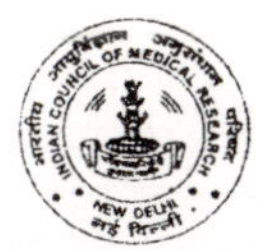

भारतीय आयुर्विज्ञान अनुसंधान परिषद
(स्वास्थ्य अनुसंधान विभाग)
स्वास्थ्य एवं परिवार कल्याण मंत्रालय
वी. रामलिंगस्वामी भवन, अंसारी नगर
नई दिल्ली - 110 029 (भारत)

Indian Council of Medical Research
(Department of Health Research)
Ministry of Health & Family Welfare
V. Ramalingaswami Bhawan, Ansari Nagar
New Delhi - 110 029 (INDIA)

Foreword

It is my pleasure to write this foreword for "Global Health Care Systems and Management". This book has chapters which deal with overview of healthcare systems around the globe, healthcare systems in India as well as other third world countries and western world including United States. There is a beautiful description of primary healthcare system. The topics on outsourcing and health tourism are contemporary and have immense value from the point of view of developing public-private partnerships and creating health infrastructure which will serve not only the needs of our population but also serve as a self-sustaining industry.

Our public health system has served very well in improving the health standards of our population. The ultimate goal of our endeavors should be to strengthen our system so as to control communicable as well as non-communicable diseases and march towards early achievement of millennium development goals. This would require a good blend of horizontal and vertical programming which has been nicely discussed in this book.

I am sure that this volume will provide useful material to the readers that will enable them in contributing better towards development of efficient healthcare systems in our country. I compliment the author and his team for this excellent effort.

(V.M. KATOCH)

Preface

Affluent sections, elite urban populations and those working in the organized sector who are covered under some form of social security such as Employee State Insurance Scheme and Central Government Health scheme, have unlimited access to medical services in India. The rural population and those working in the unorganized sector have only the tax-based public facilities to depend upon for free or subsidized care, and private facilities depending on their ability to pay. Unfortunately, 80-85% of the medical care is now based on out-of-pocket expenses. The scale of such expenses for each visit or intervention is also rising. Resultantly, poverty and indebtness on this account is also rising in the vulnerable segments of populations. This increased poverty is further impacting their health and capacity to purchase medical care. Similar situation prevails in other third world countries. Western countries spend more on their health care and their health care systems are also better organized.

The World Health Organization (WHO) defines a health system as "all the activities whose primary purpose is to promote, restore, or maintain health." The World Bank defines health systems more broadly to include factors interrelated to health, such as poverty, education, infrastructure and the broader social and political environment. Developing countries face many challenges to building robust, reliable health systems. These challenges include insufficient financing, lack of inter-agency coordination, poorly-functioning information systems, health worker shortages and supply interruptions. A nation's health care system can encompass many specialties. Interventions range from emergency care, to chronic disease management, to cancer therapy treatment. Dementia care, disability services and mental health strategies must all be accounted for too. Getting the infrastructure in place is far from easy. The politicians and officials who are more concerned with lining their own pockets rather than establishing care for the citizens, and they have held back the development of effective health care systems.

Horizontal Programming

Primary health care model emphasizes a horizontal and systematic approach—a model promoted by the Alma Ata declaration of 1978. The primary care model highlights the importance of equitable and general care for a population. It focuses on the collective needs of the community, and depends upon higher institutions for advanced health care provisions. In 2008, the WHO re-emphasized the need for a primary care approach. The main distinction between horizontal and vertical programming is that horizontal efforts emphasize a health system with comprehensive care and a primary provider at the core, while vertical programs focus on preventing or treating individual diseases or working with specific populations. There is merit to both approaches, as horizontal programs are needed to coordinate health care services and address multiple health issues, and vertical approaches can lead to dramatic progress on specific diseases. The Global Fund to Fight AIDS, Tuberculosis and Malaria, and the Global Alliance for Vaccines and Immunizations are now actively helping strengthen health systems in countries in which they work. WHO's "New Universalism" approach also combines primary care with organizational approaches and considers the specific burdens of disease in each country.

Primary Health Care (PHC)

To improve health and to reduce the global burden of disease, it is of utmost importance to strengthen PHC. The ultimate goal of primary health care is better health for all. WHO has identified five key elements to achieving that goal:

- reducing exclusion and social disparities in health, i.e. universal coverage;
- organizing health services around people's needs and expectations;
- integrating health into all sectors (public policy reforms);
- pursuing collaborative models of policy dialogue; and
- increasing stakeholder participation.

Countries with better provision of primary health care have greater patient satisfaction at lower costs and better health indicators.

India Suffers from Double Whammy

Andhra, Karnataka, W. Bengal and Punjab—represent different stages in the Indian health transition. West Bengal faces high incidence of communicable diseases. Prosperous states, such as Punjab further along the health transition are facing sharply increasing incidence of non-communicable diseases especially, in urban areas. The projections highlight that we are still operating on unreliable or incomplete data base on mortality and causes of death in the absence of vital registration statistics and know as yet little about how they differ between social classes and regions or about the dynamic patterns of change at work. It also highlights the policy dilemma of how to balance between the articulate upper middle class demand for more access to technologically advanced and subsidized clinical services and the more pressing needs of the poor for coverage of basic disease control interventions. This conflict over deployment of public resources will only get exacerbated in future.

Universal Health Care

It refers to access of health services by every citizen of a country. It could be by a combination of public and private systems. Germany, for example, has universal coverage, and social insurance plans cover the majority of people. Government only subsidizes 15 per cent of the costs of the funds. There are also 42 private insurers that cover 9 per cent of the total population, viz. those in upper income brackets who are excluded from the public social-insurance programs. Netherlands, which has a similar system, has deemed that 35 per cent of its population is ineligible for the social insurance programs due to high income.

Need for Public Health Reforms

The health care scenario is less than satisfactory all over the world, though the developed countries offer much better care than the third world countries. It is also a fact that need for primary health care (PHC) improvement is much more than tertiary care in all the countries. There is no doubt every society requires most modern infrastructure and technology for its sick to be treated, in case they fall seriously ill. However, preventive care and primary care assumes greater significance in the context of large populations. The PHC movement has seen a critical success in that it has contributed to the recognition of the social value of health systems, which has now taken hold in most countries in the world. This change of mindset has created a radically different health-policy landscape. Present-day health systems are a patchwork of components, many of which may be far removed from the goals set out 30 years ago. These same health systems are converging. Driven by the demographic, financial and social pressures of modernization, they increasingly share the aims of improved health equity, people-centered care, and a better protection of the health of their populations.

Today, it is possible to make a stronger case for health than in previous times. This is not only because of intrinsic values, such as health equity, or for the sector's contribution to economic growth, however, valid they may be, these arguments are not always the most effective—but on political grounds. Health constitutes an economic sector of growing importance in itself and a feature of development and social cohesion. Reliable protection against health threats and equitable access to quality health care when needed are among the most central demands people make on their governments in advancing societies. However, in third world countries like India, health and health care both are given back seat.

The author has presented his case for better management of health care worldwide in the following chapters:

1. Health Care Systems around the Globe; 2. Primary Health Care: Definition, Concept and Principles; 3. Health Care Systems in India; 4. Health Care in Third World Countries; 5. Health Care Systems in the

Western World; 6. United States Health Care System; 7. Universal Health Care Systems in the World; 8. Health Reforms; Good Primary Health Care is the way Forward; 9. Political commitment and Primary Health Care; 10. Outsourcing as a Health Care System: Health Tourism.

Chandigarh DR. R. KUMAR

1

Health Care Systems Around the Globe

There are several types of health care management systems in the world. Generally health care is better in the economically better-off countries and poor in the third world countries. Such inequalities are also prevalent in different regions of the same country or state and there is an urban-rural divide as well. While economic factors are important, the governance of health care and people's participation are also important. The development and industrialization of a nation usually heralds the basic improvements in public health—sanitization, immunizations, safer childbirth and universal access to health care. But even in the most developed of nations, for those with access to the greatest resources, the standard of care can vary greatly dependent on several other factors. Money does not necessarily mean quality; instead it may mean unnecessary over-intervention, especially if practitioners are incentivized on pay-for-performance models e.g. USA. And if the quest for quality is not at the core of a health care system, no amount of cash can make for safe and efficient practice.

—Dr. Sneh Khemka, Bupa International

The objectives of a health system are to respond to people's needs and expectations by providing services in a fair and equitable manner.[1] The World Health Organization defines a health system as "all the activities whose primary purpose is to promote, restore, or maintain health."[2,3] The World Bank defines health systems more broadly to include factors interrelated to health, such as poverty, education, infrastructure and the broader social and political environment.[4] Developing countries face many challenges to building robust, reliable health systems. These challenges include insufficient financing, lack of inter-agency coordination, poorly-functioning information systems, health worker shortages and supply interruptions.

- The health care worker shortage limits the ability of many countries to meet the (Millennium Development Goals) MDGs. The shortage weakens existing health care delivery systems and inhibits expansion of services. For example, in 15 countries in sub-Saharan Africa there are five or fewer physicians per 100,000 people.
- Both public and private sectors have a role to play in addressing the complex and unique challenges faced by developing countries to develop and maintain effective health systems issues. In many countries, only less than half of the population has access to public health services.
- Health systems strengthening aims to improve health by responding to people's needs and expectations, and by providing services in a fair and equitable manner. Interventions include improving leadership and governance, ensuring a steady supply of medical products and creating more effective and efficient delivery systems.[7]
- Health systems research identifies challenges in providing care and delivering interventions at all levels of health systems and provides innovative solutions to improve the delivery of care. Confronting these challenges in settings where health infrastructure is crumbling on multiple fronts requires targeted research on health systems and health policy.[8]

High-income Countries Spend more on Health Care

Health care is a huge industry, requiring vast sums of money to span preventative, primary and specialist care. Most developed nations spend at least 10 percent of their gross domestic product on health care, and this is rising every year. In the US the figure is now reckoned to be closer to 20 percent. A study published in *The Lancet* had highlighted this. The researchers compared cancer survival rates across five continents. They found that people in high-income countries that spend more on health care live longer. And it's well known that life expectancy in developing nations is frequently lower than that of richer nations.

One of the keys to good medical treatment is sanitization. It was the industrial revolution of the 19th century and the introduction of sewers and basic hygiene, followed by the subsequent discovery of antibiotics, that allowed people to survive diseases and infections that would otherwise have killed. And the necessary 'tools of the trade'—sterilization methods, disinfectants, antibiotics, even running water—aren't always available in poorer countries. Inevitably, standards of care suffer. Even when a country has the requisite hygiene procedures, the drugs needed to treat patients aren't always available. Poorer countries may simply be unable to afford them. There's a commonly held view that the pharmaceutical industry is a root cause of health care inequality. For patients to have access to any drug, someone has to manufacture them. And that costs money. Pharmaceutical companies defend their prices by citing the huge sums spent on research and development. With new drugs taking 10 to 15 years to bring to market, they argue that losses need to be recuperated. Given the recent and very real challenge of widespread counterfeit medicines being produced and distributed widely in Asia, it is fair to predict that access to effective medicines will continue to flame the fires of our health care industry.

A nation's health care system can encompass many specialties. Interventions range from emergency care, to chronic disease management, to cancer therapy treatment. Dementia care, disability services and mental health strategies must all be accounted for too. Getting the infrastructure in place is far from easy. Politicians and officials more concerned with lining their own pockets than establishing care for their citizens, and they have held back the development of effective health care systems. When incentivized in the wrong way or in a system where supply is more than demand, more is often done than is needed. Certain surgical interventions are performed not dependent on actual need, but more on surgeon preference or profit. That means that patients undergo procedures they don't need and don't want. Staying knowledgeable, seeking wide information about your own condition, keeping healthy and ultimately knowing who to go to when you do need to access health care are the keys to be a winner.

The Six Building Blocks of a Health Care System

In 2007, the World Health Organization (WHO) drafted a framework to guide efforts to strengthen health systems. This framework identifies six components needed to establish, sustain and strengthen a health system while allowing it to provide needed services, universal access to those services and universal coverage of health care benefits.

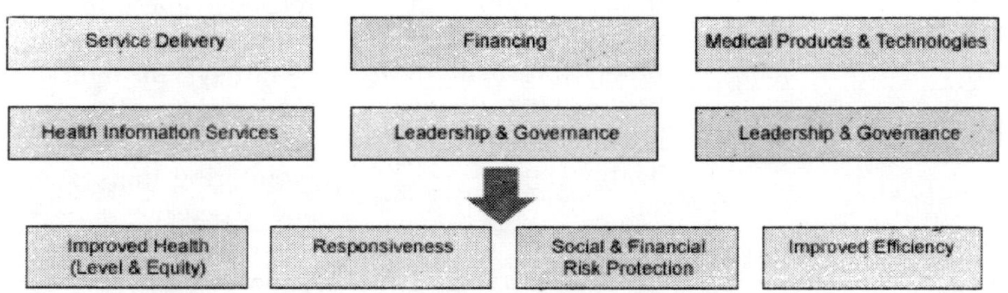

The overall goal of this framework is to provide a spectrum of needed services, provide universal access to those services, and to provide universal coverage of health care benefits. The building blocks provide means of describing the attributes needed to establish and sustain health systems. Focusing on integrating and improving these six components of a health system is, in fact, the definition of strengthening health systems.

The Goals of the Building Blocks[3,4]

Building Block	*Description*	*Goal*
Service Delivery	Effective provision of health interventions to people needing them, with a minimum waste of resources.	Improved health equity and health status, through organized and managed access to care.
Health Workforce	Adequately trained and equipped health workers that provide fair and equitable access to needed services.	Increased responsiveness by health workers and national plans to ensure quality workforce scale-up.
Financing	Adequately funded health systems that ensure service delivery and protect systems from financial disaster.	Financial risk protection while providing accessible services and sustainable scale-up.
Medical Products and Technologies	Equitable access to safe, effective and affordable drugs, supplies, tools and other products.	Increased responsiveness by providing reliable product stream and effective regulations.
Health Information System	Production, analysis, dissemination, and use of reliable and timely information on health determinants, health systems and health status.	Increased responsiveness to people by establishing health system metrics for surveying the population, monitoring the system, and disease surveillance.
Leadership and Governance	Institutes strategic, integrated policy frameworks; sets monitoring, regulative and accountability measures; and designs and coordinates coalitions and systems.	Improved efficacy, providing policy guidance and defining the government's role with regard to the other players.

Another major component of the WHO framework focuses on ensuring that components and key players in health systems and health outcome programs work effectively together:[5]

- Making sure advice to countries is provided in a "systems" context rather than in a disease-specific context.
- Providing examples of activities (programs, good practice, and building capacity) that can be integrated, providing a more sustainable program.
- Bringing together program and systems expertise—linking multiple program components.
- Extending current relationships and communicating about how to work through activities.
- Reporting information that can be used to assess both process and outcomes—monitoring and evaluating how components work together and how this impacts health outcomes.

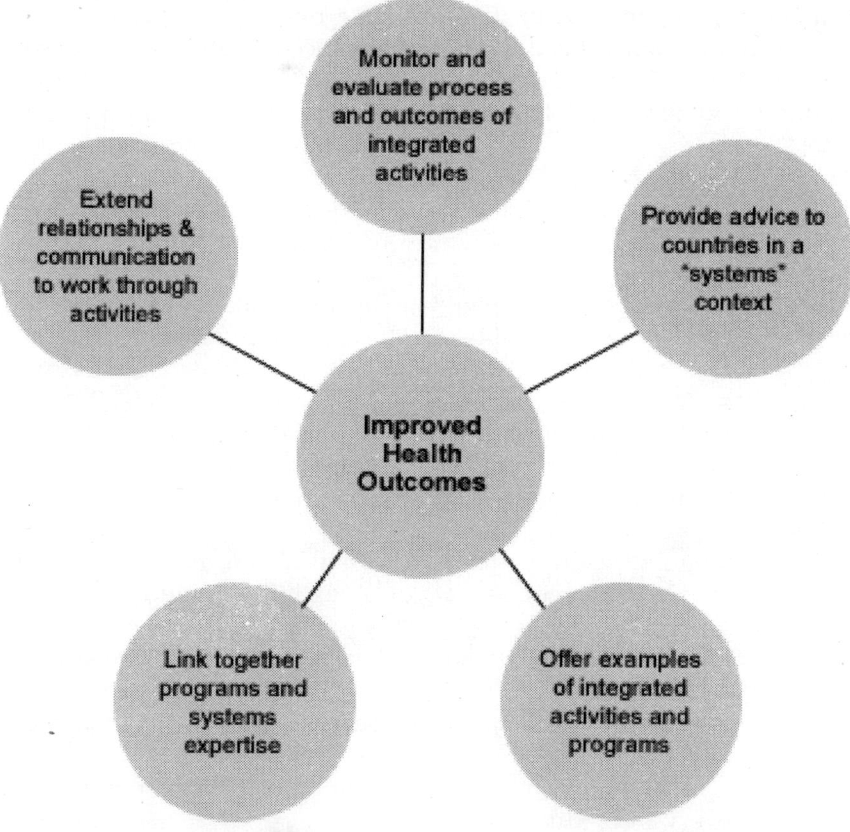

Horizontal and Vertical Programming

The main distinction between horizontal and vertical programming is that horizontal efforts emphasize a health system with comprehensive care and a primary provider at the core, while vertical programs focus on preventing or treating individual diseases or working with specific populations. There is merit to both approaches, as horizontal programs are needed to coordinate health care services and address multiple health issues, and vertical approaches can lead to dramatic progress on specific diseases. In examining a cross between the horizontal and vertical approach, The Global Fund to Fight AIDS, Tuberculosis and Malaria, and the Global Alliance for Vaccines and Immunizations Alliance are now actively helping strengthen health systems in countries in which they work. WHO's "New Universalism" approach also combines primary care with organizational approaches and considers the specific burdens of disease in each country.

The primary care model emphasizes a horizontal and systematic approach—a model promoted by the Alma Ata declaration of 1978.[6,7] The primary care model highlights the importance of equitable and general care for a population, focuses on the collective needs of the community, and depends upon higher institutions for advanced health care provision. In 2008, the WHO reemphasized the need for a primary care approach. It identified and discussed four important components of the primary care model.[8]

- *Service delivery*: increase response to community needs by increasing number and quality of community health care centers.
- *Universal coverage*: eliminate health inequalities by providing fair and accessible health care to every individual.
- *Leadership*: interactive and engaged health care leadership in all society sectors.
- *Public policy*: engage with policy-makers to increase awareness of the impact of public policy on people's health and to establish policies that positively influence health.

In evaluating health systems, accessibility is a major concern. Under the right to health, the four aspects of accessibility include:

- *Financial accessibility*: quality health services are affordable for all constituents
- *Physical accessibility*: health services are within realistic reach and distance of the population they serve.
- *Non-discrimination*: the same health services can be accessed by every individual.
- *Information accessibility*: obtaining information to educate about risks and prevention tactics for different diseases.

Assessments of primary care programs in developing countries indicated shortfalls in accessibility:

- Services were often limited for the poor, particularly in rural areas, resulting in limited use of care.
- Funding, training and equipment deficiencies made it difficult to provide even basic services.
- Services did not meet people's actual needs and services in demand were not part of the basic set of services.

The vertical or disease-specific approach focuses on the elements of health care specific to a disease or component of care, such as vaccinations.[5,9] This approach can be characterized by a single outcome focus and independent management and funding streams. For example:

- The Global Fund to Fight AIDS, Tuberculosis and Malaria is a public/private partnership that garners resources to combat three specific diseases: AIDS, malaria and tuberculosis.
- The GAVI Alliance has a single-outcome focus to improve and increase access to vaccines.

Who is most affected by Poor Health Systems

The populations that are most adversely affected from an ineffective health system are children and the elderly because they are more susceptible to illness and have limited access to resources. The lack of appropriately trained providers in countries with an increasing elderly population puts older people at risk. For example, in China, where physicians outnumber nurses, access to geriatric care is reduced because nurses play a critical role in caring for this age group.(10) To highlight the needs of children, the United Nations identified improvement in child health as one of the Millennium Development Goals. In order to strengthen child health services, WHO/UNICEF's Integrated Management of Childhood Illness (IMCI) and UNICEF's Accelerated Child Survival and Development Strategy (ACSD) combine and integrate interventions that address major contributors of childhood morbidity and mortality, including malaria, nutrition, diarrheal diseases and respiratory illnesses.

Migrant groups are also negatively affected by inadequate health systems because they tend to fall through the gaps of service provision. China, for example, has 140 million internal migrants and the decentralization of its national health policy makes it difficult for this population to access and afford health care.[11]

Impact of Trade and Poverty on Health Systems

With the dawn of globalization, trade is becomingly increasingly important to health systems through its impact on poverty and policies. Health workers, herbal medicine and pharmaceuticals are now growing commodities.[12] Trade policies and relations are directly and indirectly impacting health and health systems:

- For national health systems, pharmaceutical costs are the largest health expenditure after staff.[13,14]
- Minimizing tariffs and reducing trade measures that serve as barriers to access health commodities can contribute to the healthier populations.

Challenges of Health Care Workers

Although there are an estimated 100 million health care workers worldwide, there is a projected shortage of more than 4 million workers.[15] The World Health Organization (WHO) defines a health care worker (HCW) as anyone whose focus or activity is to improve health. This definition includes providers (e.g., doctors, paramedical staff, nurses and midwives) as well as technicians and managers.[17-19]

The nine categories of health care personnel are:[20]

1. Physicians
2. Nurses and Midwives
3. Dentists and dental assistants
4. Pharmacists
5. Laboratory scientists and technicians
6. Environment and public health workers
7. Community health workers and traditional healers
8. Other health care providers
9. Health managers and support workers

Adequate health care provision depends on the availability of resources to retain health care workers and the availability of health care workers to manage the flow of those resources. In recent years, international donors and organizations have increased attention to funding for medical supplies, technology and management. However, the shortage of health care workers is a barrier in managing the flow of these resources.[15,16.17,18,19]

- In 15 countries in sub-Saharan Africa, there are five or fewer physicians per 100,000 people—below the recommended 20 physicians per 100,000.
- In 17 countries in sub-Saharan Africa, there are 50 or fewer nurses per 100,000 people—below the recommended 100 nurses per 100,000.
- Vaccination coverage is directly linked to the density of nurses and other health-related human resources and is almost entirely independent of physicians.

- Countries with less than 2.5 HCWs per 1,000 people were unable to provide 80% coverage for measles immunizations and deliveries by skilled birth attendants.

Effective health care provision is an interdependent flow that is affected by many factors. Reasons for shortages and unbalanced skill gaps among the health care workforce are:[20]

- Migration of health care workers within and between countries.
- The growing demands of the HIV/AIDS epidemic.
- Inadequate or ineffectual governmental policies and bureaucratic systems.
- Lack of public resources.
- Unregulated private labour markets.

Millennium Development Goals (MDGs)

- The health care worker shortage compromises the inability of many countries to meet the MDGs by weakening existing health care delivery systems.[21]
- Providing essential maternal and child health interventions is particularly dependent on trained health workers.

Impact of Health Care Workers on Maternal, Child and Infant Survival

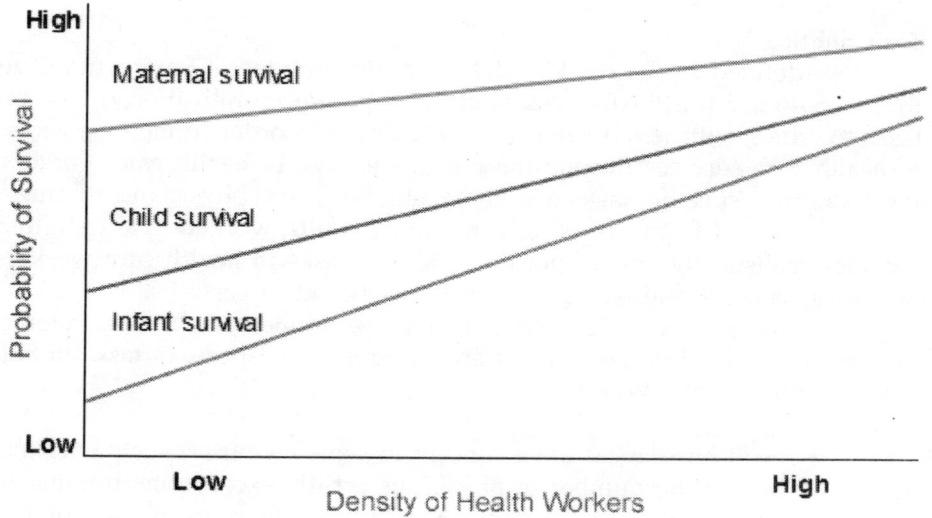

HIV/AIDS and Infectious Diseases

Emerging high-priority situations, such as the increasing treatment and care of HIV/AIDS patients, require sufficient workforce mobilization without weakening the existing primary health care systems.

- In sub-Saharan Africa, even though one medical assistant may treat as many as 200 HIV/AIDS patients per day, more than 70 percent of patients needing ARVs lack access to proper treatment.
- In some countries, the shortage of clinicians results in HIV patients waiting up to two months to start treatment.[22]
- In 17 countries with high prevalence of tuberculosis, staffing problems hindered disease control efforts and has reduced their likelihood of achieving the 2005 WHO targets.

Keys to Workforce Development

All country programs for workforce development should include involving government leaders and financial contributors, preparing for and managing an increase in workforce through policies and investments, and evaluating performance of health care workers. Raising awareness among key stakeholders is a key component of workforce development, as are policies promoting and investments in health systems. Among the players who should be involved in this process are ministers of finance, health and education; academic leaders and educational institutions; professional associations and labour unions; and non-governmental organizations.

The Global Health Workforce Alliance campaign is designed to combat health worker shortages and skill gaps. The campaign ensures that health workers have access to HIV prevention methods and funding for training and retention of health workers.[23]

Task Shifting[24]

As defined by WHO, UNAIDS and the President's Emergency Plan for AIDS Relief (PEPFAR), task shifting is the decentralization of certain tasks to others with less overall medical training in order to increase access to health care services despite the global shortage of health care workers. For example, specific tasks could be shifted from physicians to nurse practitioners and from nurses to community health workers. Task shifting includes realistically and responsibly shifting tasks to health care workers or others who are trained to deliver a specific set of services.

Adequate supervision, competency requirements, effective referral systems and patient empowerment are all important aspects of task shifting recommended by the WHO.

- Skill imbalances are a concern in some countries, such as China, where the number of physicians greatly exceeds the number of nurses. With an increasing elderly population, nurses play a critical role in geriatric care.[25] Task shifting can be used in this situation to increase geriatric services despite lower nurse density.

- Partners in Health, an organization working on health issues, describes task shifting as a "cornerstone of health care model," where community health workers will take on some physician responsibilities, among other duties. All staff in a task shifting position are financially compensated for their responsibilities.[26]

While task shifting may be optimal in some situations, there are some potential risks. Some concerns of task shifting are:[27,28]

- Standardizing task shifting instead of creating a country or community-level specific program.
- Lack of program flexibility to change with community needs and technology.
- Blurring of health professional roles leading to untrained workers in high competency positions.
- Shortage or absence of health workers to train and supervise newly trained workers.
- Taking jobs from qualified health workers; task shifting is intended to alleviate shortages.
- Inefficient shifting of tasks that reduces quality of care and slows down health systems.
- Increased responsibilities for already overburdened lower-level health workers.
- Lack of sustainable task shifting programs due to worker burnout or inadequate funding.

Internal Migration and Brain Drain

Africa is home to nearly 25 percent of the global burden of disease, but only has 3 percent of the total global health workforce. In contrast, America contain close to 40 percent of the total global health workforce, but only exhibit around 10 percent of the global burden of disease.[29]

Global Disease Burden and Health Care Workforce

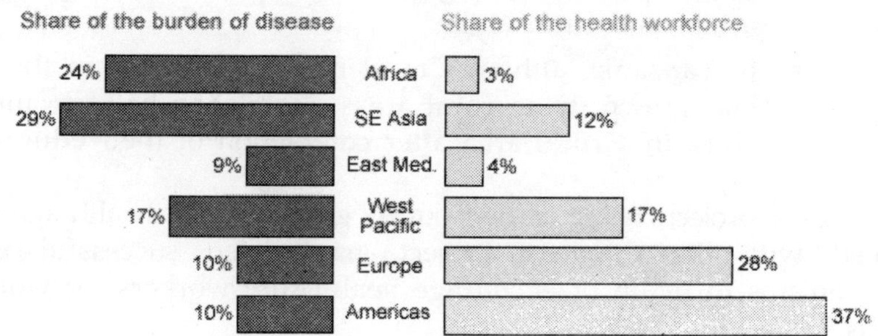

Low-income to High-income Countries

Fifty-seven of the world's poorest countries have a health care worker shortage of 2.4 million doctors, nurses and midwives. In Africa alone, there is a shortage of 1.5 million health care workers. Several high-income countries also face a shortage of health care workers. Health care workers from developing countries may leave their own countries to fill these positions, which provide better compensation and potential incentives. More than 25 percent of all doctors working in Canada, New Zealand, the United Kingdom and the United States have come from other countries; one in four physicians educated in Africa have left their home countries for a higher-income country.[30]

The Philippines is one of the world's largest exporters of health workers, making this one of the country's most important exports.[31]

- Eight out of 10 Filipino physicians plan to pursue careers overseas, mainly as nurses, in developed countries where nurses receive higher pay than a public physician in the Philippines.
- Of Filipino nursing students, 60 percent are educated professionals that have left their jobs to become nurses in other countries.
- The number of nursing schools in the Philippines has almost tripled during the past two decades.
- This shift in health workforce has been detrimental for the Filipino health system as 70 percent of the population die without the necessary health care.

Rural to Urban Areas

For developing countries, the internal migration of health care workers from rural to urban areas is a major concern, as access to health care services among rural populations is reduced. More than 75 percent of physicians, 60 percent of nurses and nearly 60 percent of other health service providers are located in urban centers. Yet over half of the global population lives in rural areas.

- In China, about 68 percent of all health professionals are located in urban areas, leaving more than a two-fold inequality between urban and rural areas.[11]
- In Tanzania, although most medical students in the final year had grown up in rural areas, more than half are unwilling to work in a rural area after completion of their education.[32]

Pilot projects being carried out by governmental health agencies; some linked with the Capacity Project, have been successful in finding mechanisms to retain or encourage health care workers for work in rural areas.[32]

- In Zambia, compensation for school costs and financial incentives for those physicians willing to work in rural areas where shown to increase the number of doctors in rural areas by 53 in two years.
- In Kenya, health worker satisfaction increased by 30 percent in 10 rural areas after the implementation of inexpensive actions to improve worker environment conditions.

Public to Private Sector

Health care workers may leave the public sector to work for a nongovernmental organization or another private entity.[33] Private sector salaries may be considerably higher than public sector wages, making it easier to support a family when employed by the private sector. In addition to low wages, public sector jobs may lack continuing education opportunities, have poor supervision and management systems and lack the basic equipment and supplies (including medications) needed to provide effective care for patients while incorporating worker safety protocols. These conditions contribute to worker dissatisfaction and fear of being infected with HIV or other diseases. Several recent initiatives, including the President's Emergency Plan for AIDS Relief and the Global Fund to Fight AIDS, Tuberculosis and Malaria, provide increased health care coordination, infrastructure and funding.

Contributing Factors to Health Worker Migration[30]

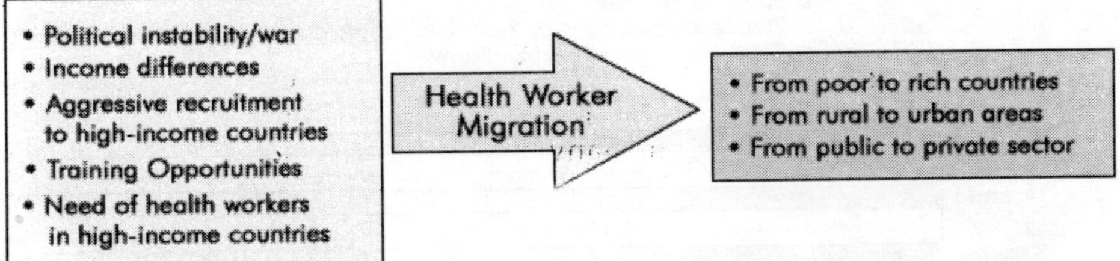

To prevent the migration of health care workers, more sustainable incentives, improved working environments, and opportunities for advanced training and certification are needed to mitigate the migration from rural areas and from developing countries. To reduce the need to import health care workers from developing countries, high-income countries need to train a greater number of health workers to meet their growing need.

Need for Private Health Care

It is increasingly apparent that health needs cannot be met through reliance on public (government) resources alone. In fact, in many counties, less than half of the population has access to public health services.[34] The private sector provides an alternative and complementary means of expanding health services, products and infrastructure. However, the private sector is not a panacea. Both public and private sector actors have roles to play in addressing the complex and unique challenges faced by developing countries to develop and maintain effective health systems issues.

Public and Private Health Expenditures in Some African Countries, Total and Percent[35]

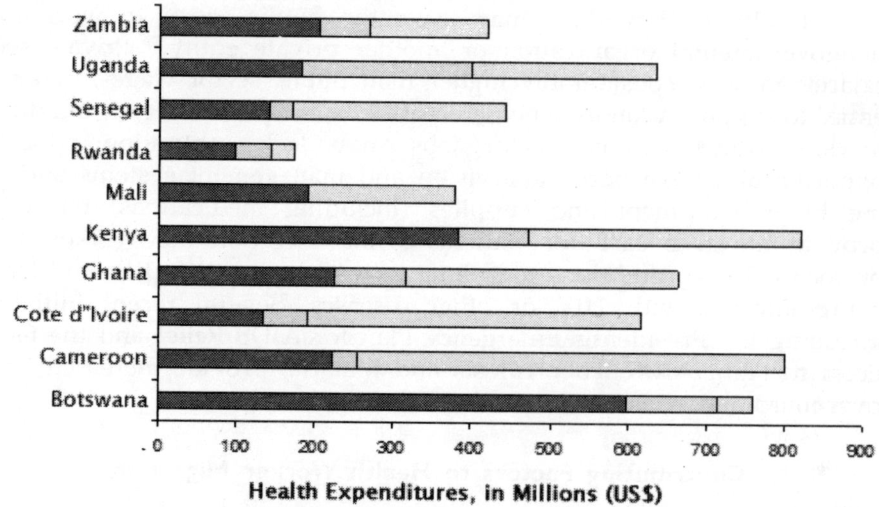

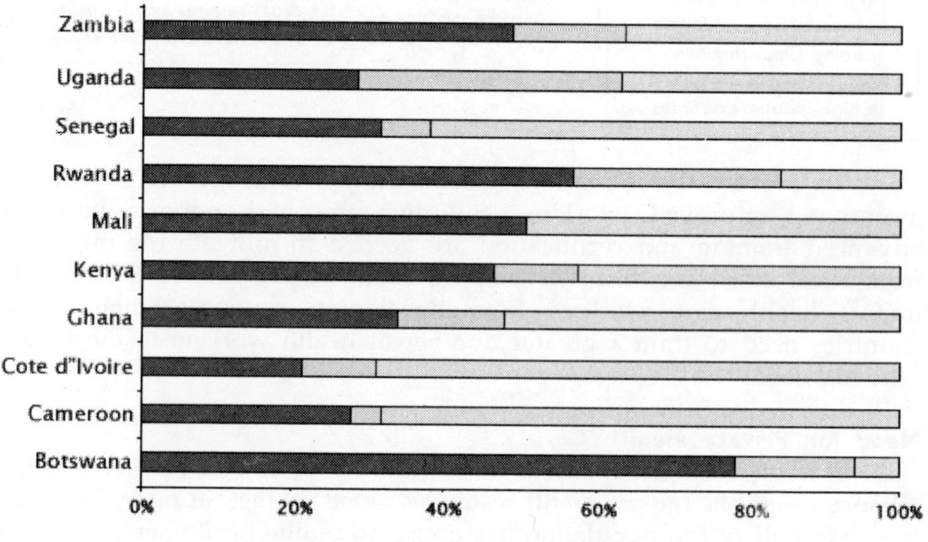

The Public Sector

The public sector has several responsibilities related to health care provision, including:

- Direct service provision;
- Regulate the health care industry and medical products; and
- Provide incentives to make services affordable, maintain a skilled workforce and ensure research and development of new products.

The public sector is responsible for providing direct goods and services to the population. In many countries, the government plays a central role in building and managing health systems, including hospitals, clinics, human resources, medical equipment, supply chains, storage facilities and general infrastructure. The largest overall use of public health funds is allocated to human resources and nearly half of total health spending is allocated to pharmaceutical companies in some developing countries.[36,37] The government also plays a key role in health care financing, by providing insurance, subsidies and conditional cash transfer programs. Increasingly, the management and supervision of health systems is becoming decentralized, with authority shifting from the centralized government to regional and district offices.

Governments play an important role in regulating and energizing the private sector. Regulatory mandates are necessary to monitor and maintain the quality of private sector services, but overregulation may stifle private sector growth. Regulation is also necessary for licensing or certifying health care providers, pharmacies, laboratories and pharmaceuticals.[38]

- Standard drug regulations and a common regulatory framework implemented by the government may also make it easier for private sector companies to register drugs and other health products.[39]
- Legal restrictions on the marketing, distribution or prescription of health care products, such as contraceptives, may also prevent private sector manufacture and distribution. For example, many countries in West Africa ban specific types of advertising for contraceptives and do not permit physicians to fill contraceptive prescriptions.[40]

The government can also provide financial incentives for private sector growth. Government and donor subsidies can encourage the private sector to provide specific services, particularly for impoverished populations.[38] Although some national tax policies and tariffs may limit private sector activities, tax breaks and monetary incentives for the purchase and distribution of essential medicines can also foster private sector growth.

The Private Sector

Composed of "all providers who exist outside the public sector, whether their aim is philanthropic or commercial and whose aim is to treat illness or prevent disease," the private sector receives funding through alternative (non-governmental) streams.[40] Although both public and private sector entities seek to improve health, other objectives of those in the private sector may differ from those in the public sector—from issues related to delivering services to developing funding streams to imposing patient fees.[41] Three forms of private sector involvement exist: for-profit, not-for-profit and social enterprises. Some examples of formal and informal private sector entities are:

- Organizations that provide health services
- Corporations
- Individual health providers
- Professional associations
- National and international non-governmental organizations (NGOs)
- Charitable entities

The private sector can be further defined to include those who contribute to health systems, including retailers, private financing agents and civil society organizations.[42]

The private sector plays a significant role in providing health care services for the poor and rural populations, more specifically in Sub-Saharan Africa.41 For example:

- Of the poorest population in Sub-Saharan Africa, more than 40 percent receive their health care services from the for-profit private sector.
- More than 50 percent of rural populations in Uganda and Nigeria access their health services through the for-profit private sector.
- When faith-based organization (FBOs) participation is included, private sector health care provision increases greatly.

Traditional Medicine as Part of the Private Sector[43]

In both developing and developed countries, traditional medicine plays a significant role in primary care and is often part of the "informal" private sector. The WHO defines traditional medicine as "the sum total of knowledge, skills and practices based on the theories, beliefs and experiences indigenous to different cultures that are used to maintain health, as well as prevent, diagnose, improve or treat physical and mental illness." Traditional medicine that is not native to a population is classified as alternative medicine.

- In parts of Asia and Africa, 80 percent of the population report frequent use of traditional medicine.
- In developed countries, nearly 80 percent have used traditional medicine services.
- Herbal medicine, a form of traditional medicine, is a billion dollar industry.
- Policies for traditional medicine exist in over 100 countries, but regulating quality and safety for patient use and sustaining knowledge and resources remain challenges.

Obstacles to Private Sector Involvement

Negative attitudes toward private sector involvement may inhibit collaboration between the public and private sectors, and between for-profit and not-for-profit entities. Concerns regarding private sector involvement in health care services, particularly in developing countries, include:[41]

- Mechanisms of generating profit that may be considered price-gouging or that disproportionately affect poor populations
- Unethical management
- Inadequate diagnostic services or care and treatment
- Unsustainable provision of services

Mechanisms of Generating Profit

Attitudes toward the private sector are shaped by the actor's perceived motive for involvement in health systems work, e.g., feelings may be more negative toward for-profit *versus* not-for-profit providers. In general, for-profit providers are perceived as driven by economic gain, with little interest in providing affordable services to the poorest people, and not-for-profit providers are perceived as motivated by public interests, with a greater commitment to health equity.[44] As a result, NGOs and FBOs are sometimes categorized as civil society organizations and considered a "third sector." This third sector includes organizations that are independent of both the state and the market.[42]

Management Systems

Elements of the private sector may not be regulated and therefore may provide inconsistent and uncoordinated services to its clients, with adverse implications for disease transmission. Some corporations may be driven by efficiency and worker productivity, adopting policies that maximize profit with little regard for workers or consumers of health care services.[45]

In most developing countries, a large proportion of the population uses private sector services, especially the poor. At a household level, the continued use of private sector services is a financial burden to many clients; households may sacrifice money for other essential services or activities to seek medical assistance from private practitioners.[7] The most impoverished often go to informal providers and pay out-of-pocket for services and treatment—a pattern more pronounced in rural or remote areas.[34] For example, in Vietnam, about 3.5 percent of the population was pushed into poverty from health expenditures in both 1993 and 1998.[46]

On the positive side, larger corporations in the private sector have extensive experience in management, distribution and marketing. Private sector infrastructure and networks are well-suited to providing services, sometimes on a large scale, and can increase service coverage, even in remote or hard-to-reach areas.[47,48]

Quality and Quantity of Care

There is general concern that private sector involvement in health systems might create inequity and compromise the public sector's ability to provide services for the poorest people.[44] The view of private sector services is mixed. In some places, private practitioners are believed to provide care of questionable quality; in other places, many people think that the private sector provides better quality, more efficient health services than the public sector.[49] The perception that the private sector is more concerned with its own financial profit rather than patients' needs is strengthened when private sector clinics and hospitals are only available to people that can afford the care.

More highly qualified private practitioners prefer to work in more affluent or urban areas where salaries are higher. Thus, care available to patients in poor areas may be provided by workers with less training and poorer supervision.[50] Some private sector providers may compromise quality of services to make a profit, supplying cheaper, less effective drugs or services to their clients for a higher price.[40] These practices may result in the development of drug resistance or an increased risk of chronic illness.[51]

Sustainable Long-term Provision of Services

Although private sector providers may be motivated to provide the best care possible to their patients, the lack of legal or moral obligation to provide comprehensive and sustained care may lead to inadequate care or an interruption of health services. Since private sector hospitals and clinics are not mandated by law to provide comprehensive care to all populations, the responsibility to provide treatment and care differ from public sector facilities. The use of multiple providers is common, with the selection of provider influenced by financial and other household factors.[47] This inconsistent and sometimes contradictory care may result in untreated illness, lack of follow-up care, and the development of chronic health conditions or drug resistant disease.[40]

Partnerships between Public and Private Sectors

Although there is debate regarding the roles and level of involvement of the private sector, there is general agreement that government services are overburdened and underfunded. Collaboration with the private sector can relieve pressure on public sector facilities and improve the quality of health care. In addition, the private sector could induce the public sector to improve their quality of care and upgrade incentive options.[44] The goal is to find the balance between public and private that works for the country by maximizing the strengths and minimizing the weaknesses of actors from both sectors.

Many organizations, providers and commercial companies are not exclusively "public" or "private." Non-governmental organizations can support and promote public interests, while being entirely or largely independent of the government.[42] Private foundations also advance public interests, but lack formal institutions of public accountability and oversight.[42] Doctors and nurses employed by the public sector may supplement their income as private providers and may refer public sector patients to private facilities.[40]

PPP Model

A public-private partnership is a joint project or program involving private and public collaboration to provide health services and health products.[52] This collaboration can assist the government by providing additional financial, human and management resources to scale up service coverage.[52] Research on this type of partnership indicates mixed results, e.g., contracting out may make service cheaper and expand coverage, but it requires appropriately structured and enforced contracts.[53]

Partnering between the public and private sectors takes many forms, including:

- Contracting with various actors in the other sector to produce and distribute health related products.
- Contracting with workers to provide additional training opportunities for public sector health professionals.
- Offering subsidies to the private sector for more consistent and coordinated care, and for the development of new programs and products.
- Franchising and co-investment in health care efforts to increase access to care.

Partnerships exist internationally and domestically, and can include a range of private sector actors to adequately address complex health sector needs. Given that partners have different governance structures, financial resources, culture and areas of expertise, the partnership establishes and adheres to a common understanding of roles and responsibilities in order to integrate successfully.[42] Due to the multitude of private sector services, governments and donors may have difficulties selecting the most appropriate private sector actors for partnership.[38]

There have been many efforts to incorporate the private sector in the national planning process in order to improve coordination and delivery of health care services. In many developing countries, the public sector is financially limited while the private sector continues to grow. Restrictions in the public sector are demonstrated by a scarcity of modern medical equipment and limited opportunity for the training of health professionals. By combining the finances and inventiveness of the private sector with the services and infrastructure of the public sector, there may be greater coordination, accessibility and overall quality of care.[41]

Strengthening the Health Systems

"Today, there is a growing consensus that better health systems are essential to achieving improved health outcomes."—World Health Organization.[54] In recent years, the global community has achieved an unprecedented level of attention to and investment in global health and strengthening health systems to deliver care. Defined by the World Health Organization (WHO) as "all the activities whose primary purpose is to promote, restore, or maintain health," health systems strengthening aims to improve health by responding to people's needs and expectations, and by providing services in a fair and equitable manner.[55]

Stronger health systems will make it easier to provide services to populations in need and to prevent disease. Fragile health systems have impeded the progress of disease-specific initiatives, such as those for HIV/AIDS, underscoring the idea that improved health infrastructure is critical for the effective control of many diseases.[56] More broadly, well-functioning health systems are recognized as a prerequisite to achieving the Millennium Development Goals by 2015. Leaders at the Group of 8 industrialized countries have called for increasing the capacity of weak health systems, particularly those in sub-Saharan Africa.

The focus of efforts to strengthen health systems is to integrate and improve the six components of a health system.[57] Although the subject of strengthening health systems is a global concern, there is not one simple model that applies to all communities. This variety in models needed to address the local context has presented a challenge in defining and operationalizing a strategy for strengthening health systems.

There are many actors in a health system, sometimes resulting in a lack of clarity about roles, management and responsibilities. The main leverage in strengthening health systems should come from governments because they are able to both control the public sector and monitor the private sector. Governments are key financial players in distribution and management of aid and finances to run effective health care systems. Some advocates have identified the G8 as a source to spur action for encouraging governments to focus on health systems improvement, especially with their most recent agenda to strengthen health systems in developing countries.[58,59] Providing a mechanism to evaluate programs is one way to ensure accountability and provide guidelines for further improvement. Yet, health systems lack standard metrics to gauge improvement of strengthening health systems and resources to conduct assessments. Currently the WHO has proposed an all-encompassing approach in which each country would be evaluated on a "dashboard" of indicators specific to that country.[57] A health system encompasses more than just delivery of health care, as poverty, water and sanitation systems, access to education, and environmental sustainability also play a role.[3] Some health system interventions extend beyond the scope of the health sector and include, for example, building or repairing roads and improving transportation methods so that people can travel to hospitals.[60]

Priorities

WHO has identified three objectives to strengthen health systems:[54]

- Improved quality and equity of health for the whole community.
- Increased responsiveness to the needs of the community and preservation of patient confidentiality.
- Ensured equity of affordable access through sufficient funding, providing health care for families with different financial backgrounds.

The WHO and the World Bank, among other institutions, have elucidated the different elements of health systems—leadership and governance, financing, health workforce, health information systems, service delivery and medical products and technologies—which serve to provide a spectrum of needed services, universal access to those services and universal coverage of all health care benefits.

Selected Interventions for Health Systems by Building Block

Leadership and Governance[56]

1. Impose regulations on standards of care or medicines.
2. Develop a plan for health systems with supportive policies and laws with monitoring and evaluation mechanisms.[60]
3. Ensure that managers have necessary training and skills for the job and are held accountable for successes or failures.
4. Leaders should ensure that the ministry of finance releases money in time for health systems to pay salaries, bills and purchase necessary pharmaceuticals.
5. Form coalitions in local governments comprised of representatives from health, agricultural and other development sectors that can enforce government accountability to its people.[56]
6. Create cross-sector public policies for development by starting with communities.[61]

Financing

1. Developing risk-pooling insurance schemes, such as community-based health financing.

2. Develop payment and other incentives for providers, e.g. reimburse private facilities for care for the poorest citizens.
3. Coordinate financing of health with other development issues.
4. Implement national health accounts that manage all public expenditures on health and development.

Health workforce

1. Develop a plan for human resources; standardize job descriptions, ensure that job duties are clear to employees.
2. Train workers properly on basic medical and nursing skills; assess knowledge, review performance.
3. Create incentives to retain workers and grant certifications that aren't easily transferable to other countries.
4. Train nurses, midwives to provide services normally provided by doctors, e.g. caesarean sections, to save more lives.

Health Information Systems

1. Track information and analyze data to implement effective interventions and measure outcomes.
2. Link patient databases of records to all departments to avoid duplication; keep information up-to-date and accessible.

Medical Products and Technologies

1. Policies and guidelines appropriate to populations served their resources and health infrastructure.
2. Ensure that supplies of blood, antibiotics, diagnostics, gloves, and other necessary commodities are always in stock.

Service Delivery

1. Mass drug administration campaigns; social-marketing methods or free government provision of goods.
2. Training and equipping village health teams to provide home-based care where no facilities exist.
3. Implement clean water and sanitation, environmental safety and health-related education programs, e.g. collaborate with schools to improve access to health and education jointly.[61]
4. Emphasize the importance of building capacity for local ownership of service delivery in communities, e.g., social microfranchise programs to distribute health products—such as oral rehydration salts, insecticide-treated nets and safe-birth kits.[62]

Based on proposals for health systems strengthening submitted to the Global Fund for AIDS, Tuberculosis and Malaria (the Global Fund), the three top needs are: human resources, health information systems development and facility and technology upgrades.[63]

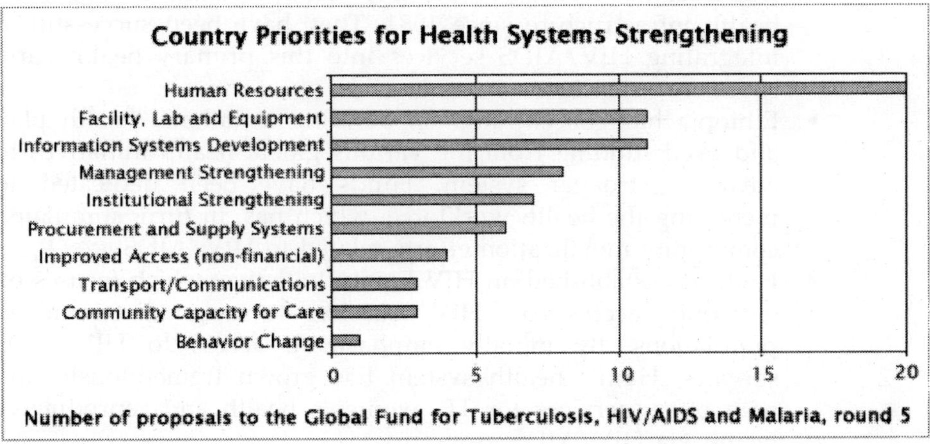

The Progress

More than 30 years ago, the Alma Ata declaration promoted the concept of a systematic approach to provide primary health care. In recent years, international organizations, governments and donors have again sought to strengthen health systems that provide essential services to all, i.e. primary health care:

- International Health Partnership and Related Activities (IHP+) is a coalition of health agencies, governments and donors committed to strengthening synergies between disease interventions and health systems.[64]
- Global AIDS Vaccine Initiative (GAVI) provides flexible, long-term funding to improve local management and leadership, infrastructure, workforce mobilization, and immunization-based systems strengthening.[65]
- The Global Fund monitors and evaluates programs' impact on health systems. Recognizing constraints on health systems, the Global Fund is considering direct funding of health systems.[66]
- U.S. Agency for International Development (USAID) focuses on policy reform, workforce development, commodity availability and appropriate use, and strengthening health information systems.[67]
- WHO and UNICEF's Integrated Management of Childhood Illness and UNICEF's Accelerated Child Survival and Development Strategy integrate interventions addressing child health problems in cohesive programs.[68]

Country-specific Improvements[63]

- Brazil's constitution includes the right to free health care for all. Recently, the Brazilian government expanded its family planning and maternal health programs.
- Dominica has focused on primary health care and an improved health infrastructure since 1981. They have been successful in integrating HIV/AIDS services into this primary health care-based infrastructure.
- Ethiopia has concentrated on building a national health plan and used funding from the various global health initiatives to create a stronger system. Funds have been dedicated to increasing the health workforce, which has, in turn, stimulated community mobilization efforts related to HIV/AIDS.
- Haiti has established an HIV Equity Initiative, which focuses on ensuring access to HIV services among discriminated populations. By initially emphasizing access to HIV/AIDS services, Haiti's health system has grown tremendously and now offers services for TB, women's health and reproductive health via HIV/AIDS programs.
- Malawi has established an Emergency Human Resource Plan to bridge the gap in funding a health workforce - resources from global health initiatives have allowed Malawi to train, task shift and pay health workers.

The Research

Weak or missing elements of the building blocks create bottlenecks to efficient and effective delivery of health care. Health systems research identifies where bottlenecks exist and provides innovative solutions to improve the delivery of care. For example, health workers need information, tools, skills and medicines to effectively deliver health care services; patients need money, subsidies or insurance to utilize them.

Practitioners and program implementers face numerous challenges in providing care and delivering interventions at all levels of health systems, but particularly at the community level. Both the need and the capacity for finding solutions are greater than ever before. Researchers, working in partnership with governments and the private sector, play an important role in developing and sustaining health systems and providing feasible solutions to systemic bottlenecks.

Select Research Needs for Health Systems by Building Block

Leadership and Governance	- On a national level, develop health priorities to guide investment and research. - At the hospital and clinic levels, examine successful interventions for management and leadership.

Financing Health Care	- Conduct long-term tests of the financial sustainability of interventions.[61,69] - Research ways to provide medical coverage for those who cannot pay out of pocket.[70,71]
Health Information Systems	- Test ways to provide accurate, reliable health information in a sustainable manner. - Research how information systems and technology investments will facilitate the management of information in all aspects of the health system and will improve the capacity for surveillance.
Health Workforce	- Train researchers across all health areas to build local capacity for research, teaching and training. - Research the impact of task shifting skills of doctors to lower-level workers on quality of care.[72]
Medical Products/ Tech.	- Research to develop effective forecasting and distribution systems for drugs and other commodities to avoid stock-outs and shortages of essential medicines.[73]
Service Delivery	- Research to identify and disseminate findings about affordable, safe and effective interventions that are widely available and to make access to health care more equitable. - Engage communities in the design of delivery mechanisms and measure results.[69]

Confronting these challenges in settings where health infrastructures are crumbling and weaknesses exist on multiple fronts requires targeted research on health systems and health policy.[74,75] Coordination and collaboration on research projects are needed to avoid duplication, maximize opportunities for data collection and comparison, and to build local capacity for health systems research in developing countries, where obstacles to care are especially problematic.

Further investigation is required to examine the impact of health systems on maternal and child mortality, access to reproductive health services and the incidence of infectious disease for Millennium Development Goals 4, 5 and 6. In addition, research is needed to establish the link and determine the impact of health systems strengthening on poverty reduction, gender equality, agricultural output and access to education, microfinance and clean water and sanitation.[60] The dissemination of research results, both positive and negative, is critical to expanding the health system in an effective and efficient manner. Improvements in the flow of information to donors, policy-makers and practitioners are needed to ensure that policy is evidence-based and to minimize the time it takes to transfer research to policy action.

A Comparison: Health Care Around the World

Healthcare comparisons

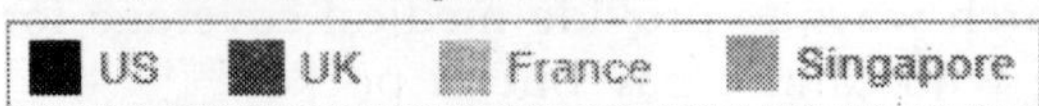

Expenditure on health % GDP

US: 16%
France: 11%
UK: 8.4%
Singapore: 3.4%

Expenditure on health, per capita US $

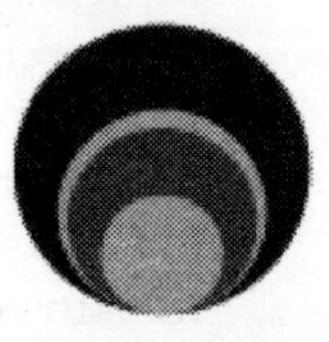

US: $7,290
France: $3,601
UK: $2,992
Singapore: $1,228

Expenditure from private sector

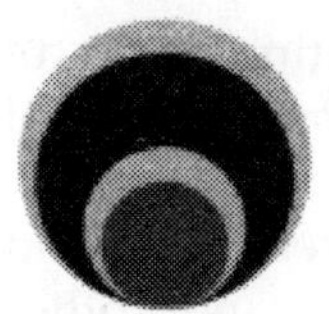

Singapore: 67.4%
US: 52.8%
France: 20.8%
UK: 12.9%

Infant mortality per 1,000 live births

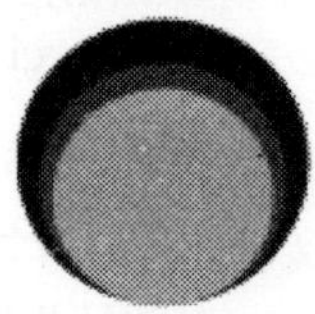

US: 6.7
UK: 4.8
France: 3.8
Singapore: 2.1

Life expectancy at birth

France	Singapore	UK	US
81 years	79.7 years	79.1 years	78.1 years

US – without health insurance

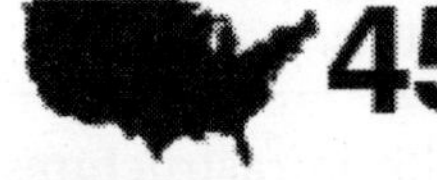

45.7 million (15.3% of population)

10.4%	19.5%	32.1%	16.8%
Of Non-Hispanic whites	Of Blacks	Of Hispanics	Of Asians

SOURCE: OECD, WHO

United States—Private System

Health sector has been funded more than half from private sources. Private health insurance is available through employer, government or private schemes. 15.3% of population (45.7 million people) do not have health insurance. Federal government is largest health care insurer—involved in two main schemes, Medicaid and Medicare, each covering about 13% of population. Medicaid—joint funded federal-state programme for certain low income and needy groups—e.g. children, disabled. Medicare is for people 65 years old and above and some younger disabled people and those with permanent kidney failure undergoing dialysis or transplant. Most doctors are in private practice and are paid through combination of charges, discounted fees paid by private health plans, public programmes, and direct patient fees. In-patient care is provided in public and private hospitals. Hospitals are paid through a combination of charges, per admission, and capitation.

UK—Universal, Tax-funded System

Public sector is funded by taxation and some national insurance contributions.

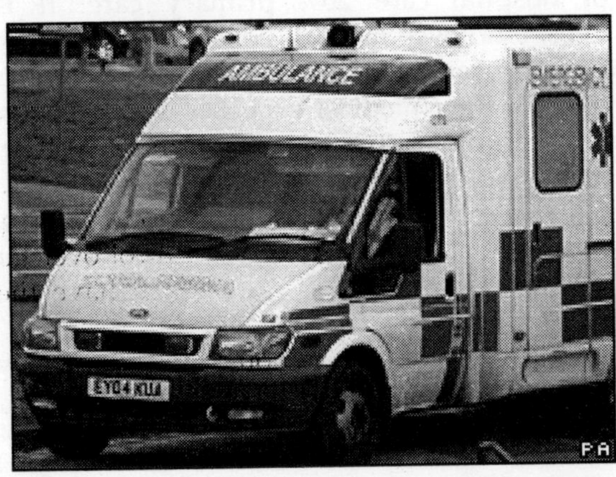

Emergency Ambulances are Part of Free NHS Service

Only about 11% people have private health insurance. Private GP services are very small. Health care is free at the point of delivery except charges for prescription drugs (except in Wales), ophthalmic services and dental services unless exempt. Exemptions include children, elderly, and unemployed. About 85% of prescriptions are exempt. Most walk-in care is provided by GP practices but also some walk-in clinics and 24-hour NHS telephone helpline. There is a free ambulance service and access to accident and emergency. In patient care is through GP referral and follow contractual arrangements between health authorities, Primary Care Trusts and the hospital. Hospitals are semi-autonomous self-governing public trusts.

France—Social Insurance System

All legal residents covered by public health insurance funded by compulsory social health insurance contributions from employers and employees with no option to opt out. Most people have extra private insurance to cover areas that are not eligible for reimbursement by the public health insurance system and many make out of pocket payments to see a doctor. Patients pay doctor's bills and are reimbursed by sickness insurance funds. Government regulates contribution rates paid to sickness funds, sets global budgets and salaries for public hospitals. In-patient care is provided in public and private hospitals (not-for-profit and for-profit). Doctors in public hospitals are salaried whilst those in private hospitals are paid on a fee-for-service basis. Some public hospital doctors are allowed to treat private patients in the hospital. A percentage of the private fee is payable to the hospital. Most out-patient care is delivered by doctors, dentists and medical auxiliaries working in their own practices.

Singapore—Dual System

Dual system is funded by private and public sectors. Public sector provides 80% of hospital care 20% primary care. It is Financed by combination of taxes, employee medical benefits, compulsory savings in the form of Medisave, insurance and out-of-pocket payments. Patients are expected to pay part of their medical expenses and to pay more for higher level of service. Government subsidizes basic health care. Public sector health services cater for lower income groups who cannot afford private sector charges. In private hospitals and outpatient clinics, patients pay the amount charged by the hospitals and doctors on a fee-for-service basis.

Sources

1. Freedman, L.P., Waldman, R.J., de Pinho, H., Wirth, M.E., Chowdhury, A.M.R., Rosenfield, A., Who's got the power? Transforming health systems for women and children. Geneva: UNDP; 2005.
2. WHO. 2008. Maximizing positive synergies between health systems and global health initiatives. Geneva.
3. WHO. Maximizing positive synergies between health systems and global health initiatives. Geneva; 2008.
4. World Bank. What is a health system? Washington, DC: World Bank; 2007.
5. World Health Organization. WHO's strategy for strengthening health systems. [cited September 12, 2007]; Available www.who.int/healthsystems/strategy/en/
6. Declaration of Alma-Ata. 1978 [cited August 1, 2007]; Available from: www.who.int/hpr/NPH/docs/declaration_almaata.pdf
7. Walley, J., Lawn, J.E., Tinker, A., Francisco, Ad., Chopra, M., Rudan, I., *et al.* Primary health care: making Alma-Ata a reality. *Lancet.* 2008;372:1001-7.
8. World Health Organization. Primary health care: now more than ever. Geneva: World Health Organization; 2008.
9. Magnussen, L., Ehiri, J., Jolly, P., Comprehensive *versus* selective primary health care: lessons for global health policy. *Health Affairs.* 2004;23(1):167-76.
10. Frenk, J., Strengthening health systems to promote security. *Lancet.* 2009;373:2181-2.
11. Hu, X., Cook, S., Salazar, M.A., Internal migration and health in China. *Lancet.* 2008;372:1717-9.
12. World Health Organization. Fact sheet: traditional medicine. Geneva: World Health Organization; 2008.
13. MacDonald, R., Horton, R., Trade and heath: time for the health sector to get involved. *Lancet.* 2009;373:273-4.
14. Perez-Casas, C., Herranz, E., Ford, N., 2001. Pricing of drugs and donations: options for sustainable equity pricing. Trop Med Int Health 6(11):960
15. Chen, L.C., Timothy, E., Anand, S., Boufford, J.I., Brown, H., Chowdhury, M., *et al.* Human resources for health: overcoming the crisis. *Lancet.* 2004;364:1984-90.
16. World Health Organization. World health report 2000: health systems: improving performance. Geneva: WHO; 2000

17. Harvard University. Human Resources for Health: overcoming the crisis: Harvard University Press; 2004.
18. Friedman Eric, A. An Action plan to prevent brain drain: building equitable health systems in Africa. Boston: Physicians for Human Rights; 2004.
19. World Health Organization. Health workforce definitions. [cited April 19, 2009]; Available from: http://apps.who.int/globalatlas/docs/HRH/HTML/Dftn.htm
20. World Health Organization. World health report 2006: working together for health. Geneva: WHO; 2006.
21. United Nations. UN Millennium Development Goals. [cited April 26, 2009]; Available from: www.un.org/millenniumgoals/
22. Medecins San Frontieres. Help wanted: confronting the health care worker crisis to expand access to HIV/AIDS treatment, the MSF experience in South Africa; 2007.
23. World Health Organization. WHO's strategy for strengthening health systems. [cited September 12, 2007]; Available from: www.who.int/healthsystems/strategy/en/
24. World Health Organization. Task shifting : rational redistribution of tasks among health workforce teams. Global recommendations and guidelines. Geneva: World Health Organization; 2008.
25. Anand, S., Fan, V.Y., Zhang, J., Zhang, L., Ke, Y., Chen, L.C. China's human resources for health: quantity, quality and distribution. *Lancet*. 2008;372:1774-81.
26. Partners in Health. Task Shifting: Sharing another piece of PIH's model with the world [cited May 2, 2009]; Available from: www.pih.org/inforesources/news/task-shifting_and_PIH_model.html
27. Joint Health Professions. Statement on task shifting. 2008 [cited February 28, 2008]; Available from: www.icn.ch/Statement_12_principles.pdf
28. Philips, M., Zachariah, R., Venis, S. Task shifting for antiretroviral treatment delivery in sub-Saharan Africa: not a panacea. *Lancet*. 2008;371:682-4.
29. World Health Organization. WHO global burden of disease (GBD) 2002 estimates (revised); 2004.
30. World Health Organization. Fact sheet: migration of health workers. Geneva: World Health Organization; 2006.
31. Cheng, M.H. The Philippines' health worker exodus. *Lancet*. 2009;373:111-2.
32. Yumkella, F. Worker retention in human resources for health: catalyzing and tracking change. Washington, D.C: USAID; 2009.
33. International Finance Corporation. The business of health in Africa: partnering with the private sector to improve people's lives Washington, D.C: World Bank; 2007.
34. Human Development Network. Private participation in health services. Washington, DC: The World Bank; 2003.
35. World Health Organization. World health report 2006: working together for health. Geneva: WHO; 2006.
36. Glassman, A., Becker, L., Makinen, M., de Ferranti, D. Planning and costing human resources for health. The *Lancet*. 2008;371:693-5.
37. World Health Organization. Why is good governance relevant to the pharmaceutical public sector? [cited 2009, July 28]; Available from: www.who.int/medicines/areas/policy/goodgovernance/why/en/index.html
38. Waters, H., Hatt, L., Axelsson, H. Working with the private sector for child health. Washington, DC: The International Bank for Reconstruction and Development/The World Bank; 2002.
39. Dowling, P. West Africa reproductive health commodity security: encouraging greater private sector participation. Alexandria: John Snow, Inc, DELIVER, for the US Agency for International Development,; 2005.
40. Mills, A., Brugha, R., Hanson, K., McPake, B. What can be done about the

private health sector in low-income countries? Bulletin of the World Health Organization,. 2002;80(4):325-30.

41. International Finance Corporation. The business of health in Africa: partnering with the private sector to improve people's lives Washington, DC: World Bank; 2007.
42. Reich, M.R., editor. Public-private partnerships for public health. Cambridge, MA: Harvard Center for Population and Development Studies; 2002.
43. World Health Organization. Fact sheet: traditional medicine. Geneva: World Health Organization; 2008.
44. Walley, J., Lawn, J.E., Tinker A, Francisco Ad, Chopra M, Rudan I, *et al.* Primary health care: making Alma-Ata a reality. *Lancet.* 2008;372:1001-7.
45. WHO. Integrating the role of the private sector in scale-up of HIV/AIDS testing and counselling to accelerate treatment access and improve prevention. [cited November 11, 2008]; Available from: www.who.int/3by5/en/concept_paper.pdf
46. Gottret, P., Schieber, G. Health financing revisited: a practitioner's guide. Washington, DC: .The World Bank; 2006.
47. USAID. Increasing the role of the private health sector: USAID; 2006.
48. Nelson, K. Stimulating research in the most neglected diseases. The *Lancet.* 2002;359:1042.
49. Palmer, N., Mills, A., Wadee, H., Gilson, L., Schneider, H. A new face for private providers in developing countries: what implications for public health? Bulletin of the World Health Organization. 2003;81(4):292-7.
50. Malmborg, R., Mann, G., Thomson, R., Squire, S. Can public-private collaboration promote tuberculosis case detection among the poor and vulnerable? Bulletin of the World Health Organization. 2006;84:752-8.
51. Brugha, R. Antiretroviral treatment in developing countries: the peril of neglecting private providers. BMJ. 2003;326:1382-4.
52. Private Sector Partnerships-One. Private sector health glossary. [cited November 11, 2008]; Available from: www.psp-one.com/section/resource/glossary
53. WHO. Working with the non-state sector to achieve public health goals; 2005.
54. WHO. Strengthened Health systems save more lives: An insight into WHO's European Health Systems' Strategy. 2001.
55. World Health Organization. World health report 2000: health systems: improving performance. Geneva: WHO; 2000.
56. Mills, A., Rasheed, F., Tollman, S. Strengthening health systems. In: D.J., J.B., A.M., Alleyne, G., Claeson, M., Evans, D., *et al.*, editors. Disease Control Priorities in Developing Countries. Washington, DC: The World Bank, Oxford Univesity Press; 2006.
57. World Health Organization. Everybody's business: strengthening health systems to improve health outcomes. WHO's framework for action. 2007.
58. Reich, M., Takemi, K. G8 and strenthening of health systems: follow-up to the Tokyo summit. *Lancet.* 2009;373.
59. Chen, L.C., Timothy, E., Anand, S., Boufford, J.I., Brown, H., Chowdhury, M., *et al.* Human resources for health: overcoming the crisis. *Lancet.* 2004;364:1984-90.
60. World Bank. What is a health system?; 2007. The Wold Bank Strategy for HNP Results. Available from: www.worldbank.org/
61. Holveck, J.C., Ehrenberg, J.P., Ault, S.K., Rojas, R., Vasquez, J., Cerqueira, M.T., *et al.* Prevention, control, and elimination of neglected diseases in the Americas: pathways to integrated, inter-programmatic, inter-sectoral action for health and development BMC Public Health. 2007;7(6).
62. Dimovska, D., Sealy, S., Bergkvist, S., H.P. Innovative Pro-Poor Health Care Financing and Delivery Models. 2009. Washington, DC: Results for Development Institute.

63. WHO. Maximizing positive synergies between health systems and global health initiatives. Geneva; 2008.

64. WHO. International Health Partnership (IHP+). [cited 2008 September 8, 2008]; Available from: www.who.in t/healthsystems/ihp/en/index.html

65. GAVI Alliance. Health systems strengthening. [cited 2008 September 9, 2008]; Available from: www.gavialliance.org/vision/policies/hss/index.php

66. Global Fund. Global Fund strategic approach to health systems strengthening. Geneva: GFATM; 2007 April 27, 2007.

67. USAID. Health systems overview. [cited 2008 September 9, 2008]; Available from: www.usaid.gov/our_work/global_health/hs/

68. UNICEF. [cited September 12, 2007]; Available from: www.unicef.org/index.php

69. Akogun, O., Audu, Z., Weiss, M., Adelakun, A., Akoh, J., Akogun, M., *et al.* Community-directed treatment of onchocerciasis with ivermectin in Takum, Nigeria. Tropical Medicine and International Health. 2001;6(3):232-43.

70. Global Health Council. Follow-up interview with Dr. Ahbay Bang. July 18, 2008. [cited October 6, 2008]; Available from: http://groups.google.com/group/ghc-research-symposium?hl=en&lnk=srg

71. Ooms, G., Derderian, K., Melody, D. Do we need a world health insurance to realise the right to health? PLoS Med. 2006;3(12):2171-6.

72. Huicho, L., Scherpbier, R.W., Nkowane, A.M., Victora, C.G., the Multi-Country Evaluation of IMCI Study Group. How much does quality of child care vary between health workers of different durations of training? An observational multi-country study. *Lancet.* 2008;372:910-6.

73. Miralles, M., Brock, T. The pillbox: where does pharmaceutical management fit into the health system? Presentation at USAID Global Health Mini University. September 12, 2008.

74. Jamison, D., Breman, J., Measham, A., Alleyne, G., Claeson, M., Evans, D., *et al*. Disease control priorities in developing countries. Washington, DC: The World Bank; 2006.

75. Lochery, P. The impact of water and sanitation on the health of children under five: Global Health Council; 2005.

2

Primary Health Care: Definition, Concept and Principles

"India is a country which claims to have high GDP but suffers from low social indicators viz. high birth and high death rates, low literacy and poor health care. Maternal mortality is one of the highest in the world, more so in the rural areas and especially in states like Bihar, Madhya Pradesh, Rajasthan, Orissa, Uttar Pradesh.

You see a mother suffering complications of labour without access to qualified support, a child missing out on essential vaccinations, an inner-city slum-dweller living in squalor. We see the absence of protection for pedestrians alongside traffic laden roads, and the impoverishment arising from direct payment for care because of a lack of health insurance. These and many other everyday realities of life personify the unacceptable and avoidable shortfalls in the performance of our health systems. There is a need for providing primary health care to all, to improve health indicators, and thus improved socio-economic indicators."

There is a growing appetite among policymakers for knowledge related to how health systems can become more equitable, inclusive and fair. Yet, despite enormous progress in health the collective failures to deliver in line with these values are obvious. You see a mother suffering complications of labour without access to qualified support, a child missing out on essential vaccinations, an inner-city slum-dweller living in squalor. We see the absence of protection for pedestrians alongside traffic laden roads, and the impoverishment arising from direct payment for care because of a lack of health insurance. These and many other everyday realities of life personify the unacceptable and avoidable shortfalls in the performance of our health systems.(Dr. Margaret Chan, Director-General, World Health Organization). India is a country which claims to have high GDP but low social indicators viz. high birth and high death rates, low literacy and poor health care. Maternal mortality is one of the highest in the world, more so in the rural areas and especially in states like Bihar, Madhya Pradesh, Rajasthan, Orrisa, Uttar Pradesh. There is a gross disparity in the women health care and there is growing incidence of female foeticide.

There is a need for providing primary health care to all, to improve health indicators, and thus improved socio-economic indicators.

Primary Health Care Definition

The ultimate goal of primary health care is better health for all. WHO has identified five key elements to achieving that goal:

- reducing exclusion and social disparities in health (universal coverage);
- organizing health services around people's needs and expectations (service delivery reforms);
- integrating health into all sectors (public policy reforms);
- pursuing collaborative models of policy dialogue (leadership reforms); and
- increasing stakeholder participation.

The concept of primary health care was defined by the World Health Organization in 1978 as both a level of health service delivery and an approach to health care practice. Remember, health care is not merely medical treatment in the event of falling sick. It entails all other components that are necessary to preserve or build health. It includes water, food, nutrients, sanitation, exercise, awareness, etc. Primary care, as the provision of essential health care, is the basis of a health care system. Seventy-five to eighty-five percent of the population seek primary health care yearly. It provides both the initial and the majority of health care services of a person or population. This is in contrast to secondary health care, which is consultative, short term, and disease oriented for the purpose of assisting the primary care practitioner. Tertiary care is for patients with unusual illness requiring highly specialized services. Primary care clinicians may be physicians, nurses, or various other health workers trained for the purpose. Countries with better provision of primary health care have greater patient satisfaction at lower costs and better health indicators.

Primary Health Care should be Available to All

While there are many definitions of primary care, the principles of accessible, comprehensive, continuous, and coordinated personal care in the context of family and community are consistent. Primary health care should be available to all people without the barriers of geography, cost, language, or culture. In primary care, all types of problems, at all ages and for both genders, are considered, including care for acute self-limited problems or injuries, the care of chronic diseases such as diabetes or AIDS (acquired immunodeficiency syndrome), the provision of preventive care services such as immunizations and family planning, and health education. Because primary health care is broad, it is information rich. Primary care clinicians coordinate care for patients among different service providers and for different patient concerns, responding to the fact that most patients have multiple problems. Continuity of care refers to the ongoing relationship between individual patients and primary care clinicians who are committed to the person, not a specific disease, body of knowledge, or specialized technique, and who recognize that physical, mental, emotional, and social concerns are related. Primary care clinicians, interested in the meaning of illness to the particular person, must negotiate care with that individual. A person's health is greatly influenced by the individual's family, culture, and community. Thus, the delivery of primary health care may be different for each individual and in different areas of the world.

The proportion of primary care physicians varies by country—for example, in Great Britain, it is 80 percent; in the United States, it is 32 percent. Primary care physicians in the United States consist of family or general practice physicians, general internists, and general pediatricians. Some primary care may be delivered by specialists, especially obstetrician-gynecologists, but it is not the focus of their practice. In the United States, primary care is also delivered by nurse practitioners and physician assistants. Considering all sources of primary care, there is still a lack of primary care providers in many areas of the country, particularly in the inner city and rural areas. (See Appendices 1 and 2 at the end of the book for more details on PHC, in the World Health Report, 2008).

Essentials of PHC: Indian Scenario

I. Equitable Distribution

The first key principle in the primary health care strategy is equity or equitable distribution of health services, i.e. health services must be shared equally by all people irrespective of their ability to pay, and all (rich or poor, urban or rural) must have access to health services. A commitment to health equity focuses not only on ensuring program inputs such as services and personnel based on need but also reducing differences in health outcomes. An equitable health system ensures that the groups or individuals with most compromised health conditions receive more health services. In practice it is inverse care, i.e. those who need the care most are able to access or afford the least. There is a clear urban-rural, rich-poor division in India. In the 42nd (1986-87), 52nd (1995-96), and 60th (2004 Jan.-June) rounds of National sample Survey Organization (NSSO), the percentage of ailing persons who got their ailments treated is found to be higher in the urban areas than in rural areas.

It was observed in 60th round of NSSO that more reliance was to public care provider than private provider by the scheduled castes in both rural and urban areas. Both in rural areas and urban areas, it was observed in 42nd, 52nd and 60th rounds of NSSO, percentage of people citing financial reason as an attribute for not attending to last spell of ailment has increased over time (In rural areas, 15% to 24% to 28% and in urban areas 10% to 20% to 28% from 42nd round, 52nd round to 60th round NSSO.) This inequity, described as the "inverse care law" has been captured through numerous studies on health status differentials between various groups and regions. For instance, IMR in the lowest wealth index group (70 per 1,000 live births) is more than twice the IMR in the highest group (29 per 1,000 live births) according to 2005-06 National Family Health Survey 3 (NFHS-3). Similarly, IMR in states like Uttar Pradesh, Chhattisgarh, Bihar, and Jharkhand is much higher than the southern states. Only one in five women from the poorest quintile have deliveries assisted by a skilled provider 1 as compared to the national average of 47%. Visits to a public health facility or camp were also higher by women from the highest quintile (42 percent) as compared to women from the lowest quintile (29 percent). Peters *et al* (2002) and Mahal *et al* (2001) analyzed that in-patient days, outpatient usage and obstetric care favours the rich whereas immunization and ante/post natal care is more equitably distributed. The poor have cited poor quality of services and financial implications as primary reasons for underutilization of public health services. A survey by National Council of Applied Economic Research (NCAER) revealed that expenses towards medical needs are the second most important cause of indebtedness among the rural poor. Indian health care plans and policies have stressed on making conscious and consistent efforts to deliver health services for "underprivileged" as a strategy for reaching "Health for all." While highlighting the continued health inequities across various groups and regions, NHP 2002 sought to craft a policy structure to allow for even access to public health services by Skilled provider includes doctor, ANM/ nurse/midwife/LHV, and other health personnel. In terms to access to health care, tribal areas in the country remain one disadvantaged and vulnerable group of population. The access and utilization of health care remain sub-optimal and health and nutrition indices in the tribal population continue to be poor

National Rural Health Mission (NRHM) and Equity

The National Rural Health Mission aims to restructure the health delivery systems towards providing universal access to equitable, affordable, and quality health care responsive to the health needs of India's population. The NRHM addresses equity concerns in a number of forms. It seeks to gather data with dis-aggregation for gender and for SC and ST. The mission promotes the health of weaker sections of the society. ASHA being women is believed to improve access of health care by women and children. Making all peripheral health facilities to become fully functional is one of the most basic ways in which social protection for the poor is provided and the health sector reaches out to hitherto underserved areas. NRHM promotes delivering services to even more remote areas through the mobile medical units and holding outreach sessions. It also seeks to exempt below poverty line families from all charges ensuring access. In Tripura, a helicopter service, to reach a particularly remote set of tribal hamlets has been sanctioned and is functional. In Andhra Pradesh, free bus passes to pregnant women for three visits for antenatal care has been attempted. In Tamil Nadu, in remote hilly and forested areas of Dharmapuri and Krishnagiri, a concept of birth resorts is introduced under the state plan-which provides for pregnant women in the last month to move to a temporary home nearer a site that can offer institutional delivery. Akha-ship of hope, is an innovative way of Assam state to provide primary health care services in riverine island through boat clinics

II. Need-based Universal Access to Care

Accessibility and availability of health services reflect the reach and coverage of primary health care facilities. According to NFHS 3, private health facilities are favoured for health care by a majority of the urban households (70%) as well as rural households (63%). However, the use of public health facilities by the lowest wealth quintile (39%) is comparatively more than the highest wealth quintile (34%). At the same time, a very negligible proportion of the sampled population (1.4%) access health care from the subcenter. Non-usage of public health facilities varies greatly across states, ranging from 8% in Sikkim to 93% in Bihar. Poor quality of care is cited as the most common reason (58%) for not using government facilities followed by lack of nearby facility (47%), long waiting period (25%), inconvenient timings (13%), and provider absenteeism (9%).

The role of grassroot health workers such as ANM, LHV, AWW, ASHA and MPW in providing health services at the community level is at the heart of the primary health care system employed by India. However, as per NFHS-3 only 17% of the women reported any contact with health workers in the three months preceding the NFHS-3 survey. Rural women reported higher contact (21%) with health workers compared to urban women (10%), and women from the lowest wealth quintile had the maximum exposure to health workers (22%). Pervasive absenteeism by health providers contributes to the ineffectiveness in delivery of primary health care services. A study by Chaudhury *et al.* (2005) revealed that 40% of the health workers were absent from their facility in India at the time of a random unannounced spot check. Similar studies quote the lack of regularity in terms of the time of day or day of the week by absentee health providers, which further serves as a disincentive to seek health care.

Health Care Facilities Inadequate in Quality and Quantity

While on the one hand the existing extensive health care system falls short of the population needs, on the other hand, essential infrastructure and equipment are lacking in most facilities. A Facility Survey covering 370 districts in 26 states of India conducted by the Department of Family Welfare in 2003, revealed that essential inputs and infrastructure were far from satisfactory in the government facilities—54% PHCs do not have a labour room and a laboratory, 80% and 77% PHCs do not have communication and transport facilities, only 58% PHCs conducted deliveries, 6% conducted MTPs, and 22% provided neonatal care. Training needs of medical and paramedical staff is acute, and only 20% of the PHCs are adequately staffed with trained personnel.

Human resource requirement under NRHM has stepped up drastically in view of renewed commitment to universal coverage. An additional 200,000 ANMs, 400,000 ASHAs, 84,000 Staff nurses, 7,200 Public Health Nurses, 15,400 Lab technicians, 4,000 Radiographers, 5,000 Gynecologists, 7,000 anesthetists. 7,800 physicians, and 8,445 public health managers are required to meet the manpower requirements. The challenges involved in training, recruitment, placement, and motivation of health workers across the country cannot be overemphasized if universal coverage is to be attained. Several alternatives are being explored to address the existing and anticipated shortfall of human resources. These include increasing retirement age to 65 years, decentralization of recruitment to district level, contractual employment of doctors on attractive salaries, incentives for rural postings, posting junior/postgraduate studentes and doctors at PHCs/CHCs for a fixed period, incentives for financial and career advancement, enabling work environment and residential facilities/ allowances, and educational incentives for children of doctors in rural areas, etc.

III. Community Participation

The Primary Health Care approach lays emphasis on health care provision by the people. It centers on peoples' participation in their own activities. Community involvement in health programmes has been tried through various approaches in India. Some of these include:

(a) Community Health Volunteers

Health care delivery in the country has utilized community volunteers from time to time in different forms to link the community with the health care system. As part of NRHM, a cadre of Accredited Social Health Activists (ASHA) is being established at the village/large habitat level in 2.5 lakh villages of 18 priority states. The ASHA is an honorary volunteer who is accountable to the community; acts as an interface between the community and the public health care system; facilitates preparation and implementation of Village Health Plan along with Anganwadi worker, community workers and ANM under the Anganwadi workers engaged by the Government to work in the Integrated Child Development Services (ICDS) which cater to the health and pre-school education needs of 0-6 year old children as also the health and nutrition needs of pregnant women, nursing mothers and adolescent girls. All 0-6 year old children, all pregnant women, nursing mothers and adolescent girls in India are entitled to access to this Service.

(b) ASHAs

She receives performance-based incentives for promoting construction of household toilets, universal immunization, referral and escort services for RCH, and other health care delivery programmes. In Chhattisgarh, the existing Mitanins are declared ASHA equivalents and they have been performing well in this slight modification of their role and support systems. In Rajasthan the Sahyoginis of the Anganwadi centers were declared ASHAs—and re-named ASHA Sahyoginis. Of the 42,000 target some 37,000 have been selected and renamed.

Primary Health Care holds much Deeper Significance

The Alma Ata Declaration Declaration recommended that primary health care should include at least: education concerning prevailing health problems and methods of identifying, preventing and controlling them; promotion of food supply and proper nutrition, and adequate supply of safe water and basic sanitation; maternal and child health care, including family planning; immunization against major infectious diseases; prevention and control of locally endemic diseases; appropriate treatment of common diseases and injuries; promotion of mental health and provision of essential drugs. It emphasized the need for strong first-level care with strong secondary- and tertiary-level care linked to it. It called for an integration of preventive, promotive, curative and rehabilitative health services that had to be made accessible and available to the people, and this was guided by the principles of universality, comprehensiveness and equity. In one sense, primary health care reasserted the role and responsibilities of the State, and recognized that health is influenced by a multitude of factors and not just the health services. It also recognized the need for a multisectoral approach to health and clearly stated that primary health care had to be linked to other sectors. At the same time, the Declaration emphasized on complete and organized community participation, and ultimate self-reliance with individuals, families and communities assuming more responsibility for their own health, facilitated by support from groups such as the local government, agencies, local leaders, voluntary groups, youth and women's groups, consumer groups, other non-governmental organizations, etc.

Initially Health Care was Fashioned in the Public Domain

During the earlier times, India's leaders envisaged a national health system in which the State would play a leading role in determining priorities and financing, and provide services to the population. 'If it were possible to evaluate the loss, which this country annually suffers through the avoidable waste of valuable human material and the lowering of human efficiency through malnutrition and preventable morbidity, we feel that the result would be so startling that the whole country would be aroused and would not rest until a radical change had been brought about' (Bhore Committee Report 1946). The emphasis of the first health report, i.e. the

Health Planning and Development Committee's Report, 1946 (popularly known as the Committee Report) on the role of the State was explicit. It was a plan equivalent to Britain's National Health Service. The Report was based on a countrywide survey in British India. It is the first organized set of health care data for India. The poor health status was attributed to the prevalence of insanitary conditions; malnutrition and undernutrition leading to high infant and maternal mortality rates; inadequacy training and health education; self-sufficiency in drugs and equipment; family planning and population control. Starting from the first plan, vertical programmes started, which became the centre of focus. The Malaria Control Programme, which was made one of the principal programmes, apart from other programmes for the control of TB, filariasis, leprosy and venereal diseases, was launched. Provision of universal, comprehensive primary health services was its goal. A large number of private and voluntary organizations who are active across the country in the health field were to support the Government in its efforts to integrate health services. GOBI-FF (growth monitoring, oral rehydration, breastfeeding, immunization, food supplements for pregnant women and children, and family planning) approach (Rifkin and Gill, 1986). Programme-driven health policies were once again the importance of a strong referral system.

The World Health Report, 2008

The report says that there has been some improvement in the health care, though there is a long way to go! The Declaration of Alma-Ata was clear about the values pursued: social justice and the right to better health for all, participation and solidarity1. If children were still dying at 1978 rates, there would have been 16.2 million deaths globally in 2006. In fact, there were only 9.5 million such deaths. This difference of 6.7 million is equivalent to 18 329 children's lives being saved every day. There have been significant improvements in access to water, sanitation and antenatal care. Knowledge and understanding of health are growing rapidly. The accelerated technological revolution is multiplying the potential for improving health and transforming health literacy in a better-educated and modernizing global society. However, the substantial progress in health over recent decades has been deeply unequal. Ageing and the effects of ill-managed urbanization and globalization accelerate worldwide transmission of communicable diseases, and increase the burden of chronic and non-communicable disorders. The factors that are at work are; long-term increases in income and population, climate change, challenges to food security, and social tensions, all with definite, but largely unpredictable, implications for health in the years ahead. In many regards, the responses of the health sector to the changing world have been inadequate and naïve. Rather than improving their response capacity and anticipating new challenges, health systems seem to be drifting from one short-term priority to another, increasingly fragmented and without a clear sense of direction.

Growing Expectations for Better Delivery: Five Common Shortcomings

1. *Inverse care*: People with the most means—whose needs for health care are often less—consume the most care, whereas those with the least means and greatest health problems consume the least. Public spending on health services most often benefits the rich more than the poor in high- and lowincome countries alike.
2. *Impoverishing care*: Wherever people lack social protection and payment for care is largely out-of-pocket at the point of service, they can be confronted with catastrophic expenses. Over 100 million people annually fall into poverty because they have to pay for health care.
3. *Fragmented care*: The excessive specialization of health care providers and the narrow focus of many disease control programmes discourage a holistic approach to the individuals and the families they deal with and do not appreciate the need for continuity in care. Health services for poor and marginalized groups are often highly fragmented and severely under-resourced, while development aid often adds to the fragmentation.
4. *Unsafe care*: Poor system design that is unable to ensure safety and hygiene standards leads to high rates of hospital-acquired infections, along with medication errors and other avoidable adverse effects that are an underestimated cause of death and ill-health.
5. *Misdirected care*: Resource allocation clusters around curative services at great cost, neglecting the potential of primary prevention and health promotion to prevent up to 70% of the disease burden. At the same time, the health sector lacks the expertise to mitigate the adverse effects on health from other sectors and make the most of what these other sectors can contribute to health.

CURRENT CONCERNS OF PHC

1. Extended access to a basic package of health interventions and essential drugs for the rural poor.
2. Transformation and regulation of existing health systems, aiming for universal access and social health protection.
3. Concentration on mother and child health.
4. Dealing with the health of everyone in the community.
5. Focus on a small number of selected diseases, primarily infectious and acute.
6. A comprehensive response to people's expectations and needs, spanning the range of risks and illnesses.

7. Improvement of hygiene, water, sanitation and health education at village level. Promotion of healthier lifestyles and mitigation of the health effects of social and environmental hazards.
8. Simple technology for volunteer, non-professional community health workers.
9. Teams of health workers facilitating access to and appropriate use of technology and medicines.
10. Participation as the mobilization of local resources and health-centre management through local health committees.
11. Institutionalized participation of civil society in policy dialogue and accountability mechanisms.
12. Government-funded and delivered services with a centralized top-down management.
13. Pluralistic health systems operating in a globalized context.
14. Management of growing scarcity and downsizing.
15. Guiding the growth of resources for health towards universal coverage.
16. Bilateral aid and technical assistance Global solidarity and joint learning.
17. Primary care as the antithesis of the hospital Primary care as coordinator of a comprehensive response at all levels.

WHO Suggested Four Sets of Reforms

1. universal coverage reforms that ensure that health systems contribute to health equity, social justice and the end of exclusion, primarily by moving towards universal access and social health protection;
2. service delivery reforms that re-organize health services around people's needs and expectations, so as to make them more socially relevant and more responsive to the changing world, while producing better outcomes;
3. public policy reforms that secure healthier communities, by integrating public health actions with primary care, by pursuing healthy public policies across sectors and by strengthening national and transnational public health interventions; and
4. leadership reforms that replace disproportionate reliance on command and control on one hand, and *laissez-faire* disengagement of the state on the other, by the *inclusive,* participatory, negotiation-based leadership indicated by the complexity of contemporary health systems.

The first of these four sets of reforms aims at diminishing exclusion and social disparities in health. Ultimately, the determinants of health inequality require a societal response, with political and technical choices that affect many different sectors. Health inequalities are also shaped by the inequalities in availability, access and quality of services, by the financial burden these impose on people, and even by the linguistic, cultural and gender-based barriers that are often embedded in the way in which clinical practice is conducted. If health systems are to reduce health inequities, a precondition is to make services available to all, i.e. to bridge the gap in the supply of services. Service networks are much more extensive today than they were 30 years ago, but large population groups have been left behind. In some places, war and civil strife destroyed infrastructure, in others, unregulated commercialization has made services available, but not necessarily those that are needed. Supply gaps are still a reality in many countries, making extension of their service networks a priority concern, as was the case 30 years ago. As the overall supply of health services has improved, it has become more obvious that barriers to access are important factors of inequity: user fees, in particular, are important sources of exclusion from needed care. Moreover, when people have to purchase health care at a price that is beyond their means, a health problem can quickly precipitate them into poverty or bankruptcy. That is why extension of the supply of services has to go hand-in-hand with social health protection, through pooling and pre-payment instead of out-of-pocket payment of user fees.

PHC does not mean Rudimentary Care

The service delivery reforms are meant to transform conventional health care delivery into primary care, optimizing the contribution of health services—local health systems, health care networks, health districts—to health and equity while responding to the growing expectations for "putting people at the centre of health care, harmonizing mind and body, people and systems." These service delivery reforms are but one subset of PHC reforms, but one with such a high profile that it has often masked the broader PHC agenda. There is a substantial body of evidence on the comparative advantages, in terms of effectiveness and efficiency, of health care organized as peoplecentred primary care. Despite variations in the specific terminology, its characteristic features (person-centredness, comprehensiveness and integration, continuity of care, and participation of patients, families and communities) are well identified. Care that exhibits these features requires health services that are organized accordingly, with close-to-client multi-disciplinary teams that are responsible for a defined population, collaborate with social services and other sectors, and coordinate the contributions of hospitals, specialists and community organizations.

Primary care provides a place to which people can bring a wide range of health problems—it is not acceptable that in low-income countries primary care would only deal with a few "priority diseases"—it is not acceptable that, in low-income countries, primary care would be reduced to a stand-alone health post or isolated community-health worker; primary care facilitates ongoing relationships between patients and clinicians, within which patients participate in decision-making about their health and health care; it builds bridges between personal health care and patients' families and communities. Primary care opens opportunities for disease prevention and health promotion as well as early detection of disease—it is not acceptable that, in low-income countries, primary care would just be about treating common ailments; primary care requires teams of health professionals: physicians, nurse practitioners, and assistants with specific and sophisticated biomedical and social skills—it is not acceptable that, in low-income countries, primary care would be synonymous with low-tech, non-professional care for the rural poor who cannot afford any better; primary care requires adequate resources and investment, and can then provide much better value for money than its alternatives- it is not acceptable that, in low-income countries, primary care would have to be financed through out-of-pocket payments on the erroneous assumption that it is cheap and the poor should be able to afford it.

Unequal Growth, Unequal Outcomes

Since 1975, the rate of decline in under-five mortality rates has been much slower in low-income countries as a whole than in the richer countries. Some countries have made great improvements and are on track to achieve the health-related MDGs. Others, particularly in the African region, have stagnated or even lost ground. Mirroring the overall trends in child survival, global trends in life expectancy point to a rise throughout the world of almost eight years between 1950 and 1978, and seven more years since: a reflection of the growth in average income per capita. As with child survival, widening income inequality is refl ected in increasing disparities between the least and most healthy. Between the mid-1970s and 2005, the difference in life expectancy between high-income countries and countries in sub-Saharan Africa, or fragile states, has widened by 3.8 and 2.1 years, respectively. The unmistakable relation between health and wealth, exists. Secondly, there is considerable variation in achievement across countries with the same income, particularly among poorer countries. In 1978, about two-thirds of the world's population lived in countries that went on to experience increases in life expectancy at birth and considerable economic growth. The most impressive relative gains were in a number of low-income countries in Asia (including India), Latin America and northern Africa, totalling 1.1 billion inhabitants 30 years ago and nearly 2 billion today. These countries increased life expectancy at birth by 12 years, while GDP per capita was multiplied by a factor of 2.6. Public expenditure on health declined in the 1990s to levels that made running a basic system virtually impossible in several countries. The contribution of rural primary care and urban health insurance to this has been well documented. With the economic reforms of the early 1980s, however, average GDP per capita increased spectacularly, but access to care and social protection deteriorated, particularly in rural areas. This slowed down improvements to a modest rate, suggesting that only the improved living conditions associated with the spectacular economic growth avoided a regression of average life expectancy.

People are more exposed and more vulnerable to environmental and other health threats that, in today's globalized world, include lifestyle threats, such as smoking, obesity and urban violence. They lack the material security required to invest in their own health and their governments lack the necessary resources and/or commitment to public investment. They are at much greater risk of war and civil conflict than richer countries. Without growth, peace is considerably more difficult and without peace, growth stagnates: on average, a civil war reduces a country's growth by around 2.3% per year for a typical duration of seven years, leaving it 15% poorer. A history of poor economic growth is also a history of stagnating resources for health. Low income countries generally allocate a smaller proportion of their GDP to health than high-income countries, while their GDP is smaller to start with and they have higher disease burdens. Higher health expenditure is associated with better health outcomes.

A Globalized, Urbanized and Ageing World

Thirty years ago, some 38% of the world's population lived in cities; in 2008, it is more than 50%, 3.3 billion people. By 2030, almost 5 billion people will live in urban areas. Most of the growth will be in the smaller cities of developing countries and metropolises of unprecedented size and complexity in southern and eastern Asia. Although on average health indicators in cities score better than in rural areas, the enormous social and economic stratification within urban areas results in significant healthinequities. One third of the urban population today—over one billion people—lives in slums: in places that lack durable housing, sufficient living area, access to clean water and sanitation, and secure tenure. Slums are prone to fire, floods and landslides; their inhabitants are disproportionately exposed to pollution, accidents, workplace hazards and urban violence. Loss of social cohesion and globalization of unhealthy lifestyles contribute to an environment that is decidedly unfavourable for health. This mobile and urbanized world is ageing fast and will continue to do so. By 2050, the world will count 2 billion people over the age of 60, around 85% of whom will be living in today's developing countries, mostly in urban areas. Contrary to today's rich countries, low- and middle-income countries are ageing fast before having become rich, adding to the challenge, changes combine to make chronic and non-communicable diseases—including depression, diabetes, cardiovascular disease and cancers—and injuries increasingly important causes of morbidity and mortality. There is a striking shift in distribution of death and disease from younger to older ages and from infectious, perinatal and maternal causes to non-communicable diseases. Traffic accident rates will increase; tobacco-related deaths will overtake HIV/AID Srelated deaths. In the industrialized world, as many as 25% of 65-69 year olds and 50% of 80-84 year olds are affected by two or more chronic health conditions simultaneously. In socially deprived populations, children and younger adults are also likely to be affected. It is insufficiently appreciated that the shift to chronic diseases or adult health has to come on top of an unfinished agenda related to communicable diseases, and maternal, newborn and child health. Efforts directed at the latter, especially in the poorest countries where coverage is still insufficient, will have to expand. Data from WHO's World Health Surveys, covering 18 low-income countries, show low coverage of the treatment of asthma, arthritis, angina, diabetes and depression, and of the screening for cervical and breast cancer: less than 15% in the lowest income quintile and less than 25% in the highest. Public-health interventions to remove the major risk factors of disease are often neglected, even when they are particularly cost effective: they have the potential to reduce premature deaths by 47% and increase global healthy life expectancy by 9.3 years. For example, premature tobacco-attributable deaths from ischaemic heart disease, cerebrovascular disease, chronic obstructive pulmonary disease and other diseases are projected to rise from 5.4 million in 2004 to 8.3 million in 2030, almost 10% of all deaths worldwide, with more than 80% in developing countries.

Hospital-centrism Approach not the Best, though Essential

For much of the 20th century, hospitals, with their technology and subspecialists, have gained a pivotal role in most health systems throughout the world Today, the disproportionate focus on hospitals and sub-specialization has become a major source of inefficiency and inequality, and one that has proved remarkably resilient. Health authorities may voice their concern more insistently than they used to, but sub-specialization continues to prevail. the experience of industrialized countries has shown that a disproportionate focus on specialist, tertiary care provides poor value for money. Hospital-centrism carries a considerable cost in terms of unnecessary medicalization and iatrogenesis, and compromises the human and social dimensions of health. It also carries an opportunity cost: Lebanon, for example, counts more cardiac surgery units per inhabitant than Germany, but lacks programmes aimed at reducing the risk factors for cardiovascular disease.

Global expenditure on medical equipment and devices has grown from US$ 145 billion in 1998 to US$ 220 billion in 2006: the United States accounts for 39% of the total, the European Union for 27%, and Japan for 16%. The industry employs more than 411 400 workers in the United States alone, occupying nearly one third of all the country's bioscience jobs. The pharmaceutical industry weighs even more heavily in the global economy, with global pharmaceutical sales expected to expand to US$ 735-745 billion in 2008, with a growth rate of 6-7%. Here, too, the United States is the world's largest market, accounting for around 48% of the world total: per capita expenditure on drugs was US$ 1141 in 2005, twice the level of Canada, Germany or the United Kingdom, and 10 times that of Mexico.

Fragmentation in Health Systems

While urban health by and large revolves around hospitals, the rural poor are increasingly confronted with the progressive fragmentation of their health services, as "selective" or "vertical" approaches focus on individual disease control programmes and projects. Originally considered as an interim strategy to achieve equitable health outcomes, they sprang from a concern for the slow expansion of access to health care in a context of persistent severe excess mortality and morbidity for which cost-effective interventions exist. Short-term advances have been short-lived and have fragmented health services to a degree that is now of major concern to health authorities. With parallel chains of command and funding mechanisms, duplicated supervision and training schemes, and multiplied transaction costs, they have led to situations where programmes compete for scarce resources, staff and donor attention, while the structural problems of health systems—funding, payment and human resources ? are hardly addressed. The discrepancy in salaries between regular public sector jobs and better-funded programmes and projects has exacerbated the human resource crisis in fragile health systems. Eventually, service delivery ends up dealing only with the diseases for which a (funded) programme exists—overlooking people who have the misfortune not to fit in with current programme priorities.

Commercialization is the Bane

Commercialization of health care has reached previously unheard of proportions in countries that, by choice or due to a lack of capacity, fail to regulate the health sector. Originally limited to an urban phenomenon, small-scale unregulated fee-for-service health care offered by a multitude of different independent providers now dominates the health care landscape from sub-Saharan Africa to the transitional economies in Asia or Europe. Commercialization often cuts across the public-private divide. Health care delivery in many governmental and even in traditionally not-for-profit NGO facilities has been *de facto* commercialized, as informal payment systems and cost-recovery systems have shifted the cost of services to users in an attempt to compensate for the chronic under-funding of the public health sector and the fiscal stringency of structural adjustment. The public-private debate of the last decades has, thus, largely missed the point: for the people, the real issue is not whether their health care provider is a public employee or a private entrepreneur, nor whether health facilities are publicly or privately owned. Rather, it is whether or not health services are reduced to a commodity that can be bought and sold on a fee for-service basis without regulation or consumer protection.

Commercialization has consequences for quality as well as for access to care. The reasons are straightforward: the provider has the knowledge; the patient has little or none. The provider has an interest in selling what is most profitable, but not necessarily what is best for the patient. Those who cannot afford care are excluded; those who can may not get the care they need, often get care they do not need, and invariably pay too much. Thus, commercialization of health care is an important contributor to the erosion of trust in health services and in the ability of health authorities to protect the public. This is what makes it a matter of concern for politicians and, much more than was the case 30 years ago, one of the main reasons for increasing support for reforms that would bring health systems more in line not only with current health challenges, but also with people's expectations.

People First

People obviously want effective health care when they are sick or injured. They want it to come from providers with the integrity to act in their best interests, equitably and honestly, with knowledge and competence. The demand for competence is not trivial: it fuels the health economy with steadily increased demand for professional care (doctors, nurses and other non-physician clinicians who play an increasing role in both industrialized and developing countries). For example, throughout the world, women are switching from the use of traditional birth attendants to midwives, doctors and obstetricians.

This has pushed people towards commercial care, which they, rightly or wrongly, perceived to be more competent, while attention was diverted from the challenge of more effectively incorporating professionals under the umbrella of PHC. They do not want to be taken advantage of by unscrupulous providers, nor do they want to be considered mere targets for disease control programmes (they may never have liked that, but they are now certainly becoming more vocal about it). In poor and rich countries, people want more from health care than interventions. Only people-centred services will minimize social exclusion and avoid leaving people at the mercy of unregulated commercialized health care, where the illusion of a more responsive environment carries a hefty price in terms of financial expense and iatrogenesis.

Participation

At the same time, however, surveys show that, as societies modernize, people increasingly want to "have a say" in "important decisions that affect their lives", which would include issues such as resource allocation and the organization and regulation of care. Experience from countries as diverse as Chile, Sweden and Thailand shows, however, that people are more concerned with having guarantees for fair and transparent processes than with the actual technicalities of priority setting. In other words, an optimum response to aspirations for a bigger say in health policy matters would be evidence of a structured and functional system of checks and balances. This would include relevant stakeholders and would guarantee that the policy agenda could not be hijacked by particular interest groups.

PHC Reforms: Driven by Demand

The core values articulated by the PHC movement three decades ago are, thus, more powerfully present in many settings now than at the time of Alma-Ata. They are not just there in the form of moral convictions espoused by an intellectual vanguard. Increasingly, they exist as concrete social expectations felt and asserted by broad groups of ordinary citizens within modernizing societies. Thirty years ago, the values of equity, people-centredness, community participation and self-determination embraced by the PHC movement were considered radical by many. Today, these values have become widely shared social expectations for health that increasingly pervade many of the world's societies - though the language people use to express these expectations may differ from that of Alma-Ata. This evolution from formal ethical principles to generalized social expectations fundamentally alters the political dynamics around health systems change. It opens fresh opportunities for generating social and political momentum to move health systems in the directions people want them to go. It moves the debate from a purely technical discussion on the relative efficiency of various ways of "treating" health problems to include political considerations on the social goals that define the direction in which to steer health systems.

Sources

Primary health care: report of the International Conference 1 on Primary Health Care, Alma-Ata, USSR, 6-12 September, 1978, jointly sponsored by the World Health Organization and the United Nations Children's Fund. Geneva, World Health Organization, 1978 (Health for All Series No. 1).

Dahlgren, G., Whitehead, M. Levelling up (part 2): a discussion paper on European strategies for tackling social inequities in health. Copenhagen, World Health Organization Regional Office for Europe, 2006 (Studies on social and economic determinants of population health No. 3).

WHO Regional Office for South-East Asia and WHO Regional Office for the Western Pacific. People at the centre of health care: harmonizing mind and body, people and systems. Geneva, World Health Organization, 2007.

Renewing primary health care in the Americas: a position paper of the Pan American Health Organization. Washington DC, Pan American Health Organization, 2007.

Saltman, R., Rico, A., Boerma, W. Primary health care in the driver's seat: organizational reform in European primary care. Maidenhead, England, Open University Press, 2006

Report on the review of primary care in the African Region. Brazzaville, World Health Organization Regional Office for Africa, 2003.

International Conference on Primary Health Care, Alma-Ata: twenty-fifth anniversary. Geneva, World Health Organization, 2003 (Fifty-sixth World Health Assembly, Geneva, 19-28 May 2003, WHA56.6, Agenda Item 14.18).

The Ljubljana Charter on Reforming Health Care, 1996. Copenhagen, World Health Organization Regional Office for Europe, 1996.

World Health Statistics 2008. Geneva, World Health Organization, 2008.

Hart, T. The inverse care law. *Lancet*, 1971, 1:405-412.

World development report 2004: making services work for poor people. Washington DC, The World Bank, 2003.

Filmer, D. The incidence of public expenditures on health and education. Washington DC, The World Bank, 2003 (background note for World development report 2004—making services work for poor people).

Hanratty, B., Zhang, T., Whitehead, M. How close have universal health systems come to achieving equity in use of curative services? A systematic review. *International Journal of Health Services*, 2007, 37:89-109.

Xu, K. *et al*. Protecting households from catastrophic health expenditures. *Health Affairs*, 2007, 6:972-983.

Starfield, B. Policy relevant determinants of health: an international perspective. *Health Policy*, 2002, 60:201-218.

Moore, G., Showstack, J. Primary care medicine in crisis: towards reconstruction and renewal. *Annals of Internal Medicine*, 2003, 138:244-247.

Shiffman J. Has donor prioritization of HIV/AIDS displaced aid for other health issues? *Health Policy and Planning*, 2008, 23:95-100.

Kohn, L.T., Corrigan, J.M., Donaldson, M.S., eds. To err is human: building a safer health system. Washington DC, National Academy Press, Committee on Quality of Care in America, Institute of Medicine, 1999.

Fries, J.F. *et al*. Reducing health care costs by reducing the need and demand for medical services. *New England Journal of Medicine*, 1993, 329:321-325.

The World Health Report, 2002—Reducing risks, promoting healthy life. Geneva, World Health Organization, 2002.

Sindall, C. Intersectoral collaboration: the best of times, the worst of times. *Health Promotion International*, 1997, 12(1):5-6.

Stevenson, D. Planning for the future—long-term care and the 2008 election. *New England Journal of Medicine*, 2008, 358:19.

Blendon, R.J. *et al*. Inequities in health care: a fi ve-country survey. *Health Affairs*, 2002, 21:182-191.

Tarimo, E., Webster, E.G. Primary health care concepts and challenges in a changing world: Alma-Ata revisited. Geneva, World Health Organization, 1997 (Current concerns ARA paper No. 7).

Everybody's business: strengthening health systems to improve health outcomes: WHO's framework for action. Geneva, World Health Organization, 2007.

Dans, A. *et al*. Assessing equity in clinical practice guidelines. *Journal of Clinical Epidemiology*, 2007, 60:540-546.

Primary care. America's health in a new era. Washington DC, National Academy Press, Institute of Medicine 1996.

Starfield, B. Primary care: balancing health needs, services, and technology. New York, Oxford University Press, 1998.

Ståhl, T. *et al*, eds. Health in all policies. Prospects and potentials. Oslo, Ministry of Social Affairs and Health, 2006.

The Paris declaration on aid effectiveness: ownership, harmonisation, alignment, results and mutual accountability. Paris, Organisation for Economic Co-operation and Development, 2005.

Nussbaum, M.C., Sen, A., eds. The quality of life. Oxford, Clarendon Press, 1993.

Further Readings

Smith, R. Oman: leaping a cross the centuries. *British Medical Journal*, 1988, 297:540-544.

Sultanate of Oman: second primary health care review mission. Geneva, World Health Organization, 2006.

Primary health care performance. Muscat, Sultanate of Oman. Directorate General of *Health Affairs*, Department of Primary Health Care, 2006.

Infante, A. The post-military government reforms to the Chilean health system. A case study commissioned by the Health Systems Knowledge Network. Paper presented in the Health Services Knowledge Network Meeting, London, October 2006. Geneva, World Health Organization, Commission on the Social Determinants of Health, 2007.

Pathmanathan, I., Dhairiam, S. Malaysia: moving from infectious to chronic diseases. In: Tarimo, E., ed. Achieving health for all by the year 2000: midway reports of country experiences. Geneva, World Health Organization, 1990.

Biscaia, A. *et al.* Cuidados de saúde primários em Portugal: reformar para novos sucessos. Lisbon, Padrões Culturais Editora, 2006.

Pongsupap, Y. Introducing a human dimension to Thai health care: the case for family practice. Brussels, Vrije Universiteit Brussel Press, 2007.

Barros, P., Simões, J. Portugal: health system review. Geneva, World Health Organization Regional Office for Europe on behalf of the European Observatory of Health Systems and Policies, 2007

Bentes, M., Dias, C.M., Sakellarides, C., Bankauskaite, V. Health care systems in transition: Portugal. Copenhagen, World Health Organization Regional Office for Europe on behalf of the European Observatory on Health Systems and Policies, 2004 (Health Care Systems in Transition No. 1; Ferrinho, P., Bugalho, M., Miguel, J.P. eds. For better health in Europe, Vol. 1. Lisbon, Fundação Merck Sharp and Dohme, 2004.

World Health Statistics 2008. Geneva, World Health Organization, 2008.

Murray, C.J.L. *et al.* Can we achieve Millennium Development Goal 4? New analysis of country trends and forecasts of under-5 mortality to 2015. *Lancet,* 2007, 370:1040-1054.

The Millennium Development Goals Report, 2007. New York, United Nations, 2007.

Levels and trends of contraceptive use as assessed in 2002. New York, United Nations, Department of Economic and Social Affairs, Population Division, 2004 (Sales No. E.04.XIII.9).

World contraceptive use 2007, wall chart. New York, United Nations, Department of Economic and Social Affairs, Population Division, 2008 (Sales No. E.08.XIII.6).

Sedgh, G. *et al.* Induced abortion: estimated rates and trends worldwide. *Lancet,* 2007, 370:1338-1345.

Koblinsky, M. *et al.* Going to scale with professional skilled care. *Lancet,* 2006, 368:1377-1386.

Goesling, B., Firebaugh, G. The trend in international health inequality. Population and Development Review, 2004, 30:131?146.

Preston, S. The changing relation between mortality and level of economic development. *Population Studies,* 1975, 29:231-248.

The state of the world's children, 2008. Paris, United Nations Children's Fund, 2008.

Cutler, D.M., Deaton, A., Lleras-Muney, A. The determinants of mortality. Cambridge, MA, National Bureau of Economic Research, 2006 (NBER Working Paper No. 11963).

Deaton, A. Global patterns of income and health: facts, interpretations, and policies, WIDER Annual Lecture, Helsinki, September 29th, 2006. Princeton NJ, Princeton University Press, 2006.

Field, M., Shkolnikov, V. Russia: socioeconomic dimensions of the gender gap in mortality. In: Evans, *et al.* Challenging inequities in health: from ethics to action. New York, Oxford University Press 2001. WHO mortality database: tables [online database]. Geneva, World Health Organization, 2007 http://www.who.int/healthinfo/morttables/en/index.html.

Suhrcke, M., Rocco, L., McKee, M. Health: a vital investment for economic development in eastern Europe and central Asia. European Observatory on Health Systems and Policies, 2008.

Banister, J., Zhang, X. China, economic development and mortality decline. *World Development*, 2005, 33:21?41.

Banister, J., Hill, K. Mortality in China, 1964-2000. *Population Studies*, 2004, 58:55?75.

Ikpe, E. Challenging the discourse on fragile states. Conflict, Security and Development, 2007, 77:84-124.

Collier, P. The bottom billion: why the poorest countries are failing and what can be done about it. New York, Oxford University Press, 2007.

Coghlan, B. *et al.* Mortality in the Democratic Republic of Congo: a nationwide survey. *Lancet*, 2006, 367:44-51.

World development indicators 2007. Washington DC, The World Bank, 2007.

Van Lerberghe, W, De Brouwere, V. Etat de santé et santé de l'Etat en Afrique subsaharienne [State of health and health of the state in sub-Saharan Africa], Afrique Contemporaine, 2000, 135:175-190.

National health accounts country information for 2002-2005. Geneva, World Health Organization, 2008

WHO global burden of disease estimates: 2004 update. Geneva, World Health Organization, 2008.

State of world population, 2007. Unleashing the potential of urban growth. New York, United Nations Population Fund, 2007.

Montgomery, M., Hewett, P.C. Urban poverty and health in developing countries: household and neighbourhood effects demography. New York, The Population Council, 2004 (Policy Research Division Working paper No. 184).

Satterthwaite, D. Coping with rapid urban growth. London, Royal Institution of Chartered Surveyors, 2002 (RICS Leading Edge Series; POPLINE Document No. 180006).

Garenne, M., Gakusi, E. Health transitions in sub-Saharan Africa: overview of mortality trends in children under 5 years old (1950-2000). *Bulletin of the World Health Organization*, 2006, 84:470-478.

Strong, K., *et al.* Preventing chronic diseases: how many lives can we save? *Lancet*, 366:1578-1582.

Ezzati, M., *et al.* Comparative risk assessment collaborating group. Estimates of global and regional potential health gains from reducing multiple major risk factors. *Lancet*, 2003, 362:271?280.

Moran, M. Governing the health care state. A comparative study of the United Kingdom, the United States and Germany. Manchester, Manchester University Press, 1999.

Starfield, B. Primary care. Balancing health needs, services and technology. New York, Oxford University Press, 1998.

Pongsupap, Y. Introducing a human dimension to Thai health care: the case for family practice. Brussels, Vrije Universiteit Brussel Press, 2007.

Brotherton, S.E., Rockey, P.H., Etzel, S.I. US graduate medical education, 2004-2005: trends in primary care specialties. *Journal of the American Medical Association*, 2005, 294:1075-1082.

Starfield, B., Shi, L. Policy relevant determinants of health: an international perspective. *Health Policy*, 2002, 60:201-218.

Schoen, C. *et al.* 2006 US health system performance: a national scorecard. *Health Affairs*, 20 September 2006 (Web Exclusive, w457-w475).

Aid effectiveness and health. Making health systems work. Geneva, World Health Organization, 2007 (Working Paper 9; Ferrinho, P. *et al.* Pilfering for survival: how health workers use access to drugs as a coping strategy. *Human Resources for Health*, 2004, 2:4.

McIntyre, D., *et al.* Commercialisation and extreme inequality in health: the policy challenges in South Africa. *Journal of International Development*, 2006, 18:435-446.

Sakboon, M., *et al.* Case studies in litigation between patients and doctors. Bangkok, The Foundation of Consumer Protection, 1999.

Ammar, W. Health system and reform in Lebanon. Beirut, World Health Organization Regional Office for the Eastern Mediterranean, 2003.

Macintosh, M. Planning and market regulation: strengths, weaknesses and interactions in the provision of less inequitable and better quality health care. Geneva, World Health Organization, Health Systems Knowledge Network, Commission on the Social Determinants of Health, 2007.

Marmot, M. Achieving health equity: from root causes to fair outcomes. *Lancet*, 2007, 370:1153-1163.

Health care: the stories we tell. Framing review. Oakland CA, American Environics, 2006 (http.www.americanenvironics.com, accessed 2 July 2008).

Garland, M., Oliver, J. Oregon health values survey, 2004. Tualatin, Oregon Health Decisions, 2004.

Mullan, F., Frehywot, S. Non-physician clinicians in 47 sub-Saharan African countries. *Lancet*, 2007, 370:2158-2163.

Lee, K. Globalisation and the need for a strong public health response. The European *Journal of Public Health*, 1999 9:249-250.

McKee, M., Figueras, J. Setting priorities: can Britain learn from Sweden? *British Medical Journal*, 1996, 312:691-694.

Daniels, N. Accountability for reasonableness. Establishing a fair process for priority setting is easier than agreeing on principles. *BMJ*, 2000, 321:1300-1301.

Martin, D. Fairness, accountability for reasonableness, and the views of priority setting decision-makers. *Health Policy*, 2002, 61:279-290.

3

Health Care Systems in India

"In recent times though India has eradicated mass famines, half of children in India are underweight, one of the highest rates in the world. Water supply and sanitation continue to be a challenged, only one of three Indians has access to improved sanitation facilities such as toilet. India's HIV/AIDS epidemic is a growing threat. 2.47 million People in India are estimated to be HIV positive. India is one of the four countries worldwide where polio has not as yet been successfully eradicated and one-third of the world's tuberculosis cases are in India. Cholera epidemics are not unknown. The maternal mortality in India is the second highest in the world. On the top of infections and malnutrition the epidemic of lifestyle diseases is raising its ugly head, threatening the already fragile health care in the country. Vehicular accidents, drug abuse and sexually transmitted ailments are also settling in Indian society with the changed social scenario. Providing health care and disease prevention to India's growing population of more than a billion people has become challenging in the face of increased competition for resources."

It was the India of antiquity which was the first state to give its citizens national health care. However, now the public health care system is crumbling. While infectious diseases remain un-eradicated, a large proportion of population is in the grip of obesity-related ailments. There are 2.47 million people in India, who are estimated to be HIV positive. India is one of the four countries worldwide where polio has not as yet been successfully eradicated and one-third of the world's tuberculosis cases are in India. According to the World Health Organization 900,000 Indians die each year from drinking contaminated water and breathing in polluted air. As India grapples with these basic issues, new challenges are emerging, for example, there is a rise in chronic adult diseases such as cardiovascular illnesses and diabetes as a consequence of changing lifestyles. There are vast disparities in people's health even among the different states across the country largely attributed to the resource allocation by the state governments where some states have been more successful than others. Better efforts are needed by the local governments to ensure that the health services provided are actually reaching the poor in worst-affected areas. (See Appendix 3 at the end of the book for India's Health Care Vision, 2020).

However, at the same time, India's health care system also includes entities which are world class. The Apollo set of hospitals are considered amongst Asia's most advanced hospitals. Thus, India's health care system has progressed and is a leader in South East Asia.

Essential Points

- India has the largest number of medical colleges in the world.
- India produces among largest number of doctors in the developing world. These doctors are exported to many other countries, and are considered among the best in the world.
- This country gets 'Medical tourists' from many developed countries reflecting the high standard of medical skill and expertise here. They seek care in its state-of-the-art, high-tech hospitals which compare with the best in the world.
- This country is the fourth largest producer of drugs by volume in the world and is among the largest exporter of drugs in the world.
- Despite all these resources, the majority of citizens has very limited access to quality Health care, and has poor health indicators
- There are low levels of immunization—in fact less than half of the children are completely immunized (added to this, complete immunization coverage has declined in recent years).
- Similarly, the minimum of three checkups during pregnancy remains unavailable for half of all pregnant women.
- There are massive inequities in access to health care—while the rich avail of most modern and expensive health services, the poor, especially in rural areas do not get even rudimentary health care. But the rich may also be denied the optimum care, since they may be fleeced with un-necessary surgery, tests, etc.
- Incredibly, hospitalization rates among the well off are six times higher than rates among the poor
- Despite such a large drug industry which exports medicines across the globe, about two-thirds of the population lack access to essential drugs.
- This is a country of paradoxes where women from well off families suffer due to unnecessary cesarean operations—in some urban centers close to half of deliveries are done by operation—

while poorer rural women frequently die during childbirth due to lack of access to the same cesarean operation at time of genuine need.

- Although people spend a lot on health care (the poorest spend one-eighth of their total income on health care), the government spends much less. Of the total health spending in the country, all levels of government make less than one-fifth, while the remaining major portion is shelled out by ordinary citizens from their pockets. This makes the health care system in this country one of the most privatized systems in the world.
- Taking loans or selling assets pays for two out of five hospitalization episodes. The proportion of people who are unable to access any form of treatment due to inability to pay is quite large and increasing.

Mixed Health Care System

In India, the hospitals are run by government, charitable trusts and by private organizations. The government hospitals in rural areas are called the primary health centre (PHC)s. Major hospitals are located in district head quarters or major cities. The Modern System of Medicine is regulated by Medical Council of India, whereas the Alternate systems recognized by Government of India are regulated by Department of AYUSH (an acronym for Ayurveda, Yunani, Siddha and Homeopathy) under Ministry of Health, Government of India. PHC's are existent in most places, but due to poor pay and scarcity of resources, patients generally prefer private health clinics. However, most of the private clinics, esp. in rural areas may be manned by unqualified doctors or equipped with spurious medicines. These days some of the major corporate hospitals are attracting patients from neighbouring countries such as Pakistan, countries in the Middle East and some European countries by providing quality treatment at low cost. In 2005, India spent 5% of GDP on health care, or US$36 per capita. Of that, approximately 19% was government expenditure. Despite the increase in spending, health care is often unaffordable for many individuals. Many individuals do not seek physician care or hospitalization when needed since they cannot afford this care. In both countries, provinces and states with higher levels of GDP per capita have better health care outcomes than provinces and states with lower levels of GDP per capita.

Health Care Delivery is Abysmal

While, China has maintained public ownership over most health facilities, India has followed a policy of benign neglect and allowed entrance into and expansion of the private sector to fill in the gaps, with little effective regulation or enforcement. In India, the government pays for most of the care in public facilities, but prices are generally low or below cost. The government, however, allows public practitioners to run private practices, which means that many providers try to divert their patients to their higher margin, private practice. Yip and Mahal claim that in this environment, "supplier-induced demand is prevalent." In India, providers are well known for systematically over-prescribing drugs and tests (this is where they make their money). Counterfeit drugs are often used in rural areas. In India, it has been shown that even licensed doctors generally provide poor-quality service. Smaller hospitals in India lack basic medical equipment and trained personnel. "The public sector, too, is inefficient, with shortages of drugs and consumables and frequent absenteeism."

So what is the remedy for all that ails the health care system?

A Few Suggestions may be Considered

1. Develop and implement national standards for examination by which doctors, nurses and pharmacists are able to practice and get employment.
2. Rapidly develop and implement national accreditation of hospitals; those that do not comply would not get paid by insurance companies. However, a performance incentive plan that targets specific treatment parameters would be a useful adjunct.
3. Obtain proposals from private insurance companies and the government on ways to provide medical insurance coverage to the population at large and execute the strategy. It is healthy to have competition in health care, and provide health insurance to the millions who cannot afford it.
4. Utilize and apply medical information systems that encourage the use of evidence-based medicine, guidelines and protocols as well as electronic prescribing in inpatient and outpatient settings. This is possible though the implementation of the EHR; this will, in time, encourage health care data collection, transparency, quality management, patient safety, efficiency, efficacy and appropriateness of care.
5. Perverse incentives between specialists, hospitals, imaging and diagnostic centers on the one hand and referring physicians on the other need be removed and a level of clarity needs to be introduced.
6. Develop multi-specialty group practices that have their incentives aligned with those of hospitals and payers. It is much easier to teach the techniques of sophisticated medical care to a group of employed physicians than it is to physicians as a whole. It is also important that doctors are paid adequately for what they do.
7. Encourage business schools to develop executive training programmes in health care, which will effectively reduce the talent gap for leadership in this area.
8. Revise the curriculum in medical, nursing, pharmacy and other

schools that train health care professionals, so that they too are trained in the new paradigm.

9. Develop partnerships between the public and private sectors that design newer ways to deliver health care. An example of this would include outpatient radiology and diagnostic testing centers.
10. The government should appoint a commission which makes recommendations for the health care system and monitors its performance.

This System is not Sustainable

The present system is not sustainable due to its inefficiency and a lack of aligned incentives for improving performance. A country that has leapfrogged from rotary phones to a ubiquitous presence of mobile phones must make a similar change in health care. India has achieved substantial improvement in its health care. Life expectancy has increased, infant mortality rate, maternal mortality has declined. However, this progress is uneven. Lack of accountability is plaguing the system. Public-private partnership (PPP), which has become a buzz word, does not imply privatization.

Poverty, geography and poor infrastructure mean that India faces perhaps the world's heaviest disease burden, ranging from infectious diseases, the traditional scourge of the poor, to diseases of affluence such as diabetes and hypertension. The public sector has been overwhelmed, which is not surprising considering how little India's government spends on health as a share of national income. Accordingly, nearly four-fifths of all health services are supplied by private firms and charities-a higher share than in any other big country.

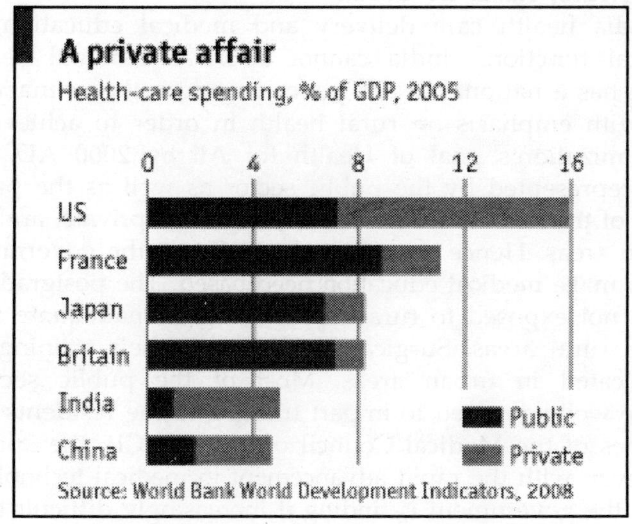

Techno-pak Health care, a consulting firm, expects spending on health care in India to grow from $40 billion in 2008 to $323 billion in 2023. In part, that is the result of the growing affluence of India's emerging middle classes. Another cause is the nascent boom in health insurance, now offered both by private firms and, in some cases, by the state. In addition, the government has recently liberalized the industry, easing restrictions on lending and foreign investment in health care, encouraging public-private partnerships and offering tax breaks for health investments in smaller cities and rural areas.

System Needs Revamping

India's health care system needs to be decentralized and revamped to cater to people in both urban and rural areas. "There is a need to decentralize our health system. Local bodies and panchayats, rather than the central government, should have control over government hospitals and primary health care centers. They should have the right to hire or fire a medical practitioner based on his performance," said Srinath Reddy, chairman of the Public Health Foundation, India. Reddy said the country's health system should be brought into public domain by involving NGOs, activists and local bodies. "We need to improve our management capacity and the health system should not be doctor dependent. We should focus on task-shifting, where nurses and paramedics are trained to handle work efficiently," Reddy maintained. "The government has been an absolute failure in providing health care facilities to the people of the country." "We need more public-private partnerships in the country to strengthen our health care system. We have to increase our investment in the sector to provide good facilities to people," said Jihnu Das, a senior economist with the World Bank.

Public *v/s* Private, Rural *v/s* Urban

In India health care delivery and medical education are largely governmental functions. India cannot afford a national health service. However, it has a national health policy based on the primary health care approach, with emphasis on rural health in order to achieve the World Health Organization's goal of Health for All by 2000 AD. Health care delivery is represented by the public sector as well as the private sector. Nearly 80% of the health facilities, both public and private, are concentrated in the urban areas. Hence despite its best efforts, the government has not been able to make medical education need-based. The postgraduate surgical trainees are not exposed to rural work owing to inadequate facilities and resources in rural areas. Surgical residents get their training in teaching hospitals located in urban areas. Most of the public sector teaching hospitals are well equipped to impart training to the residents according to the guidelines of the Medical Council of India (MCI), the apex governing body. However, with the rapid advancement in medical technology over the last decade, the government is finding it increasingly difficult to keep these teaching hospitals up-to-date. Of late, some of the sophisticated private sector hospitals are therefore sharing the onus of surgical education, especially at the sub-specialty level. Thus despite the good intentions of government planning a two class system of health care delivery has come into being and a two class system of medical education is foreseeable.

There are a wide variety of health care systems around the world. In some countries, the health care system has evolved and has not been planned, whereas in others a concerted effort has been made by governments, trade unions, charities, religious, or other coordinated bodies to deliver planned health care services targeted to the populations they serve. However, health care planning has often been evolutionary rather than revolutionary. World Health Report, 2000—Health systems: improving performance (WHO, 2000), are good health, responsiveness to the expectations of the population, and fair financial contribution. Duckett (2004) proposed a two dimensional approach to evaluation of health care systems: quality, efficiency and acceptability on one dimension and equity on another.

High GDP: Low Health Care

The Indian economy is witnessing phenomenal growth, currently at 8.5% of Gross Domestic Product—a fiery pace that most analysts predict is sustainable and likely to accelerate further, making it one of the fastest growing economies in the world. The last decade has seen the health care sector transition from a static and seemingly inconspicuous industry to an increasingly dynamic and significant industry today. A decade ago in India, health care sector was not usually considered as a key driver of national economic performance. However, over the years, there has been a fundamental change to this paradigm, with incontrovertible evidence from the world over firmly establishing that improved health leads to better economic performance. The direct as well as unquantifiable benefits from health care have become too large to be ignored. Small wonder that health care planning and investment have become the buzzwords for corporate planners the world over.

Health is influenced by general economic prosperity and social cohesion, and economic and social inequalities, said Nobel Laureate Amartya Sen. Drawing parallels between India and China to highlight his point on the role of economic prosperity in facilitating good health, the Nobel Laureate said China had managed to achieve astounding progress in general health and longevity along with economic growth. Those parts of India that had high life expectancy by 1979, partly because of following the Chinese model of social commitment,—particularly Kerala and now Himachal—have continued to have high rates of longevity and mortality reduction. Ensuring health coverage for all as a part of the human right need not await the distant possibility of the disappearance of inequalities in income and wealth.

High Burden of Global Disease

We have 21 percent of global burden of disease. Twenty-five percent of all maternal deaths take place in our country and same may be true for neonatal mortality. Politics influence health systems in significant manner. The goals, priorities, and the strategies, variations in the commitment are largely decided through the political contingencies. There are competing demands on the health systems. The evolution of the health systems is largely shaped by the culture, history, and norms. We don't have firm handle in terms of what are the client satisfaction level with private services. Client satisfaction also depends on non-clinical aspects of care. One would expect that the customer satisfaction would largely depend on the clinical outcomes of care, but non-clinical outcomes of care do influence the customer satisfaction and that's what the health system have to worry about. Financial risk protection is another goal of health systems. We need to start thinking about how health systems are covering for the financial contingencies and financial risk. Are people protected against the high cost of medical care? So any health system should see to it that the financial protection is extended against the catastrophic illnesses and the poor people who are really worst affected with the high cost, are not constrained to seek care. We also have high mortality and the burden of disease amongst the poor. Several studies have indicated that poor don't seek care on account of poor purchasing power.

How much are we Spending on Health?

Last decade has been witness to phenomenal growth in numbers of the medical colleges, nursing colleges and other similar training institutions. However, the quality of training and learning left a lot to be desired. It will be useful to see as how we are doing in terms of spending? Overall, Government spending is 0.9% of GDP, which is very low. WHO has pointed that we are really in the bottom quintile in the world in terms of public sector spending in the health care? The policy documents are explicit for increasing public spending to 2% and then 5% within next 10 years. In terms of expenditures 80 percent of all spending is on health from the private side, it's kind of out-of-pocket expenditures because the health insurance is yet to catch imagination of masses. Out-of-pocket expenditure includes risk of falling in debts after hospitalization.

Strategic opportunities for foreign investment and collaboration mark the sector, as leading Indian players draw out global expansion plans. A quick look at the estimated numbers fuelling growth:

- o 15,000 hospitals
- o 875,000 hospital beds
- o 500,000 doctors
- o 737,000 nurses
- o 170 medical colleges
- o 350,000 retail chemist outlets
- o 18,000 new doctors every year

The central administration provides co-ordination and direction to a network of health ministries that exists in each state for actual implementation. The Central Council of Health and Family Welfare (CCHFW) that includes the health ministers and secretaries from all Indian states is the primary advisory and policy-making body for health care in the country. The CCHFW is supported by the Planning Commission's Health Cell. This Cell also prepares the Plan-financed schemes for the sector. The budgetary outlay for health services has increased at over 15 per cent per year. Many state governments have sought external funding assistance for upgrading health infrastructure.

- o The Health care Delivery market is estimated at US$ 18.7 billion. Nearly 65 per cent of the health care services market has been captured by the private sector.
- o The industry is growing at about 13 per cent annually and is expected to grow at 15 per cent over the next four to five years.
- o A recent CII—McKinsey and Co. study forecasts growth from US$ 18.7 billion to around US$ 45 billion—equivalent to 8.5 per cent of GDP by 2012. Private health care is expected to account for 75 per cent of this spending.

The Confederation of Indian Industry's (CII) Indian Health Care Federation estimates that fresh investments of US$ 25 billion over the next 8-10 years to establish facilities will put the sector on the global health care map. With US$ 12-15 billion expected in domestic investments, the Indian health care sector represents a US$ 10 billion opportunity for foreign investors. Over the past two decades, a number of Indian private sector companies have set-up hospital facilities and clinics. Prominent examples include Apollo, Max, Fortis, Escorts and Wockhardt; out of an estimated total of 150 that represent a rapidly growing number of high-end facilities that offer top-of-the-line medical treatment.

- o Private hospitals account for over 32 per cent of hospital beds in India. Besides providing basic health and medical care services, these corporate hospitals often undertake complex surgeries like bone-marrow transplants, open-heart surgeries and kidney transplants.
- o Another area witnessing increasing corporate presence is diagnostic services. Premier Indian players in this segment include SRL-Ranbaxy, Metropolis Health Services and Dr. Lal's Pathlabs. The emergence of corporate hospitals on a larger scale is an important development. It has added the much needed infrastructural capacity, and, more importantly, been a catalyst in the professionalisation of hospital management. In turn, it has also facilitated impressive growth in the hospital management education industry.

Foreign Alliances

Since liberalization in 1991, a growing number of Indian companies have formed alliances with foreign firms. Most have aimed at leveraging the international partners' skills, knowledge and experience in devising and implementing improved medical care services; not relying only on capital invested. India's first geriatric hospital, the Heritage Hospital of Hyderabad has formed a joint venture with US-based United Church Homes to recruit, train and provide placement to registered Indian nurses in USA. Over the next two years, USA is likely to face a shortage of 450,000 nurses and of almost a million nurses by 2010. To cater to this shortage they have formed 2 legal entities, namely, UCH Heritage Health Care Inc. and UCH Heritage Health Care India Private Limited. Max Health Care and Singapore General Hospital (SGH) have entered into collaboration for medical practice, research, training and education in health care services. Apollo-Gleneagles Hospitals Ltd., a 50:50 joint venture between Apollo Hospitals Ltd. and Parkway Group of Singapore planned two more hospitals in India, after the first one was recently set-up at Kolkata. The joint venture is also looking at business opportunities overseas in West Asia and North Africa. Apollo Hospitals has also entered into a partnership with Yemen's Hayel Saeed Anam Group to provide advisory services to the latter's hospital project. Apollo will provide consultancy to set-up a 160-bed super specialty hospital at Taiz, Yemen.

Use of Information Technology

An important and positive development in the Indian health care sector is the use of information technology for upgrading the delivery of health care services and improving efficiency levels. Some examples include:

- o Computerization of medical records
- o Networking of various departments in a hospital
- o Providing tele-medicine services

Online reporting of laboratory and radio-diagnostic results over a Local Area Network (LAN) introduced by some medical colleges has significantly reduced reporting lag and patient movement. It has made the following partnerships possible: Wockhardt and Harvard Medical International Inc., USA. Fortis Health Care and Partners Health Care System, USA. Birla Heart and Research Centre And Cleveland Clinic Foundation, USA.

Top Corporate Hospitals

Apollo Group of Hospitals

Apollo Hospitals has emerged as the single largest private hospital group in south Asia. It operates hospitals, dispensaries, clinics and laboratories. Specialty services provided by the group include open-heart surgery, angioplasty surgery and renal transplants. The company has several firsts to its credit. It was the first hospital to obtain ISO 9002 and ISO 14001 quality certification in India. It was the first to set-up a health insurance administration company. It was the first to introduce preventive health care in India. It was the first Indian hospital to introduce new techniques in coronary angioplasty, sterio-tactic radiotherapy and radio-surgery. Apollo Hospitals got accredited with the Joint Commission International (JCI), an arm of the US-based Joint Commission on Accreditation of Health Care Organisations (JCAHO).

Escorts Heart Institute (EHIRC)

The Escorts Group has a presence in specialized cardiac treatment and multi-specialty care hospitals providing a whole gamut of specialized medical services. Escorts operates ten hospitals across India. The group is also reputed for tertiary care services such as neurology, neurosurgery, plastic surgery andurology. Escorts Heart Institute and Research Centre (EHIRC) has introduced innovative techniques of minimally invasive and robotic surgery. EHIRC is a 325 bed tertiary care institute, with 9 operation theatres, 5 cath labs, 2 heart command centres and world class facilities. It has carried out over 80,000 angiographies, 17,000 angioplasties and 43,000 cardiac surgeries over the past fifteen years—which is a world record. It is an ISO 9001 approved facility, which was recently adjudged the best cardiac care hospital in the country.

Fortis Health Care

It is a company founded by the promoters of the Indian pharmaceutical major, Ranbaxy Laboratories, started operations in 2001. Fortis Health Care has ambitious growth plans in the hospitals segment. The company aims to have a number of multi-specialty Fortis Health Care centres over the next three to five years through an investment of close to US$ 217 million. The company is focusing on increasing its capacity to 4,000 beds in 10 hospitals, up from the existing 600 beds in 4 hospitals. As part of this initiative, Fortis will be setting-up a medicity at Gurgaon in Haryana based on the John Hopkins Medical Centre in the US. To be known as Fortis International Institute of Medical and Biosciences (FIIMBS), it will house a medical college, an attached hospital, an allied sciences institute and a referral centre, among other facilities.

Max Health Care

Max Health Care, a fully owned subsidiary of the highly diversified Max Group, is focusing on becoming the largest health care player in northern India with a chain of clinics and hospitals with a bed capacity of 1200. On an average, Max Health Care treats 30,000 patients every month, with 200 new patients visiting the facilities every day. Max has a presence in all three verticals of the health care delivery segment (Primary,

Secondary and Tertiary Care). The institute has developed a three-tier business model for delivering health care services. This is a hub and spokes model, where the hub is the super specialty hospital and the spokes are its own clinical and diagnostic centres. The model comprises Dr Max Clinics at the primary level, Max Med-centers at the secondary level and Max Devki Devi Hospital at the higher end. Max Health Care has announced its plans to invest US$ 92 million during 2004-05 for setting up six hospitals in northern India. The company also plans to open around 18 primary health care clinics in the region.

Wockhardt Group

It is among India's leading pharmaceutical and health care companies. Since inception in 1989, the Wockhardt Hospital and Heart Institute has become a renowned tertiary level heart centre providing cardiac care to patients of all age groups including newborns. It has earned the recognition of a "Centre of Excellence" in cardiac care and has become a treatment destination for cardiac patients from neighbouring countries. It has an international alliance with Harvard Medical International, and has tie-ups with many global health insurance giants, including the BlueCross BlueShield.

Aravind Eye Hospital

This hospital in south India is the single largest provider of eye surgery in the world. In 1998, its hospitals saw 1.2 million outpatients and performed 183,000 cataract surgeries. It costs about US$ 10 to conduct a cataract operation. It costs hospitals in the United States about US$ 1,650 to perform the same operation. Since opening in 1976, Aravind has given sight to more than 1 million people in India. Aravind's surgeons are so productive that the hospital has a gross margin of 40 per cent. This is despite the fact that 70 per cent of the patients pay nothing or close to nothing, and the hospital does not depend on donations. The Hospital has maintained its enviable success by constantly cutting costs, increasing efficiency, and building its market. The Aravind Eye Hospital business model is taught as a case study at the Harvard Business School. The hospital's own Aurolab, started in 1992, pioneered the production of high-quality, low-cost intraocular lenses. Aurolab produces 700,000 lenses per year, a quarter of which are used at Aravind. The rest are exported all over the world.

The Jaipur Foot, named after its birthplace, the capital of the Indian state of Rajasthan, is an extraordinary prosthesis, or artificial limb, and has revolutionized life for millions of land-mine amputees. According to the *Time Magazine*, which profiled its founders as one of fifteen 'Heroes of Medicine', "The beauty of the Jaipur foot is its lightness and mobility—those who wear it can run, climb trees and pedal bicycles, and its low price. While a prosthesis for a similar level of amputation can cost several thousand dollars in the US, the Jaipur Foot costs only US$ 28 in India. The US-based Atlas Medical Software, which specializes in developing software solutions for the health care industry, has set-up its operations in India. Bayer Diagnostics, one of the largest diagnostic businesses in the world, with a presence in more than 100 countries is represented in India through Bayer Diagnostics India Limited (BDIL) in which Bayer AG of Germany owns 32.67 per cent of the stake. In India, it is mainly into the manufacture of chemical and immuno chemical test systems, medical diagnostic equipment (blood analyser and serum analyser) and electrolyte serum analyzer.

German medical instruments major Drager Medical AG, a joint venture between Dragerwerk AG and Siemens AG, is keen to enter India through a wholly owned subsidiary. Drager Medical manufactures a range of medical products like anesthesia equipment, monitoring equipment, ventilation equipment, pediatrics and medical emergency equipment, oxygen and aerosol therapy equipment. GE-BEL, a joint venture between GE and Bharat Electronics Limited is the only manufacturer of X-ray and CT tubes in South Asia. Global Technology Operations-India (GTO) is an ISO 9001 certified Software Development Centre that designs and develops products and solutions for GE Medical Systems using the latest computer platforms. GE Medical Systems Information Technology is a joint venture between GE and Citadel Health Ltd. of Hyderabad, for HIRePSTMa state-of-the-art Hospital Information System. UK-based iSOFT Group plc (iSOFT), one of the world's leading suppliers of application systems for hospitals and health care organisations, will be investing U$100 million over the next three years in its Offshore Development Centre (ODC) in Chennai in southern India, which was set-up in 2001. Philips has set a target of emerging as a distinct number two in the Indian medical systems market in another four to five years. The company today sells about US$ 43-49 million worth of medical systems in India. The aim is to take it to US$ 100 million. Philips is also looking at tele-medicine, with its DisHA (Distance Health Care Advancement) initiative to be piloted in two states. Philips will work with state governments, hospitals and other partners to provide affordable, accessible health care through mobile vans equipped with medical equipment under DisHA.

The US-based health care products major, Proton Health Care is making an entry into India with its range of digital health monitoring devices such as digital blood pressure monitors, ultrasonic nebulisers, body fat scales and thermometers. Proton has entered into a strategic tie-up with the Delhi-based SM Logistics for distributing its products in the Indian market. Siemens is a leading manufacturer of medical equipment with a market share of more than 30 per cent in India. The range of products includes X-ray systems, intensive care systems, hearing instruments, ultrasound instruments and equipment for nuclear medicine, among others.

Wipro GE Medical Systems, a joint venture between GE Medical Systems and Wipro Corporation, is India's largest medical systems sales and service provider. Wipro GE, which manufactures and exports products to global markets, pioneered the manufacture of Ultrasound and CT Scanner systems in India for global markets.

India is becoming a competitive outsourcing destination for high-end laboratory and diagnostic testing. For hospitals in the United Kingdom, United States and West Asia, it is Cheaper to outsource laboratory and diagnostic tests to India.

The industry's big players are Metropolis Health Services, SRL Ranbaxy and Dr. Lal's Pathlabs, to name a few. Some of these pathology laboratories are partnering hospital chains overseas. For example, Metropolis Health Services has already tied up with Gulf Medical College Hospital in the UAE and is in talks with hospitals in the US and UK. Outsourcing of laboratory testing and diagnostic services is set to become big business in India. According to a study on the Indian health care industry, the US$ 864 million diagnostics and pathology laboratory testing business is growing at a CAGR of 20 per cent. As part of its cost-cutting efforts, Britain may contemplate shipping blood and urine samples from National Health Service (NHS) patients to India for clinical tests and get the test results over the Internet.

Health Care: Outsourcing of Accessory Services from US

It could potentially be a US$ 4.5 billion opportunity for India by 2008, offering employment to about 200,000 people. It includes offshoring of processes such as medical billing, disease coding, forms processing and claims adjudication. Already, over a dozen companies are either consolidating operations or have kicked-off pilots in this space. These include Indian companies such as Apollo Health Street (AHS), iHealth care, Paramount Health Care, Hinduja TMT, Ajuba, Affiliated Computer Services, Cognizant Technology Solutions and Vision Healthsource. As health care BPO players mature, other businesses like claims repricing, medical diagnosis and actuarial work are expected to gain momentum. The opportunity is being driven by the US$ 1.4 trillion US health care industry, trying to rationalise costs. The American Health Care Association estimates that the profitability of US hospitals fell from 6.1 per cent, six years ago to 2.8 per cent in 2002. Almost 40 per cent of the US hospitals make losses. State-owned insurer Medicare has US$ 20 million in liabilities. Hospitals need to offshore the US$ 350 billion administrative functions and US$ 50 billion billing and coding tasks to be able to bring down their costs.

Haryana Jiva International, a health care venture on the outskirts of Delhi, is implementing a novel plan that takes medical care right inside rural India by using a GPRS enabled Java application available with Nokia's 6800 model. The "Teledoc" project won the World Summit Award for eHealth, at the World Summit on Information Society (WSIS) held in Geneva, Switzerland. Teledoc competed and won against technology entries from 136 countries. The Massachusetts Institute of Technology, has also been sufficiently impressed by Teledoc. Nicholas Negroponte, the MIT legend, personally visited Haryana villages in northern India to see the project at work, and Alex Pentland, Head of MIT Labs Asia, is now in the process of preparing a case study as part of the institute's social enterprise course.

PAUCITY OF HIGHLY TRAINED MANPOWER

The health care industry of India will face a shortage of 45,000 doctors by 2012 and 3,50,000 nurses for primary and secondary care by 2015, with quality of services offered by the sector expected to deteriorate further, industry body Ficci has said. Telemedicine is an answer to patient's treatment in inaccessible area in India with fewer medical facilities. The exponential growth in the ICT (information and communication technologies) sector and the reducing telecom costs are making India highly competitive in Telemedicine. There are around 120 Telemedicine centers across the country. "Teleradiology' is a means of electronic transmission of radiological images such as X-rays, CTs and MRIs from one location to another for the purposes of interpretation and/or consultation. The demand for radiology services is growing rapidly, while there is a shortage of radiologists the world over. In India there is an abundance of radiologists. By outsourcing Teleradiology to India, overseas hospitals can be assured of competent and trained professionals, time zone adherence to HIPAA (Health Insurance Portability and Accountability Act) mandates and round the clock services. According to an estimate, approximately 50 percent of the 6,000-odd hospitals in the US still do not have the technology for Teleradiology, and this represents a huge potential market to be tapped. The Indian health imaging market is expected to double from the existing US$ 350 million by 2010. X-ray, ultrasound, CT and MRI are expected to collectively account for 68.6 percent of the health imaging market.

Economics and Health

It is service-based jobs and industrial jobs that comprise the majority of India's GDP (51.4% and 28.1% respectively. This has created an imbalance of economy and of opportunity. Urban India, despite having a smaller percentage of the overall workforce, is driving the economy and therefore controls where new opportunities in technology, lifestyle, and health are placed. In fact, 75% of the health infrastructure and medical personnel in India are concentrated in urban areas (Patil). This has translated into different health scenarios for rural *vs.* urban India. When measuring health, the three factors that are considered most informative about standards of living are mortality, morbidity and life expectancy. These measures allow us to examine rate of life, death and disease in an area and draw conclusions about the population health in those areas.

	Rural	*Urban*	*Reference Year*
Population (%)	72.2	27.8	2001
Birth Rate	26.4	19.8	2003
Death Rate	8.7	6.0	2003
Infant Mortality Rate	66	38	2003

Source: *SRS Bulletin*, April 2005, Sample Registration System, Registrar General, India.

Surprisingly, birth rates nearly triple death rates in both rural and urban India. This tells us that the population is growing very quickly all across the country. The population in rural India continues growing larger, and they are also dying at a greater rate than urban India. The death rate there is almost 50% greater in rural India, and Infant Mortality is nearly twice as much. Maternal mortality rates (MMR) are also significantly high at 407 deaths/100,000 live births. In fact, MMR has actually risen over the last decade (Deogaonkar). There are many reasons for this, some of which are outlined below (Patil):

- 51% of deliveries are conducted at home by an untrained attendant.
- 75% of women have their first pregnancy before they turn 18.
- Only 67% of women complete their antenatal checkup.
- Only 30% of women get postnatal check-ups.

The good news out of all of this is that most rural deaths are preventable. They arise from infections and communicable, parasitic and respiratory diseases (Patil). The bad news is that mortality and morbidity rates in rural India have not shown significant improvement over time. Health care delivery in India comes in three major forms.

Public Health Systems

While the network exists to serve rural and poor areas, these centers are grossly under funded and understaffed. Then there is a real problem of absenteeism of the health staff.

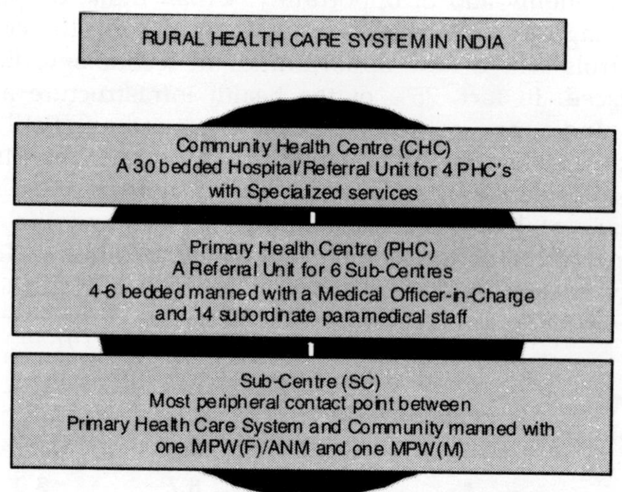

Source: *Bulletin on Rural Health Statistics in India*, 2006.

Primary Health Centers (PHCs)

Each PHC has five to six sub-centers located closer to rural villages that are managed by an Auxiliary Nurse. Each sub-center is meant to serve three to four villages. Overall, one PHC can serve anywhere from 25,000 to 48,000 people. The National Health Policy report of 2002 found that the current infrastructure of public health needs to increase by 16% in order to adequately serve the population (Ministry of Health and Family Welfare).

Rural areas already have much fewer staff and beds than urban areas. Doctor to patient ratio's are six times lower in rural areas, and doctor to bed ratios are fifteen times lower (Deogaonkar). A 2004 health survey in rural Udaipur found that each PHC served over 45,000 people and had on average of 5.8 medical personnel and 1.5 doctors appointed (Banerjee). Having such few staff serve such large populations no doubt contributes to their inefficiencies. Unfortunately, 80% of general practitioners practice allopathic medicine without proper training (Patil). The same is true of the private health care. A survey found that the average distance to a public health facility was 2.09 km and to a PHC was 6.7 km (Banerjee). For many rural people, who don't have transportation, traveling 6.7 km to closest doctor when ill is a great distance and could be a factor in their choosing unqualified private practitioners who are closer. The rural Udaipur survey showed that the people chose to go to private doctors almost twice as much as public facilities. In fact Patil tells us that 70% of rural families spend 60% of their annual income on health. The rural health survey supported this data by finding that only 37.7% of private doctors had an MBBS (qualifications to practice allopathic medicine) or higher specialty degree. 13.9% of "private doctors" in this survey had no formal qualifications and 36% did not have a college degree in any subject.

Indicators of Health Status of the Indian Population

Annual incidence of cataract, the cause of 80 percent of blindness, is 3.8 millions of cases. The total potential for surgical cataract removal is 1.75 million cases per year. The total number of cancer cases in India was estimated at 924,790 in 2001. This is projected to increase to 1,229,968 by 2011 and to 1,557,800 by 2021. The mortality rate due to cardiac arrest and related causes was estimated at 2.4 million in 1990. With increasing urbanization the problem is on the rise. Malaria is projected to increase from 2.03 million cases in 2001 to 2.62 million cases in 2021. Hypertension, diabetes and renal diseases; stress and lifestyle related disorders are on the rise. The diabetic population in India is projected to increase from 40 million of 2001 to 47 million people in 2010. Hypertension is lower in rural areas but on an increase in urban cities. Prevalence rate in Delhi alone is 17.34 percent. Both hypertension and diabetes further cause renal disorders. The current prevalence rate for neurological disorders is 15 to 20 people per thousand. The most common ailments are epilepsy, migraine, cerebrovascular disorders, Parkinson's disease and peripheral neuropathies. It is estimated that 1 percent of the population is suffering from serious psychiatric illnesses, 10-15 percent have neuro-disorders, and 2.5 percent are mentally retarded. (*Source*: ICRA report on Indian Health Care.)

Reduction in child mortality involves as much attention to protecting children from infection as in ensuring nutrition and calls for a holistic view of mother and child health services. The cluster of services consisting of antenatal services, delivery care and post mortem attention and low birth weight, childhood diarrhoea and ARI management are linked priorities. Programme of immunization and childhood nutrition seen in better performing stats indicate sustained attention to routine and complex investments into growing children as a group to make them grow into persons capable of living long and well. Often interest fades in pursuing the unglamorous routine of supervised immunization and is substituted by pulse campaigns, etc. which in the long-run turn out counter-productive.

As part of rural Primary health care network alone, a total of 1.6 lakh sub-centers, (with 1.27 lakh.' ANMa in position) and 22975 PHCs and 2935 CHCs (with over 24000 doctors and over 3500 specialists to serve in them) have been set-up. To promote Indian systems of medicine and homeopathy there are over 22000 dispensaries 2800 hospitals Besides 6 lakh angawadis serve nutrition needs of nearly 20 million children and 4 million mothers. The total effort has cost the bulk of the health development outlay, which stood at over Rs. 62.500 crores or 3-64% of total plan spending during the last fifty years. On any count these are extraordinary infrastructural capacities created with resources committed against odds to strengthen grass roots. There have been facility gaps, supply gaps and staffing gaps, which can be filled up only by allocating more funds and determined will to ensure good administration and synergy from greater congruence of services. It has got more firmly established at the periphery/sub-center level and dedicated to RCH services only. At PHC and CHC levels this has further been compounded by a weak referral system. PHCs and CHCs are funded by States, several of whom are unable to match Central assistance offered and hence these centers remain inadequate and operate on minimum efficiency.

The Disease Burden Affects the Wage Earning Capacity

The disease burden affects the wage earning capacity as well as productivity. It also entails expenditure on medical treatment, travel, attendants and the unfortunate premature death. A study shows that sixty percent of morbidity is due to infectious diseases and common tropical diseases, a quarter due to life-style disorders and 13% due to potentially preventable per-natal conditions. We were able to control smallpox and guinea worm diseases. It has now been proposed to eliminate or control the following diseases.

- o Polio Yaws and leprosy which seems distinctly feasible though the removal of social stigma and reconstructive surgery and other rehabilitation arrangements in a decade.

- o Kalaazar by 20I0 and Filalriasis by 2010 which also seems feasible due to its localized prevalence and the possibility of greater community based work.
- o Blindness prevalence to 0.5% by 2010 sees less feasible due to a graying population.
- o AIDS reaching zero growth by 2007 appears to be problematic as there are disputes even about base data on infected population.

Eleven out of thirteen diseases recommended by the Bhore Committee were infectious diseases and at least three of them may well continue to be with us for the next two decades, i.e. TB Malaria and Aids to which diarrhoea in children and complicated and high risk maternity should be added in view of their pervasive incidence and avoidable mortality among the poorer and under served sectors,

Tuberculosis

It is estimated that about 14 million persons are infected, from radiological active tuberculosis. More than 300 000 deaths occur every year. The prevalence among working age adults (15-59) is even higher. TB is a widespread disease of poverty among women living and working in ill ventilated places and other undernourished persons in urban slums. No universal screening is possible. Drugs are prescribed on the basis of fever and shadows as a result incomplete cure becomes common and delayed tests only prove the wrong diagnosis. Treatment costs in case of drug resistance can soar close to ten times the normal level of Rs. 3000 to 4000 per person treated.. There is reason to hope that DOTS programs would prove a greater success over time with increased community awareness. With commitment and full use of infrastructure it will be possible to arrest further growth in absolute numbers of TB cases keeping it at below 1.5 million till 2010 even though the population will be growing. Once that is done TB can be brought down to less than a million, i.e. within internationally accepted limits and disappears as a major communicable disease in India by 2020.

Malaria

At present India has a large manpower fully aware of all aspects of malaria but often low in motivation. There is evidence of reemergence with focal attacks of malaria with the virulent falciparum variety especially in tribal areas. About 2 million cases of malaria are recorded all over India every year with seasonal high incidence local failures of control. Drug resistance in humans and insecticide resistant strains of mosquitoes present a significant problem. There is growing interest and community awareness of biological methods of control of mosquito growth. As regards a vaccine, there seems to be no sufficient incentive for international R&D to focus on a relatively lower priority or research. The search for a vaccine continues but has little likelihood of immediate success. It is necessary that routine tasks like timely spraying and taking blood slides testing and their analysis and organic methods of reducing mosquito spread are carried out diligently. Malaria can certainly be reduced by a third even upto a half in ten years, and there is a prospect of near freedom from malaria for most of the country by 2020.

AIDS

The Draft NHP 2001 seeks to stop further infection by educating and counseling and condom supplies. Further such awareness efforts must be followed by multi-pronged and culturally compatible techniques of public education that go beyond segments easier to be convinced or behaviour changed. In about a decade vaccine development may possibly be successful and drugs may by more effective but they may not always be affordable nor can be given free. A recent analysis reveals that the three drug regimen recommended will cost $10000 per person per year from Western companies and the treatment will be life long. Three Indian companies are offering to Central Government anti retro; viral drugs at $600/(Rs. 30,000) per person per year and to an international charity at an even lower price $ 350/(Rs. 13,000) per year. It has been public policy in Brazil that the drug is supplied free to all AIDS patients.

Child Health and Nutrition

There is a issue of infant and child mortality, (70 out of 1000 dying in the first year and 98 before five years) and low birth weight (22% UW at birth ands 47% EJW at below 3 years). Most mortality occurs from diarrhea and the stagnation in IMR in the last few year is bound to have a negative effect on population stabilization goals. At the same time, more streamlined RCH services are getting established as part of public systems and through private partnerships. Therefore, there is every reason to hope that the NPP 2000 target of 30 per thousand live births by 2010 will be met barring a few pockets of inaccessible and resource lean areas with stubborn persistence of poverty and dominantly composed of weaker sections.

As regards childhood diarrhoea, deaths are totally preventable with simple community action and public education by targeting children of low birth weights and detecting early those children at risk from malnutrition through proper low cost screening procedure. The success can be built upon till 2025 for reaching levels comparable to China.

Mild and moderate malnutrition still prevalent in over half of our young population can be halved if food as the supplemental pathway to better nutrition becomes a priority both for self reliance and lower costs. There has been a tendency for micro nutrient supplementation to overwhelm food derived nourishment. This trend is assisted by foreign aid but over a long-run may prove unsustainable. By engaging the adolescents into proper nutrition education and reproductive health awareness we can seamlessly weave into the nutritional security system of our country a corps of informed interconnected and imaginative ideas can be tried out.

For the sake of comparison, let us look at some other countries of the world; some poor and others rich.

Niger

It is one of the poorest health care system in the world. Health care system of Niger suffers from a chronic lack of resources and a small number of health providers relative to population. Some medicines are in short supply or unavailable. There are government hospitals in Niamey, Maradi, Tahoua, Zinder and other large cities, with smaller medical clinics in most towns. Medical facilities are limited in both supplies and staff, with a small government health care system supplemented by private, charitable, religious, and Non-government organisation operated clinics and public health programs (such as Galmi Hospital near Birnin Konni and Maradi). Government hospitals, as well as public health programmes, fall under the control of the Nigerien Ministry of Health. The total expenditure on health per capita in 2005 was Intl. $25. There were 377 Physicians in Niger in 2004, a ratio of 0.03 per 10,000 population. In 2003, 89.2 percent of individual expenditures on health care were "out-of-pocket" (paid by the patient).

Pakistan

Pakistan's health indicators, health funding, and health and sanitation infrastructure are generally poor, particularly in rural areas. About 19 percent of the population is malnourished—a higher rate than the 17 percent average for developing countries—and 30 percent of children under age five are malnourished. Leading causes of sickness and death include gastroenteritis, respiratory infections, congenital abnormalities, tuberculosis, malaria, and typhoid fever. The United Nations estimates that in 2003 Pakistan's human immunodeficiency virus (HIV) prevalence rate was 0.1 percent among those 15-49, with an estimated 4,900 deaths from acquired immune deficiency syndrome (AIDS). AIDS is a major health concern, and both the government and religious community are engaging in efforts to reduce its spread. In 2003 there were 68 physicians for every 100,000 persons in Pakistan. According to 2002 government statistics, there were 12,501 health institutions nationwide, including 4,590 dispensaries, 906 hospitals with a total of 80,665 hospital beds, and 550 rural health centers with a total of 8,840 beds. According to the World Health Organization, Pakistan's total health expenditures amounted to 3.9 percent of gross domestic product (GDP) in 2001, and per capita health expenditures were US$16. The government provided 24.4 percent of total health expenditures, with the remainder being entirely private, out-of-pocket expenses.

Afghanistan

Afghanistan's military conflict destroyed the health system of Afghanistan. Most medical professionals left the country in the 1980s and

1990s, and all medical training programs ceased. In 2004 Afghanistan had one medical facility for every 27,000 people, and some centers were responsible for as many as 300,000 people. In 2004 international organizations provided a large share of medical care. An estimated one-quarter of the population had no access to health care. In 2003 there were 11 physicians and 18 nurses per 100,000 populations, and the per capita health expenditure was US $ 28.

Bhutan

Bhutan's health care system development accelerated in the early 1960s with the establishment of the Department of Public Health and the opening of new hospitals and dispensaries throughout the country. By the early 1990s, health care was provided through twenty-nine general hospitals, forty-six dispensaries, sixty-seven basic health units, four indigenous-medicine dispensaries, and fifteen malaria eradication centers. The major hospitals were the National Referral Hospital in Thimphu, and other hospitals in Geylegphug, and Tashigang. Hospital beds in 1988 totaled 932. There was a severe shortage of health care personnel with official statistics reporting only 142 physicians and 678 paramedics, about one health care professional for every 2,000 people, or only one physician for almost 10,000 people.

Japan

In Japan, services are provided either through regional/national public hospitals or through private hospitals/clinics, and patients have universal access to any facility, though hospitals tend to charge higher for those without a referral. Public health insurance covers most citizens/residents and pays 70% or more cost for each care and each prescribed drug. Patients are responsible for the remainder. The monthly insurance premium is 0-50,000 JPY per household. Supplementary private health insurance is available only to cover the co-payments or non-covered costs, and usually makes a fixed payment per days in hospital or per surgery performed, rather than per actual expenditure. In 2005, Japan spent 8.2% of GDP on health care, or US $ 2,908 per capita. Of that, approximately 83% was government expenditure.

Malaysia

Health care in Malaysia is divided into private and public sectors. Doctors are required to perform 3 years of service with public hospitals throughout the nation, ensuring adequate coverage of medical needs for the general population. Foreign doctors are encouraged to apply for employment in Malaysia, especially if they are qualified to a higher level. Malaysian society places importance on the expansion and development of health care, putting 5% of the government social sector development budget into public health care—an increase of more than 47% over the previous figure. This has meant an overall increase of more than RM 2 billion. With a rising and aging population, the Government wishes to improve in many areas including the refurbishment of existing hospitals, building and equipping new hospitals, expansion of the number of polyclinics, and improvements in training and expansion of telehealth. There is still a shortage in the medical workforce, especially of highly trained specialists. The majority of private hospital facilities are in urban areas and, unlike many of the public hospitals, are equipped with the latest diagnostic and imaging facilities.

People's Republic of China

The effective public health work and dramatic improvements in nutrition greatly improved the health and life expectancy of the Chinese people. The 2000 WHO World Health Report—Health systems: improving performance found that China's health care system before 1980 performed far better than countries at a comparable level of development, since 1980 ranks much lower than comparable countries. The end of the famed "barefoot doctor" system was abolished in 1981. The New Rural Co-operative Medical Care System (NRCMCS) is a new 2005 initiative to overhaul the health care system, particularly intended to make it more affordable for the rural poor. Under the NRCMCS, the annual cost of medical cover is 50 yuan (US$7) per person. Of that, 20 yuan is paid in by the central government, 20 yuan by the provincial government and a contribution of 10 yuan is made by the patient. As of September 2007, around 80% of the whole rural population of China had signed up (about 685 million people). If patients go to a small hospital or clinic in their local town, the scheme will cover from 70-80% of their bill. If they go to a county one, the percentage of the cost being covered falls to about 60%. And if they need specialist help in a large modern city hospital, they have to bear most of the cost themselves; the scheme would cover about 30% of the bill.

In rural areas the first tier was made up of barefoot doctors working out of village medical centers. They provided preventive and primary care services, with an average of two doctors per 1,000 people. At the next level were the township health centers, which functioned primarily as out-patient clinics for about 10,000 to 30,000 people each. These centers had about ten to thirty beds each, and the most qualified members of the staff were assistant doctors. The two lower-level tiers made up the "rural collective health system" that provided most of the country's medical care. Only the most seriously ill patients were referred to the third and final tier, the county hospitals, which served 200,000 to 600,000 people each and were staffed by senior doctors who held degrees from 5-year medical schools. Health care in urban areas was provided by paramedical personnel assigned to factories and neighbourhood health stations. If more professional care was necessary the patient was sent to a district hospital, and the most serious cases were handled by municipal hospitals.

Singapore

Health care in Singapore is mainly under the responsibility of the Singapore Government's Ministry of Health. Singapore generally has an efficient and widespread system of health care. It implements a universal health care system, and co-exists with private health care system. Infant mortality rate: in 2006 the crude birth rate stood at 10.1 per 1000, a very low level attributed to birth control policies, and the crude death rate was also one of the lowest in the world at 4.3 per 1000. In 2006, the total fertility rate was only 1.26 children per woman, the 3rd lowest in the world and well below the 2.10 needed to replace the population. Singapore was ranked 6th in the World Health Organization's ranking of the world's health systems in the year 2000.

Singapore has a universal health care system where government ensures affordability, largely through compulsory savings and price controls, while the private sector provides most care. Overall spending on health care amounts to only 3% of annual GDP. Of that, 66% comes from private sources. Singapore currently has the lowest infant mortality rate in the world and among the highest life expectancies from birth, according to the World Health Organization. Singapore has "one of the most successful health care systems in the world, in terms of both efficiency in financing and the results achieved in community health outcomes," according to an analysis by global consulting firm Watson Wyatt. Singapore's system uses a combination of compulsory savings from payroll deductions (funded by both employers and workers) a nationalized catastrophic health insurance plan, and government subsidies, as well as "actively regulating the supply and prices of health care services in the country" to keep costs in check; the specific features have been described as potentially a "very difficult system to replicate in many other countries." Many Singaporeans also have supplemental private health insurance (often provided by employers) for services not covered by the government's programs. Patients are free to choose the providers within the government or private health care delivery system and can walk in for a consultation at any private clinic or any government polyclinic. For emergency services, patients can go at any time to the 24-hour Accident and Emergency Departments located in the government hospitals. Singapore's medical facilities are among the finest in the world, with well qualified doctors and dentists, many trained overseas. Singapore has medical savings account system known as Medisave.

Thailand

In 1995, Thailand had 0.3 physicians and 1.9 hospital beds per 1,000 population. In 2002 annual spending on health care amounted to US $ 321 per person in purchasing power parity (PPP). Total expenditures represented about 4.4 percent of the gross domestic product (GDP); of this amount, 57.1 percent came from public sources and 42.9 percent from private sources. Some 85 percent of the population had access to potable water in 2002, and 99 percent had access to sanitation. Human immunodeficiency virus/acquired immune deficiency syndrome (HIV/AIDS) is a serious problem in Thailand. The government has begun to improve its support to persons with HIV/AIDS and has provided funds to HIV/AIDS support groups. Major infectious diseases in Thailand also include bacterial diarrhea, hepatitis, dengue fever, malaria, Japanese encephalitis, rabies, and leptospirosis.

Thailand introduced universal coverage reforms in 2001, becoming one of only a handful of lower-middle income countries to do so. People joining the scheme receive a gold card which allows them to access services in their health district, and, if necessary, be referred for specialist treatment elsewhere. The bulk of finance comes from public revenues, with funding allocated to Contracting Units for Primary Care annually on a population basis. According to the WHO, 65% of Thailand's health care expenditure in 2004 came from the government, 35% was from private sources.

United Arab Emirates

Standards of health care are considered to be generally high in the United Arab Emirates, resulting from increased government spending during strong economic years. According to the UAE government, total expenditures on health care from 1996 to 2003 were US $ 436 million. According to the World Health Organization, in 2004 total expenditures on health care constituted 2.9 percent of gross domestic product (GDP), and the per capita expenditure for health care was US $ 497. Health care currently is free only for UAE citizens. Effective January 2006, all residents of Abu Dhabi are covered by a new comprehensive health insurance program; costs will be shared between employers and employees. The number of doctors per 100,000 (annual average, 1990-99) is 181. The UAE now has 40 public hospitals. The Ministry of Health is undertaking a multimillion-dollar program to expand health facilities viz. hospitals, medical centers, and a trauma center in the seven emirates. A state-of-the-art general hospital has opened in Abu Dhabi with a projected bed capacity of 143, a trauma unit, and the first home health care program in the UAE. To attract wealthy UAE nationals and expatriates who traditionally have traveled abroad for serious medical care, Dubai is developing Dubai Health Care City, a hospital free zone that will offer international-standard advanced private health care and provide an academic medical training center; completion is scheduled for 2010.

Vietnam

The overall quality of health in Vietnam is regarded as good, as reflected by 2005 estimates of life expectancy (70.61 years) and infant mortality (25.95 per 1,000 live births). However, malnutrition is still common in the provinces, and the life expectancy and infant mortality rates are stagnating. In 2001 government spending on health care corresponded to just 0.9 percent of gross domestic product (GDP). Government subsidies covered only about 20 percent of health care expenses, with the remaining

80 percent coming out of individuals' own pockets. Inadequate funding has led to delays in planned upgrades to water supply and sewage systems. As a result, almost half the population has no access to clean water, a deficiency that promotes such infectious diseases as malaria, dengue fever, typhoid, and cholera. Inadequate funding also has contributed to a shortage of nurses, midwives, and hospital beds. In 2000 Vietnam had only 250,000 hospital beds, or 14.8 beds per 10,000 people, a very low ratio among Asian nations, according to the World Bank.

Zimbabwe

Zimbabwe now has one of the lowest life expectancies on Earth-44 for men and 43 for women, down from 60 in 1990. The rapid drop has been ascribed mainly to the HIV/AIDS pandemic. Infant mortality has risen from 59 per thousand in the late 1990s to 123 per 1000 by 2004. The health system has more or less collapsed: By the end of November 2008, three of Zimbabwe's four major hospitals had shut down, along with the Zimbabwe Medical School and the fourth major hospital had two wards and no operating theatres working. Due to hyperinflation, those hospitals still open are not able to obtain basic drugs and medicines. The ongoing political and economic crisis also contributed to the emigration of the doctors and people with medical knowledge. In August 2008, large areas of Zimbabwe were struck by the ongoing cholera epidemic.

Sources

Winnie Yip and Ajay Mahal, (2008): "The Health Care Systems Of China And India: Performance And Future Challenges", *Health Affairs*, 27(4): 921-932.

Aggarwal, A.K.: Public health and public-private partnership, *Indian Journal of Community Medicine*, Vol. 33, Issue 2, April 2008.

Getting there from here New Yorker article. Jan. 2009.

Johns Hopkins University President William Brody (2008) proposed another set of criteria for evaluating the US health systems: Cost, Coverage, Consistency, Complexity and Chronic Illness.

How Private Insurance Works: A Primer by Gary Claxton, Institution for Health Care Research and Policy, Georgetown University, on behalf of the Henry J. Kaiser Family Foundation.

Afghanistan country profile. Library of Congress Federal Research Division (May 2006). This article incorporates text from this source, which is in the public domain.

Rais Akhtar; Health Care Patterns and Planning in Developing Countries, Greenwood Press, 1991. p. 264.

Ronald J. Vogel; Financing Health Care in Sub-Saharan Africa Greenwood Press, 1993. p. 18.

Ronald, J. Vogel; Financing Health Care in Sub-Saharan Africa Greenwood Press, 1993. pp. 1-18.

Ronald J. Vogel; Financing Health Care in Sub-Saharan Africa Greenwood Press, 1993. pp. 101-02.

Felicia Monye; 'An Appraisal of the National Health Insurance Scheme of Nigeria', *Commonwealth Law Bulletin*, 32:3, 415-27.

WHO World Health report, 2000—Health systems: improving performance.

The reform of the rural cooperative medical system in the People's Republic of China: interim experience in 14 pilot counties. Authors: Carrin, G.1.; Ron, A.; Hui, Y.; Hong, W.; Tuohong, Z.; Licheng, Z.; Shuo, Z.; Yide, Y.; Jiaying, C.; Qicheng, J.; Zhaoyang, Z.; Jun, Y.; Xuesheng, L. *Source*: *Social Science and Medicine*, Volume 48, Number 7, April 1999, pp. 961-972(12).

Bribes for basic care in Romania. *The Guardian Weekly* (March 26th, 2008).

"The Singapore health system - achieving positive health outcomes with low expenditure", *Watson Wyatt Health Care Market Review*, October 2004.

G20 Health Care: "Health Care Systems and Health Market Reform in the G20 Countries." Prepared for the World Economic Forum by Ernst and Young. January 3, 2006.

Hughes, D., Leethongdee, S. (2007). "Universal coverage in the land of smiles: lessons from Thailand's 30 baht health reforms". *Health Affairs*, 26(4): 999-1008. doi:10.1377/hlthaff.26.4.999. PMID 17630443.

"Income, Poverty, and Health Insurance Coverage in the United States:2007" (PDF). U.S. Census Bureau. http://www.census.gov/prod/2008pubs/p60-235.pdf233.pdf. Retrieved 2008-08-26.

.Jackson, David (August 1, 1993). "Pursuit of ideas primes research institute; Conservative Dallas organization is part of movement to shape national politics".

Goodman, John (2006), "Consumer Driven Health Care", Networks Financial Institute Policy Brief, Indiana State University.

Further Readings

Banerjee, Abhijit, Angus Deaton and Esther Duflo. "Health Care Delivery in Rural Rajasthan". *Economic and Political Weekly*. February 28, 2004. V. 39, iss. 9. pp. 944-949.

Express Health Care Management. Rural Health Care. 16th August 2005. http://www.expresshealth caremgmt.com/20050831/ruralhealth care01.shtml.

Patil, Ashok V., K.V. Somasundaram, and R.C. Goyal. "Current Health Scenario in Rural India". *Australian Journal of Rural Health*. January 2002. pp. 129-53.

Deogaonkar, Milind. "Socio-economic inequality and its effect on health care delivery in India: Inequality and health care". *Electronic Journal of Sociology*. 2004. http://www.sociology.org/content/vol18.1/deogaonkar.html.

CIA. CIA World Fact Book 2002. 2002. CIA. 1 January 2002. http://www.faqs.org/docs/factbook/geos/in.html.

Bardhan, Pranab. "Globalization and Rural Poverty". *World Development*. December 2005.

Government of India. Ministry of Health and Family Welfare, National Rural Health Mission Document. 2005.

Government of India. Ministry of Health and Family Welfare, *Bulletin on Rural Health Statistics in India*, 2006. 2006. http://mohfw.nic.in/dofw%20website/Bulletin%20on%20RHS%20-%2006%20-%20PDF%20Files/bulletin_on_rural_health_statistics.htm

Government of India. Ministry of Health and Family Welfare, *National Health Policy-2002*. 2002. http://mohfw.nic.in/np2002.htm.

Health Care Systems in Third World Countries

"Common characteristics of third world countries are poverty, high birthrates, and economic dependence on the advanced countries. Most of these nations are plagued by problems of under nutrition and a host of infections. Epidemics of diarrheal diseases provide a rough guide to the poor sanitation of the community. Safe drinking water is a dream for millions even now. The private sector is interested only in curative medicine and these hospitals and clinics are necessarily run with a profit motive. Services rendered to people are generally abysmally poor, especially in a rural setting. In fact it is understood that the third world countries have third rate health care! The developing and underdeveloped countries in the world look to the west as the model of development. However, the state of Kerala in southern India has achieved health indices which are comparable to the west. This achievement which is known as the "Kerala model" was attained with a GDP much less than the national average. Kerala boasts of universal literacy for 100% of its citizens and its robust health status is simply a reflection of education of the people especially among women."

The developed countries have in place many systems by which health care is provided to their needy citizens. It may be state owned health care delivery as in the case of NHS in UK or managed care services offered by health insurance firms as in the US. It may be noted that even developed countries are shying away from supporting health care delivery by public sector. However, Public health institutions are the only hope for the underprivileged people in the developing countries like India, also called third world countries.

Third World Countries give Back Seat to Health

The government pumps in some money to keep the system afloat, but the Many programmes aimed at the prevention of communicable disease are run in under developed countries with the help of the WHO. Even these programmes have not had the desired effect due to faulty implementation. It is revealing to note that the custodian of world health has started disbelieving cooked up reports of programme implementation by corrupt officials and has instead started on site status checking by their own independent teams. The reasons for the failure of these national health programmes are multi-factorial. The most important among these are the lackadaisical approach by the government officials involved in implementing the programmes. Apart from the half hearted involvement of government in these programmes, the money gets diverted to construction of buildings, purchase of vehicles and equipments. Very often the beneficiaries receive less than 1% worth of what is envisaged in the programme. Who is to blame?

The rural people, who are the beneficiaries, should change their role from meek passive observer status beneficiaries into active decision makers in the planning and implementation of the programmes in their locality. Major strategies regarding fund allocation and implementation can always be made centrally by bureaucrats and experts but the people in the periphery should have a very decisive role in health development. They should know the allocation for their region in terms of money, personnel and other resources. The officials concerned should interact with the local people not in a "we give thou" style but in a way that the people feel part of these programmes. The print and visual media should take a proactive role in health matters rather than painting a dismal picture of a weak system, which is on the verge of collapse. Major irregularities are to be exposed, but not at the expense of public losing faith in these programmes. Any unwarranted and destructive criticism of public health system will be beneficial only to the private sector. Representation from all sections of society without political overdose must be ensured in such public participation programmes. The Nobel laureate, Amartya Sen wanted to call it "Kerala phenomenon". Kerala had a system of public schools started by the local rulers and education of girls was ensured by royal decree. Successive governments in Kerala with socialist approach to education and health care have sustained this momentum. (see Appendices 1 and 2 for excerpts of world health report 2008, attached at the end of the book).

The rulers should recognize that the best asset and strength of the nation is its population, which is healthy and vibrant.

What is Third World?

The term 'Third World Country' was used in reference to the economically underdeveloped countries of Asia, Africa, Oceania, and Latin America, and were considered as an entity with common characteristics, such as poverty, high birthrates, and economic dependence on the advanced countries. A First World Country is one that is industrialized and has generally accepted the concepts of capitalism and world trade, a Second World Country is an industrialized nation that had rejected capitalism, in favour of Communism or Marxism. The Third World Countries were those that did not fit either of these two. The key features used to define a Third World Country are its lack of industrialization, a very low GNP, a high population and a high level of poverty.

A quick look at the Third World countries shows that income maldistribution is very much with us: Comparing the top 20% income group with the bottom 20% (1995) shows that in China the gap was 7 times higher, in Thailand it was 9%; in Malaysia 11%; in The Philippines 7%, and in Vietnam 5%.

Third World Countries and Third Rate Health Care!

It is believed that rich countries use around 7% of their income on health and poor countries are using around 10-11%. Yet, in 2003, the average spending on health care in all developing countries worldwide was US $ 11/capita. (It is deemed this amount must be increased to $60). Households are the main source of financing health care services, i.e. close to 80% in many countries in Asia. Against this background, the disease burden of the poorest quintile is roughly threefold that of the richest, their life expectancy is around 10 years shorter, and their infant mortality rate is twice as high. Close to one third of the patients who need hospitalization fail to be hospitalized: around 80% due to financial constraints. There is also evidence that poor patients abscond due to lack of money to pay hospital bills. In many countries, unofficial payments to hospital staff and doctors are estimated to be about 15 times higher than official payments for hospital services. People think these payments—formal as well as informal—are necessary for receiving proper treatment. Unfortunately, close to 60% of the people self-medicate!! Medical expenditures are now one of the main causes of why people become poor (the 'medical poverty trap').

It is not exaggerated to estimate that a good 80% of private practitioners are primarily employed in the pubic health care sector. But they are not making a decent living from the salaries, so, now, even a big part of their monthly take-home wages have to be generated locally through fee-for-service regimes. The problem is sometimes so acute that even traditionally preventive health care facilities have had to start providing curative services to make money. See Appendix attached to this chapter for 'Quality Assessment and Improvement: Experiences in Developing Countries'.

Fee for Service

The charging of fees in public health facilities is inconsistent with equity objectives; revenues from it only cover about 10% of all health expenditures. These fees thus only marginally contribute in terms of overall HCF—and they grossly increase inequality. In the user fee system (a regressive tax), the sick pay more; the poor pay more; children and the elderly pay more. The fee for service system increases the burden on the sick, especially the rural. It has weakened the structure of preventive care, because it has decreased funding for it causing a loss of preventive care staff with the ones left having poor skills. We are witnessing an "under-the-table" commercialization of public health services. On the other hand, there is NO positive relationship between high user charges and good quality of care—for either the rich or the poor. Under the fee for service regime, providers tend to over-provide costly services (e.g., extra diagnostic tests and costly treatments) neglecting the needs for regular services of the rest of the population. This clearly gives priority to the more profitable, paying segment of the health care market.

User Charges have Worsened the Lot of Poorer Citizens

In response to shrinking budgets and growing demands, many developing countries have adopted formal or informal user fees in government health facilities. While they raise revenue, in the absence of special provisions user fees may hurt equity and efficiency. This paper reviews the success of two such provisions—waivers and exemptions. Waivers enable the poor to obtain free health care while exemptions enable all people to receive certain services for free. The dilemma is how to preserve user fees without hurting equity and efficiency.

Scenario in Seven Developing Countries

Let us look at the experience of seven developing countries—Cambodia, Chile, Ghana, Indonesia, Kenya, Thailand, and Zimbabwe—with waivers and exemptions, and draw lessons for countries wishing to introduce such mechanisms. The review is chiefly concerned with (1) the degree to which waivers reduce out-of-pocket spending by the poor; (2) the increase in utilization resulting from waivers and exemptions; and (3) the enabling factors of successful waiver and exemption systems. Ricardo Bitran and Ursula Giedion prepared this note based on their paper "Waivers and Exemptions for Health Services in Developing Countries", 2003. Social Protection Discussion Paper No. 0308, World Bank, Washington, D.C. Those that carefully designed and implemented their waiver systems—such as Thailand and Indonesia—have had much greater success in terms of benefits incidence than those countries—such as Ghana, Kenya, and Zimbabwe—that took a more improvised approach. The key to a waiver system's success is adequate financing. Systems—such as those in Thailand, Indonesia, and Cambodia—that compensate providers for the revenue they must forego in granting waivers and exemptions have been more successful than those, i.e. Kenya—which expect providers to absorb the cost of waivers and exemptions.

Medicines: How much of a Culprit?

Drugs account for up to 70% of overall health expenditures. Drug vendors in the private sector are the relief providers of choice and they are

NOT health providers. Why do people choose them? Because of the limited access they have to professional health care services: the poor often have no choice; self-medication is thus a major item of household expenditure. Otherwise, private health care providers earn a large share of their income selling drugs in their private offices. This is as unethical as it is dangerous, causing losses to society that end up wasting money on unnecessary, useless or dangerous drugs. The focus is to be on decreasing poly-pharmacy and the use of antibiotics, injections, steroids and vitamins,, i.e. controlling the irrational use of drugs.

Cross-subsidization may Help

Ideally, in the population, the healthy should subsidize the sick, the rich should subsidize the poor, the working should subsidize the dependent. One option to keep in mind is for private for profit hospitals to be taxed at levels that will secure cross-subsidization to public hospitals. To universalize access to health services, one needs to subsidize the poor using both local and outside funds coming both from inside and outside the health sector. [In Vietnam, it has been proposed that, in rural areas: The government should end up paying 75% of all health care costs; the community 10%; foreign aid 10%; and user fees 5%. In urban areas: taxes should cover 50-60% of the costs; health insurance 20-25%; fees 10%; and foreign aid 5%. Insurance schemes cannot replace a national publicly financed health care system; they can only contribute to it. Subsidies will thus be required even for well-designed and efficiently run public insurance schemes. There is a need that the public sector takes the lead and exerts an effective controlling role over the private sector. Also, the government has to increase its health spending. But it has to gear it to pro-poor interventions, e.g., preventive services and services directed at the diseases of poverty; it is these that have to be fully financed. As part of strategy, measures have to be taken to have all health resources used more effectively. Exemptions are nevertheless needed for all cases of public health importance such as TB, malaria, STDs, HIV/AIDS.

Community-based Health Insurance (CBHI)

CBHI is a household responsibility system; it is meant for people in the informal sector, mostly the rural and urban poor; as any insurance, it is based on risk sharing and resources pooling; it is more viable where the community is already organized for other purposes. A CBHI system assures a highly equitable coverage, a potentially more egalitarian geographical access, a greater equity in the financing of its operations, a potential for health care cost controls and an increased efficiency in the use of resources, as well as good financial sustainability and a chance for improved quality of care. It provides a greater latitude compared with pure tax financing of health care. To begin with, three major policy changes are deemed necessary: 1. legislation for a community tax of 1.5-2% of income; 2. an additional central government tax support of 0.2-0.5 of GDP; and 3. changes in the personnel compensation system allowing for bonus payments. A fully voluntary CBHI system will inevitably lead to an adverse selection problem (with mostly the sicker and the elderly wanting to join). A compulsory system will also not work. The main challenge will ultimately be to convince people that what is proposed is for them to reduce their 'envelope (under-the-table) payments', and, instead, start paying a clearly identified local health tax. Once the community accepts to join, people get together and make a pre-payment (an investment, really, since they will not have a financial burden at the time of illness). At this time, communities can also determine exemption mechanisms to be applied.

Poverty breeds poor health

The poorest of the poor, around the world, have the worst health. Those . . the bottom of the distribution of global and national wealth, those marginalized and excluded within countries, and countries themselves disadvantaged by historical exploitation and persistent inequity in global institutions of power and policy-making present an urgent moral and practical focus for action. But focusing on those with the least, on the 'gap' between the poorest and the rest, is only a partial response.... In rich countries, low socioeconomic position means poor education, lack of amenities, unemployment and job insecurity, poor working conditions, and unsafe neighbourhoods, with their consequent impact on family life. These all apply to the socially disadvantaged in low-income countries in addition to the considerable burden of material deprivation and vulnerability to natural disasters. So these dimensions of social disadvantage—that the health of the worst off in high-income countries is, in a few dramatic cases,

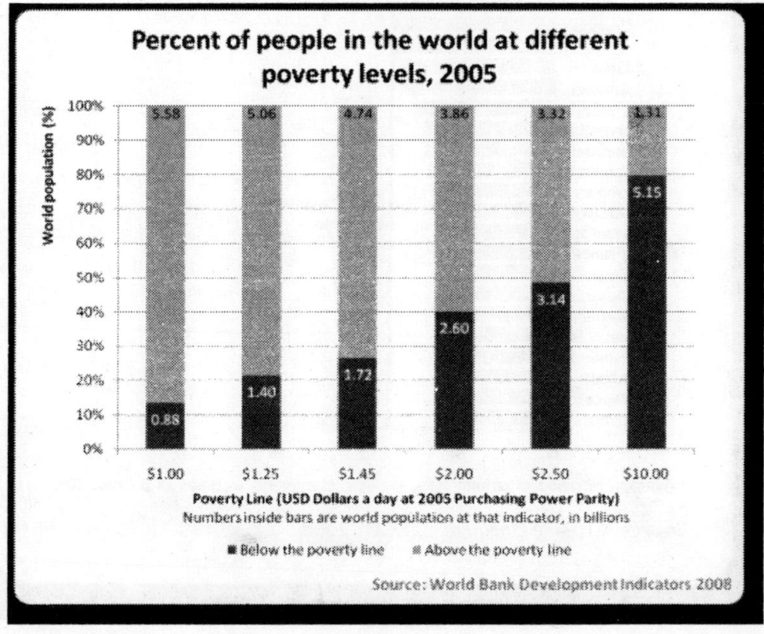

worse than average health in some lower-income countries—are important for health.

The health services in these countries have been modeled on the systems available in developed countries and meet the needs of the affluent sections of the population who control government policy. But these services are beyond the reach of the poor. There are wide disparities between the health indicators of the rich and poor consumers in the Third World. To provide adequate health services to the poor, there should be a re-allocation of resources away from high technology and hospital based curative services to preventive and promotive health services. It is often argued that low income countries cannot expect the health of all their inhabitants without first increasing productivity. Evidence from selected Third World countries indicates, however, that visible improvements in the health status of the poor are quite feasible with low per capita GNPs if there is the political will to implement progressive policies in health and certain non-health sectors. The latter include policies on land reform and education, particularly education of women.

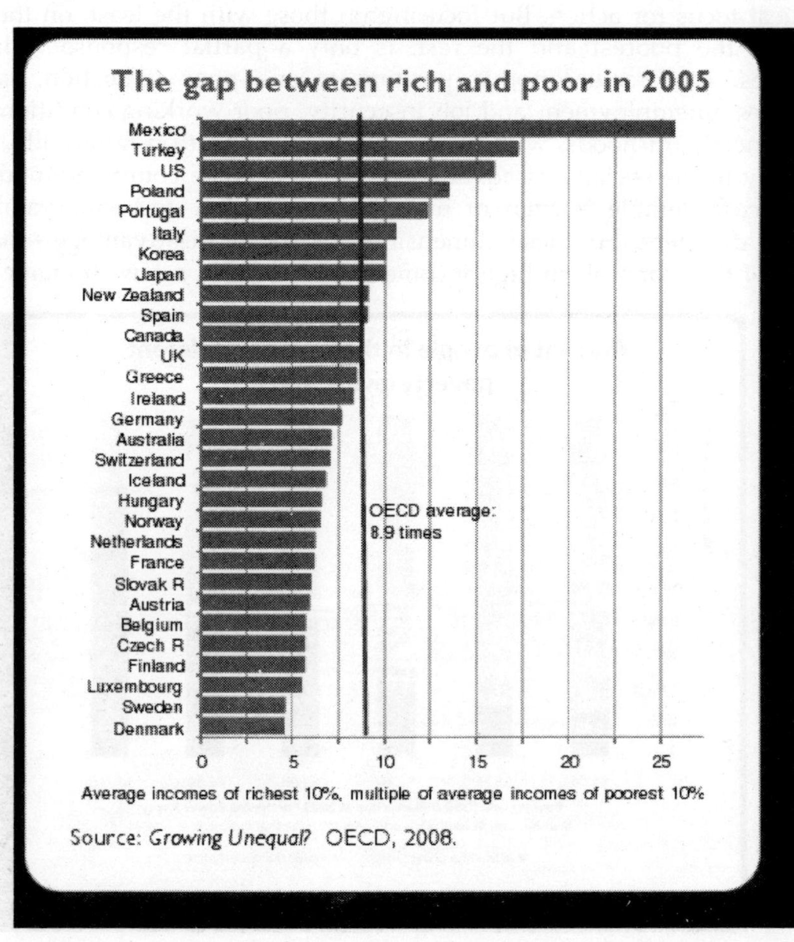

Source: *Growing Unequal?* OECD, 2008.

Indices of the Health Inequality between Poor and other Australians

- Indigenous/poor women are three times more likely to die while pregnant, during labour or up to six weeks after giving birth than non-indigenous women, a figure that has not changed since statistics started being kept in the early 1990s.
- Babies born to indigenous women weigh on average 217 grams less than those born to non-indigenous women. In the NT almost 17 babies died out of 1,000 births, more than three times the rate for the rest of the Australian population in 2005.
- Respiratory illnesses in Aboriginal children aged 1 to 5 years are widespread and account for more than 15 percent of all NT Aboriginal hospital admissions. The rate of bronchiectasis amongst Aboriginal children in central Australia is one of the highest in the world.
- Aboriginal children in the NT have high rates of growth faltering and anaemia, while skin infections, such as scabies and streptococcal pyoderma, are commonplace in remote communities. Up to half the children are infected.
- Diabetes is about three-and-a-half times more common among indigenous people than other Australians, with deaths from the disease 10 times higher.
- Eye-conditions affecting the indigenous population, including cataracts, trachoma and diabetic retinopathy, are endemic. Up to 30 percent of indigenous children in the Northern Territory suffer infectious trachoma.
- A recent Alice Springs Hospital survey found that Aboriginal people are 11 times more likely to die with an infectious disease than non-indigenous patients, a rate far higher than most third-world countries. Tuberculosis infection rates are 10 times higher; and haemophilus influenzae, which causes otitis media, conjunctivitis and sinusitis, 14 times higher in indigenous children under 5 years of age.
- End-stage renal disease is 25 times more common for indigenous people than for non-indigenous people, with the death rate from kidney disease at least 10 times higher. Some medical experts estimate that indigenous Australians in the Central Desert region are 30 to 50 times more likely to need dialysis than the national average.
- Indigenous people live 17 years less than the rest of total population and only 3 percent live to 65 years, the official retirement age. In central Australia, the average life expectancy difference is 24 years.

Poverty Affects Health of Women and Young Children more

It has been discovered that household living standards have a substantial influence on three measures of health: unmet need for modern contraception; attendance of a trained provider at childbirth; and children's height for age. According to the United Nations (2000), by the year 2030 the world's population will exceed today's total by 2.06 billion persons, of whom some 1.94 billion will be added to the urban areas of Africa, Asia, and Latin America. The first of the above mentioned needs, the unmet need for contraception, is closely linked to unintended pregnancy; birth attendance is a measure of the protection given mothers and children at the time of delivery; and height for age is an often-used indicator of the state of child health. Taken together, these measures describe a relatively high-risk period in the lives of women and their children.

Estimates by UN-HABITAT (United Nations Human Settlements Programme) suggest that some 38 percent of the population of developing-country cities live in slums, with total slum populations numbering 126 million persons in Africa, 433 million in Asia, and 87 million in Latin America (Herr and Karl, 2002; Herr and Mboup, 2003). "The key determinants of health of individuals and populations are the circumstances in which people are born, grow, live, work and age," he says. "And those circumstances are affected by the social and economic environment. They are the cause premature of disease and suffering; that's unnecessary. And that's why we say a toxic combination of poor social policies, bad politics and unfair economics are causing health and disease on a grand scale", Marmot says. Even within a country such as the UK, then, the report finds that the average life-span can differ by some 28 years, depending on whether you are in the poorer or wealthier strata of society.

Third World Countries have Huge Reservoir of Infections

Infectious diseases are the #1 killer in the developing world. Among infectious diseases, Acute Respiratory Infections such as influenza and pneumonia are the #1 killer. However, for the rapidity and lethality of its spread, AIDS is rightly claimed "the worst pandemic since the 14th century's Black Plague."

The failure of developing countries to cope with the AIDS epidemic, particularly in sub-Saharan Africa, is symptomatic of fundamental inadequacies in their health care delivery systems. Handicapped by limited resources, these nations' ability to fight AIDS and a host of other killer diseases is compromised by poor infrastructure, famine and malnutrition, cultural attitudes and practices, ignorance, and inadequate public health systems. Political leaders in many countries lack the will to confront their nation's health care needs. The papers that follow describe health care conditions in the world's poorest nations, discuss ongoing anti-AIDS efforts in the developing world, and address the many barriers to care.

The Key Points

- HIV/AIDS afflicts some 42 million people worldwide and about

29.4 million in Africa. AIDSrelated diseases kill more than three million people every year. Its reach now extends into India, China, Eastern Europe and Latin America.

- Even without AIDS, developing world health systems would be overwhelmed. Other infectious diseases killed roughly nine million people in developing nations last year—about three times as many as died from AIDS.
- Significant percentage of developing world populations has virtually no access to meaningful health care, largely because of poor infrastructure, especially transportation. Public health systems are grossly underfunded and often concentrated in cities.
- Famine and malnutrition exacerbate disease and complicate treatment, not to mention undercut maintenance of basic health. Effects of ignorance and stigma abound.
- Developing world governments must make fighting AIDS a priority.
- In recognition of conditions in the developing world, the pharmaceutical industry has supported humanitarian efforts there for many years—providing more than $1.9 billion in financial assistance and donated medicines over the last four years alone.

Inequality Fueled by many Factors

Various things can create inequality. Most common generalizations will be things like greed, power, and money. But even in societies where governments are well-intentioned, policy choices and individual actions (or inactions) can all contribute to inequality. In wealthier nations, the political left usually argue for addressing inequality as a matter of moral obligation or social justice, to help avoid worsening social cohesion and a weakening society. While ideological debates will always continue on the causes of inequality, both the political left and right agree that social cohesion (social justice or family values, etc.) is suffering, risking the very fabric of society if it gets too out of control.

Common people don't have basic health facilities under their reach or either these facilities are expensive and costly. In case of any disaster there is no local management system to cope up with it and often under such conditions the locals depend upon the foreign aid. In case of any calamity, epidemic diseases spread all over and due to absence of basic health facilities, the death toll is usually high. Clean drinking water and sanitation facilities are out of reach for majority of the population in the Third world countries. Third world countries are mostly agriculture-based economies and usually in need of water for production however they face dearth of water reserves. "Water scarcity in countries of South Asia and Sub-Saharan Africa is growing concern for agricultural productivity, health and sanitation". The poor health conditions also resulted from the rising prices of commodities, which have emerged a hesitating trend among the people from buying health friendly food. "A study in East Asian setting a 50 persent increase in price of food will lead to the decline of iron intake by 30 percent"

Crime and unhappiness stalk unequal societies. In the UK the bottom 50% of the population now owns only 1% of the wealth: in 1976 they owned 12%. Our economic system's incentive structure, instead of "trickle-down", is causing a "flood-up" of resources from the poor to the rich. Inequality leads to instability, the last thing the country or world needs right now. "The widening gaps between rich and poor within nations" is "morally outrageous, economically wasteful and potentially socially explosive".

The Wealthy Elbow out the Poor in All Societies

In the developing world, there is a pattern of inequality caused by the powerful subjugating the poor and keeping them dependent. Outside influence is often a large factor and access to trade and resources is the usual cause. It is often asked why the people of these countries do not stand up for themselves. In most cases when they do, they face incredible and often violent oppression from their ruling elites and from outsiders who see their national interests threatened. Everyone has the right to work, to just and favourable conditions of work and to protection for himself and his family and an existence worthy of human dignity ... Everyone has the right to a standard of living adequate for the health and well being of himself and his family, including food, clothing, housing and medical care. - Universal Declaration of Human Rights, 1948.

While it is recognized that strong institutions, a functioning and non-corrupt democracy, an impartial media, equitable distribution of land and a well structured judicial system (and other such factors), etc. all help in realizing a successful nation and society, a lack of any of these things can lead to a marginalization of a sector of people. Often, it can be a very large sector. For example, those likely to lose out in such an equalizing effect are the rich, elite power holders. As a result of their ability to own and/or influence one of these above-mentioned things, they affect the lives of millions. This is a pattern seen throughout history. Take for example the medieval days of Europe where the wealthy of the time controlled land via a feudal ruling system and hence impoverished the common people intentionally. The poor are elbowed out of the health care system, as well.

The Situation is Set to Get Worse

In a statement released by the World Bank, it estimated that between 200,000 and 400,000 more babies could die each year between now and 2015 if the global economic crisis persists. Already, 11 million children die each year because of lack of health care, sanitation, food and clean water, according to the statement. However, with an estimated 53 million more people living on US $ 2 a day in 2009, the last thing that is needed is yet another development assistance package steeped in First World bureaucracy and profiteering. The devastating global poverty that billions suffered even before the current economic crisis hit reveals that not only is capitalism a failed system when it comes to meeting people's needs, but that the institutions that grow out of it (such as the World Bank and IMF) are inevitably flawed as well. When a square peg doesn't fit in a round hole, it's usually time to pick up another block.

Rather than simply aid from First World countries, what is required is a break from the policies promoted by institutions like the IMF and World Bank, which work to increase the exploitation of the Third World by multinationals and help ensure that the underdeveloped and poor stay that way. The Third World needs control over its own resources, markets and industries, in order to promote sustainable development that can tackle the needs of the poor.

Infant Mortality Rates in Third World Countries

Although the past century has seen dramatic advances in the fields of health services and education, infant mortality and third world countries continues to be a source of heartache and grief. The great strides that medicine has made in the twentieth century have not made their way to most third world nations and infant mortality rates reflect this demoralizing fact. Infant mortality rates are based on the birth of 1,000 infants. So a rate of seven, which the United States currently experiences, means that out of every one thousand babies born, seven will die before its first birthday. Currently, the United States ranks thirtieth among the wealthier nations for its infant mortality rates. Infant mortality and third world countries have alarming statistics. For example in Afghanistan the infant mortality rate is 165 deaths for every thousand babies born. With 182 infants, out of 1000 born, dying before their first birthdays, the infant mortality rate in Sierra Leone are even more alarming. In Angola, 170 babies out of every thousand born, and in Niger the rate is 166 deaths, and in Liberia the infant mortality rate is 157 babies out of every thousand born. Infant mortality rates in other third world countries range from 95 in Madagascar to 144 in Mali. With the highest rates occurring in the sub-Saharan countries, there appears to be a direct tie-in between poverty rates and infant mortality rates. With droughts, famines, civil war and rebellions, ravaging their countries poverty runs rampant. When this poverty is combined with poor overall health care, it is little wonder why infant mortality and third world countries have such high rates of infant deaths.

According to the World Health Organization, the 10 leading causes of death in 2002 were:

1. 12.6% Ischaemic heart disease
2. 9.7% Cerebrovascular disease
3. 6.8% Lower respiratory infections
4. 4.9% HIV/AIDS

5. 4.8% Chronic obstructive pulmonary disease
6. 3.2% Diarrhoeal diseases
7. 2.7% Tuberculosis
8. 2.2% Malaria
9. 2.2% Trachea/bronchus/lung cancers
10. 2.1% Road traffic accidents

Causes of death vary greatly between first and third world countries.

Third World Countries in Terms of Human Development Index

The Human Development Index (HDI) is published annually by the UN. It measures the average achievements in a country in three basic dimensions of human development: A long and healthy life as measured by life expectancy at birth. Knowledge as measured by the adult literacy rate (with two-thirds weight) and the combined primary, secondary and tertiary gross enrolment ratio. A decent standard of living as measured by GDP per capita (PPP US$).

Below is given the list of 20 countries with the lowest Human Development Index (HDI)

Country, Life expectancy at birth, Adult literacy rate, Combined gross enrolment, GDP per capita (PPP US$), Life expectancy Index, Education index, GDP index, HDI, GDP rank minus HDI rank.

157 Senegal 52.7 39.3 38 1,580 0.46 0.39 0.46 0.437 -11 158 Timor-Leste 49.3 58.6 75 .. 0.41 0.64 0.26 0.436 19 159 Rwanda 38.9 69.2 53 1,270 0.23 0.64 0.42 0.431 -6 160 Guinea 48.9 41.0 29 2,100 0.40 0.37 0.51 0.425 -30 161 Benin 50.7 39.8 52 1,070 0.43 0.44 0.40 0.421 -5 162 Tanzania 43.5 77.1 31 580 0.31 0.62 0.29 0.407 12 163 Cote d'Ivoire 41.2 49.7 42 1,520 0.27 0.47 0.45 0.399 -16 164 Zambia 32.7 79.9 45 840 0.13 0.68 0.36 0.389 3 165 Malawi 37.8 61.8 74 580 0.21 0.66 0.29 0.388 9 166 Angola 40.1 42.0 30 2,130 0.25 0.38 0.51 0.381 -38 167 Chad 44.7 45.8 35 1,020 0.33 0.42 0.39 0.379 -8 168 Congo, Dem.Rep. 41.4 62.7 27 650 0.27 0.51 0.31 0.365 4 169 Central African Rep. 39.8 48.6 31 1,170 0.25 0.43 0.41 0.361 -15 170 Ethiopia 45.5 41.5 34 780 0.34 0.39 0.34 0.359 -1 171 Mozambique 38.5 46.5 41 1,050 0.22 0.45 0.39 0.354 -14 172 Guinea-Bissau 45.2 39.6 37 710 0.34 0.39 0.33 0.350 -1 173 Burundi 40.8 50.4 33 630 0.26 0.45 0.31 0.339 0 174 Mali 48.5 19.0 26 930 0.39 0.21 0.37 0.326 -11 175 Burkina Faso 45.8 12.8 22 1,100 0.35 0.16 0.40 0.302 -20 176 Niger 46.0 17.1 19 800 0.35 0.18 0.35 0.292 -8 177 Sierra Leone 34.3 36.0 45 520 0.16 0.39 0.28 0.273 -1

Source: UN Human Development Report, 2004.

Successful development can imply many things, such as:

- An improvement in living standards and access to all basic needs such that a person has enough food, water, shelter, clothing, health, education, etc.;

- A stable political, social and economic environment, with associated political, social and economic freedoms, such as (though not limited to) equitable ownership of land and property;
- The ability to make free and informed choices that are not coerced; and
- Be able to participate in a democratic environment with the ability to have a say in one's own future.

Yet, for a variety of reasons, these "full rights" are not available in many segments of various societies from the richest to the poorest. When political agendas deprive these possibilities in some nations, how can a nation develop? Is this progress?

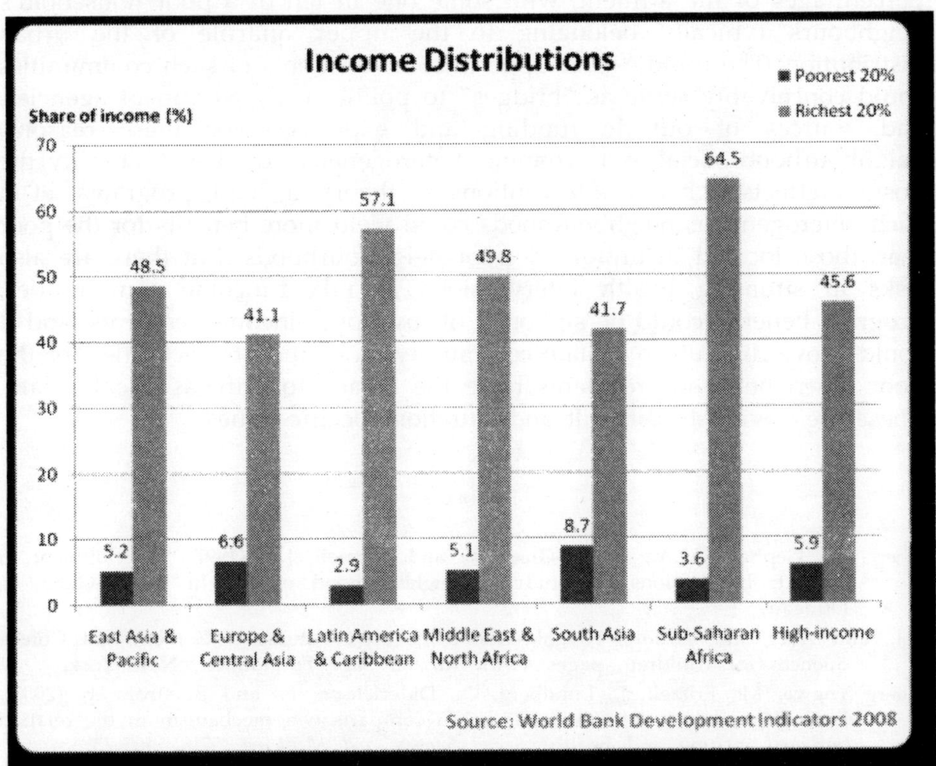

Living Standards and Health

Very few studies of developing-country cities have examined the issue of health in relation to living standard. A paper by Mark R. Montgomery and Paul C. Hewett investigates whether in these cities the health of women and young children is influenced by both household and neighbourhood standards of living. They found that as a rule, poor urban households do not tend to live in uniformly poor communities; indeed, about one in ten of a poor household's neighbours is relatively affluent, belonging to the upper quartile of the urban distribution of living standards. Do household and neighbourhood living standards influence health? Yes, household living standards have a substantial influence on three measures of health: unmet need for modern contraception; attendance of a trained provider at childbirth; and children's height for age.

They have found strong evidence that household living standards exert substantial influence on the unmet need for modern contraception, birth attendance, and children's height for age. It seems that the health of poor households can depend not only on their own standards of living, but also on the economic composition of their neighbourhoods. Their analyses have shown, the neighbourhoods of poor urban households often contain considerable percentages of non-poor households, and even appreciable percent-ages of the affluent, with some one in ten of a poor household's neighbours typically belonging to the upper quartile of the urban distribution. The middle- and upper-income residents of such communities could conceivably serve as "bridges" to politicians, government agencies, and sources of outside funding and expertise. For these reasons, neighbourhood social and economic heterogeneity could well amplify the positive effects of health interventions. In theory, at least, programs set in such heterogeneous neighbourhoods could yield more benefits for the poor than those located in uniformly poor neighbourhoods. But there are also risks in situating health interventions in mixed-income communities. Program benefits could be siphoned off by upper-income residents, and it could prove difficult to sustain community motivation for activities for the poor when better-off residents have the means to purchase health care. These are obviously difficult and situation-specific issues.

Sources

Aber, J.L., Gephart, M.A., Brooks-Gunn, J., and Connell, J.P. (1997). Development in context: Implications for studying neighbourhood effects. In Brooks-Gunn, J., Duncan.

G.J., and Aber, J.L., editors, Neighbourhood Poverty, volume I: Context and Consequences for Children, pages 44-61. Russell Sage Foundation, New York.

Aberg Yngwe, M., Fritzell, J., Lundberg, O., Diderichsen, F., and Burström, B. (2003). Exploring relative deprivation: Is social comparison a mechanism in the relation between income and health? *Social Science and Medicine*, 57(8):1463-73.

African Population and Health Research Center (2002). Population and Health Dynamics in Nairobi's Informal Settlements: Report of the Nairobi Cross-Sectional Slums Survey

(NCSS) 2000. African Population and Health Research Center, Nairobi.

Astone, N., Nathanson, C.A., Schoen, R., and Kim, Y.J. (1999). Family demography, social theory, and investment in social capital. *Population and Development Review*, 25(1):1-31.

Behrman, J., Kohler, H.-P., and Watkins, S. (2001). Social networks, family planning, and worrying about AIDS. Paper presented at the 2001 Annual Meetings of the Population Association of America, Washington, DC, 29-31 March.

Bollen, K. (1989). Structural Equations with Latent Variables. John Wiley and Sons, New York.

Caldeira, T.P.R. (1999). Fortified enclaves: The new urban segregation. In Holston, J., editor, Cities and Citizenship, pages 114-138. Duke University Press, Durham and London.

Caldeira, T.P.R. (2000). City of Walls: Crime, Segregation, and Citizenship in S˜ao Paulo. University of California Press, Berkeley, CA.

Casterline, J.B., editor (2001). Diffusion Processes and Fertility Transition: Selected Perspectives. National Academies Press, Washington, DC.

Casterline, J.B., Montgomery, M.R., Agyeman, D.K., Aglobitse, P., and Kiros, G.-E. (2001). Social networks and contraceptive dynamics in southern Ghana. Paper presented at the 2001 Annual Meetings of the Population Association of America, Washington, DC, 29-31 March.

Casterline, J.B. and Sinding, S.W. (2000). Unmet need for family planning in developing countries and implications for population policy. *Population and Development Review*, 26(4):691-723.

Coleman, J.S. (1988). Social capital in the creation of human capital. *American Journal of Sociology*, 94 (supplement): S95-S120.

Coulton, C., Korbin, J., Chan, T., and Su, M. (1997). Mapping residents' perceptions of neighbourhood boundaries: A methodological note. Working Paper, Center on Urban Poverty and Social Change. Case Western Reserve University, Cleveland, OH.

Drukker, M., Kaplan, C., Feron, F., and van Os, J. (2003). Children's health-related quality of life, neighbourhood socio-economic deprivation and social capital. A contextual analysis. *Social Science and Medicine*, 57(5):825-841.

Ferguson, B.D., Tandon, A., Gakidou, E., and Murray, C.J.L. (2003). Estimating permanent income using indicator variables. Global Programme on Evidence for Health Policy Discussion Paper No. 42. World Health Organization, Geneva.

Filmer, D. and Pritchett, L. (1999). The effect of household wealth on educational attainment: Evidence from 35 countries. *Population and Development Review*, 25(1):85-120.

Filmer, D. and Pritchett, L. (2001). Estimating wealth effects without expenditure data or tears: An application to educational enrolments in states of India. *Demography*, 38(1):115-132.

Freedman, R. and Takeshita, J.Y. (1969). Family Planning in Taiwan: An Experiment in Social Change. Princeton University Press, Princeton, NJ.

Furstenberg, F.F. (1993). How families manage risk and opportunity in dangerous neighbourhoods. In Wilson, W.J., editor, Sociology and the Public Agenda, pages 231-258. Sage Publications, Newbury Park, CA.

Furstenberg, F.F. and Hughes, M.E. (1997). The influence of neighbourhoods on children's development: A theoretical perspective and a research agenda. In Brooks-Gunn, J., Duncan, G.J., and Aber, J.L., editors, Neighbourhood Poverty, volume II: Policy Implications in Studying Neighbourhoods, pages 23-47. Russell Sage Foundation, New York.

Gilson, L. (2003). Trust and the development of health care as a social institution. *Social Science and Medicine*, 56(7):1453-1468.

Ginther, D., Haveman, R., and Wolfe, B. (2000). Neighbourhood attributes as determinants of children's outcomes: How robust are the relationships? *Journal of Human Resources*, 35(4):603-633.

Harpham, T. and Tanner, M., editors (1995). Urban Health in Developing Countries: *Progress and Prospects*. St. Martin's Press, New York.

Heckman, J.J. (1981). Statistical models for discrete panel data. In Manski, C.F. and McFadden, D., editors, *Structural Analysis of Discrete Data with Econometric Applications*, pages 114-178. MIT Press, Cambridge, MA.

Herr, H. and Karl, G. (2002). Estimating global slum-dwellers: Monitoring the Millennium Development Goal 7, Target 11. Monitoring Systems Branch, Global Urban Observatory. UN-HABITAT, Nairobi.

Herr, H. and Mboup, G. (2003). Slum-dweller estimation methodology. Unpublished paper (in progress). UN-HABITAT, Nairobi.

Jöreskog, K.G. (2000). Latent variable scores and their uses. Unpublished paper, available at http://www.ssicentral.com/lisrel.column6.pdf.

Jöreskog, K.G. (2002). Structural equation modeling with ordinal variables using LISREL. Unpublished paper, available at http://www.ssicentral.com/lisrel/corner.htm.

Kaufman, C.E., Clark, S., Manzini, N., and May, J. (2002). How community structures of time and opportunity shape adolescent sexual behaviour in South Africa. Policy Research Division Working Paper No. 159. Population Council, New York.

Kravdal, D. (2003). Community mortality in India: Individual and community effects of women's education and autonomy. East-West Center Working Papers, Population Series, No. 112. East-West Center, Honolulu, HI.

Lawley, D.N. and Maxwell, A.E. (1962). Factor analysis as a statistical method. *Statistician,* 12(3):209-229.

Massey, D.S. (1990). American apartheid: Segregation and the making of the underclass. *American Journal of Sociology,* 96(2):329-357.

Massey, D.S. (1996). The age of extremes: Concentrated affluence and poverty in the twenty-first century. *Demography,* 33(4):395-412.

McCulloch, A. (2003). An examination of social capital and social disorganisation in neighbourhoods in the British household panel study. *Social Science and Medicine,* 56(7):1425-1438.

McDade, T.W. and Adair, L.S. (2001). Defining the 'urban' in urbanization and health: A factor analysis approach. *Social Science and Medicine,* 53(1):55-70.

Montgomery, M.R., Gragnolati, M., Burke, K.A., and Paredes, E. (2000). Measuring living standards with proxy variables. *Demography,* 37(2):155-174.

Montgomery, M.R., Lloyd, C., Hewett, P.C., and Heuveline, P. (1997). The consequences of imperfect fertility control for children's survival, health, and schooling. Demographic and Health Surveys Analytical Reports No. 7. Macro International, Inc., Calverton, MD.

Panel on Urban Population Dynamics (2003). Cities Transformed: Demographic Change and Its Implications in the Developing World. National Academies Press, Washington, DC. Montgomery, M.R., Stren, R., Cohen, B., and Reed, H., editors.

Pebley, A.R., Goldman, N., and Rodr?guez, G. (1996). Prenatal and delivery care and childhood immunization in Guatemala: Do family and community matter? *Demography,* 33(2):231-247.

Pebley, A.R. and Sastry, N. (2003). Concentrated poverty *vs.* concentrated affluence: Effects on neighbourhood social environments and children's outcomes. Paper presented at the 2003 Annual Meetings of the Population Association of America, *Minneapolis*, MN, 1-3 May.

Press, W.H., Teukolsky, S.A., Vetterling, W.T., and Flannery, B.P. (1992). Numerical Recipes in FORTRAN: The Art of Scientific Computing. Cambridge University Press, New York.

Press, W.H., Teukolsky, S.A., Vetterling, W.T., and Flannery, B.P. (1996). Numerical Recipes in Fortran 90: *The Art of Parallel Scientific Computing,* Volume 2. Cambridge University Press, New York.

Sahn, D.E. and Stifel, D.C. (2000). Poverty comparisons over time and across countries in Africa. *World Development,* 28(12):2123-2155.

Sampson, R.J., Morenoff, J.D., and Gannon-Rowley, T. (2002). Assessing 'neighbourhood effects': Social processes and new directions in research. *Annual Review of Sociology,* 28:443-478.

Sastry, N. (1996). Community characteristics, individual and household attributes, and child survival in Brazil. *Demography*, 33(2):211-229.

Sastry, N., Pebley, A., and Zonta, M. (2002). Neighbourhood definitions and the spatial dimension of daily life in Los Angeles. Paper presented at the 2002 Annual Meetings of the Population Association of America, Atlanta, GA, 9-11 May.

Szwarcwald, C.L., de Andrade, C.L.T., and Bastos, F.I. (2002). Income inequality, residential poverty clustering and infant mortality: A study in Rio de Janeiro, Brazil. *Social Science and Medicine*, 55(12):2083-2092.

Tandon, A., Gakidou, E., Murray, C.J.L., and Ferguson, B. (2002). Cross-population comparability and PPPs: Using micro-data on indicators of consumer durables. Evidence and Information for Policy Cluster draft paper. *World Health Organization*, Geneva.

Timæus, I.M. and Lush, L. (1995). Intra-urban differentials in child health. *Health Transition Review*, 5(2):163-190.

United Nations (2000). World Urbanization Prospects: The 1999 Revision: Data Tables and Highlights. United Nations, Department of Economic and Social Affairs, Population Division, New York.

van den Eeden, P. and Hüttner, H.J.M. (1982). Multi-level research. Current Sociology, 30(3):1-182.

Wellman, B. and Leighton, B. (1979). Networks, neighbourhoods, and communities: Approaches to the study of the community question. *Urban Affairs Quarterly*, 14(3):363-390.

Wen, M., Browning, C.R., and Cagney, K.A. (2003). Poverty, affluence, and income inequality: Neighbourhood economic structure and its implications for health. *Social Science and Medicine*, 57(5):843-860.

Westoff, C.F. and Bankole, A. (1995). Unmet Need 1990-1994. Demographic and HealthSurveys Comparative Studies. Macro International, Inc., Calverton, MD.

Westoff, C.F. and Pebley, A.R. (1981). Alternative measures of unmet need for family planning in developing countries. *International Family Planning Perspectives*, 7(4):126-136.

White, M.J. (2001). Residential concentration/segregation, demographic effects of. In Smelser, N.J. and Baltes, P.B., editors, International Encyclopedia of the Social and Behavioural Sciences, Volume 19, pages 13250-13254. *Elsevier Science*, Oxford.

Wilkinson, R.G. (1996). Unhealthy Societies: The Afflictions of Inequality. Routledge, London.

Wilson, W.J. (1987). The Truly Disadvantaged: The Inner City, the Underclass and Public Policy. University of Chicago Press, Chicago, IL.

APPENDIX

QUALITY ASSESSMENT (QA) AND IMPROVEMENT: EXPERIENCES IN LOW DEVELOPING COUNTRIES (LDC)

Despite the importance of quality, to date there have been few sustained QA efforts in developing countries. Many evaluations have focused on measuring changes in mortality and morbidity, or on measuring coverage rates. Few have emphasized the quality of services or the process of service delivery. Further, systematic efforts to improve quality based on findings about the delivery process have been extremely rare. In recent years several studies have focused on service quality, revealing widespread deficiencies in health care services and management systems in LDCs. For example, the A.I.D.-sponsored Primary Health Care Operations Research (PRICOR) Project designed and implemented methods for quality assessment and problem-solving in LDC systems. After developing comprehensive lists of essential activities and tasks for seven child survival interventions, PRICOR supported comprehensive quality assessment studies in twelve countries.

The project used service delivery observation as the assessment method, and experimented with simulations and role plays to study the care process. PRICOR conducted more than 6,000 observations of health worker-client encounters, discovering highly prevalent, serious program deficiencies in areas such as diagnosis, treatment, patient education, and supervision. PRICOR also found that supervision systems, which are part of most LDC health systems, were essential to quality improvement. The project worked with district-level supervisors to develop data-based supervisory methods and to address problems detected through low-cost operations research studies. Under PRICOR, local managers and researchers conducted 109 operations research studies, many of which produced successful, low-cost interventions.[1]

In other efforts, WHO's Diarrheal Disease Control Program has developed a protocol employing the same methods for evaluating oral rehydration therapy. The Center for Disease Control's Combatting Communicable Childhood Diseases (CCCD) used a similar methodology to uncover deficiencies in immunization programs and in diarrhea and malaria treatment. An increasing number of health programs in developing countries are applying such simple tools. These include observation checklists and job aids to assess and improve quality.

II. Is Quality Assurance in LDCs Feasible?

At first glance, high-quality health services may appear to be a luxury beyond the budgetary limits of most LDC health systems. However, improving quality often does not cost, it pays. Attention to quality is essential to the success of primary health care programs, a fact that health managers with restricted budgets cannot afford to ignore.

Besides evaluating population coverage and the technological merit of health interventions, health providers must assess the quality of services compared with prescribed standards.

Suppose, for example, that a measles immunization campaign meets its target coverage rates, but close examination reveals that many vaccines were ineffective due to poor cold chain maintenance. In such a case, the intervention's impact is compromised and resources are wasted. Similarly for tuberculosis treatment, the initial drug dosages will be ineffective and the advantage of early treatment lost if the quality of counseling is poor and patients default.

When symptoms recur the patient must be treated again, resulting in duplication of care and an increased risk of drug resistance. In both examples, attention to quality would have helped to reduce waste.

Health care providers and the community are expected to cooperatively assess health needs and to select a cost-effective health care approach. QA promotes confidence, improves communication, and fosters a clearer understanding of community needs and expectations. If providers do not offer quality services, they will fail to earn the population's trust, and clients will turn to the health system only when in dire need of curative care. This scenario is particularly unfortunate in developing countries, where the success of lifesaving preventive care, such as immunization, growth monitoring, family planning, and antenatal care, depends on the willing participation of communities. Moreover, as primary health care programs adopt cost-recovery strategies, the quality of service must be sufficient to attract the population to the clinic on a fee-for-service basis.

QA efforts also offer health workers an opportunity to excel, thereby increasing their job satisfaction and status in the community. Severe resource constraints limit the capacity of most developing countries health care systems to offer salary increases and professional advancement as rewards for high performance; but these are not always necessary to improve quality.

Very often, quality is a reward by itself. QA is a systematic approach for conveying the importance of excellence to individuals and teams. It provides the health team with tools that gauge current performance levels and facilitate continuous improvement. With the interest and active involvement of the organization's leadership, health workers can better meet and surpass performance standards, solve problems, and serve their clients' needs. Increased health worker satisfaction and motivation start a continuous cycle of improved health care and heightened effectiveness.

QA has the potential to improve primary health care programs without requiring additional supplies, logistical support, or financial and human resources. In fact, a legitimate QA objective is to maximize effectiveness and efficiency from current systems. Thus, QA affords donors, governments, health care providers, and communities the chance to realize more benefits from existing investments in health care.

III. What is Quality?

Quality of care must be defined in the light of the provider's technical standards and patients' expectations. While no single definition of health service quality applies in all situations, the following definitions are helpful guides:

The quality of technical care consists in the application of medical science and technology in a way that maximizes its benefits to health without correspondingly increasing its risks. The degree of quality is, therefore, the extent to which the care provided is expected to achieve the most favourable balance of risks and benefits.

—(Avedis Donabedian, M.D., 1980-82)

...proper performance (according to standards) of interventions that are known to be safe, that are affordable to the society in question, and that have the ability to produce an impact on mortality, morbidity, disability, and malnutrition.

—M.I. Roemer and C. Montoya Aguilar, WHO, 1983

The most comprehensive and perhaps the simplest definition of quality is that used by advocates of total quality management: "Doing the right thing right, right away."

A. Dimensions of Quality

Quality is a comprehensive and multifaceted concept. Experts generally recognize several distinct dimensions of quality that vary in importance depending on the context.

QA activities may address one or more dimensions, such as technical competence, access to services, effectiveness, interpersonal relations, efficiency, continuity, safety, and amenities. These dimensions of quality are a useful frame-work that helps health teams to define and analyze their problems and to measure the extent to which they are meeting program standards. The eight dimensions discussed in detail in this section have been developed from the technical literature on quality, and synthesize ideas from various QA experts. We feel that these dimensions are relevant to LDC settings; however, not all eight deserve equal weight in every program. Each should be considered in the light of specific programs and should be defined according to the local context. These dimensions of quality are as appropriate for clinical care as for management services that support service delivery.

1. Technical Competence

Technical competence refers to the skills, capability, and actual performance of health providers, managers, and support staff. For example, to provide technically competent services, a village health worker must have the skills and knowledge (capability) to carry out specific tasks and to do so consistently and accurately (actual performance). Technical competence relates to how well providers execute practice guidelines and standards in terms of dependability, accuracy, reliability, and consistency. This dimension is relevant for both clinical and nonclinical services. For health providers, it includes clinical skills related to preventive care, diagnosis, treatment, and health counseling. Competence in health management requires skills in supervision, training, and problem-solving. The requisite skills of support staff depend on individual job descriptions. For instance, a technically competent receptionist must be able to respond to information requests, while a pharmacist might be expected to possess competence in logistics and inventory management. Technical competence can also refer to material resources: for example, an X-ray machine must produce radiation that consistently meets accepted standards. A lack of technical competence can range from minor deviations from standard procedures to major errors that decrease effectiveness or jeopardize patient safety.

2. Access to Services

Access means that health care services are unrestricted by geographic, economic, social, cultural, organizational, or linguistic barriers. Geographic access may be measured by modes of transportation, distance, travel time, and any other physical barriers that could keep the client from receiving care. Economic access refers to the affordability of products and services for clients. Social or cultural access relates to service acceptability within the context of the client's cultural values, beliefs, and attitudes. For example, family planning services may not be accepted if they are offered in a way that is inconsistent with the local culture. Organizational access refers to the extent to which services are conveniently organized for prospective clients, and encompasses issues such as clinic hours and appointment systems, waiting time, and the mode of service delivery. For example, the lack of evening clinics may reduce organizational access for day labourers. Where travel is difficult, lack of home visits or village-based services may create an access problem. Linguistic access means that the services are available in the local language or a dialect in which the client is fluent.

3. Effectiveness

The quality of health services depends on the effectiveness of service delivery norms and clinical guidelines. Assessing the dimension of effectiveness answers the questions, "Does the procedure or treatment, when correctly applied, lead to the desired results?" and "Is the recommended treatment the most technologically appropriate for the setting in which it is delivered?" Effectiveness is an important dimension of quality at the central level, where norms and specifications are defined. Effectiveness issues should also be considered at the local level, where managers decide how to carry out norms and how to adapt them to local conditions. When selecting standards, relative risks should be considered. For example, more frequent use of cesarean section might be warranted in a population with many high-risk pregnancies, despite the associated risks. To determine this strategy's effectiveness, the procedure's potential harm must be compared with its potential net benefits.

4. Interpersonal Relations

The dimension of interpersonal relations refers to the interaction between providers and clients, managers and health care providers, and the health team and the community. Good interpersonal relations establish trust and credibility through demonstrations of respect, confidentiality, courtesy, responsiveness, and empathy. Effective listening and communication are also important. Sound interpersonal relations contribute to effective health counseling and to a positive rapport with patients. Inadequate interpersonal relations can reduce the effectiveness of a technically competent health service. Patients who are poorly treated may be less likely to heed the health care provider's recommendations, or may avoid seeking care.

5. Efficiency

The efficiency of health services is an important dimension of quality because it affects product and service affordability and because health care resources are usually limited. Efficient services provide optimal rather than maximum care to the patient and community; they provide the greatest benefit within the resources available. Efficiency demands that necessary or appropriate care is provided. Poor care resulting from ineffective norms or incorrect delivery should be minimized or eliminated. In this way, quality can be improved while reducing costs. Harmful care, besides causing unnecessary risk and patient discomfort, is often expensive and time-consuming to correct. It would be misleading, however, to imply that quality improvements never require additional resources. But by analyzing efficiency, health program managers may select the most cost-effective intervention.

6. Continuity

Continuity means that the client receives the complete range of health services that he or she needs, without interruption, cessation, or unnecessary repetition of diagnosis or treatment. Services must be offered on an ongoing basis. The client must have access to routine and preventive care provided by a health worker who knows his or her medical history. A client must also have access to timely referral for specialized services and to complete follow-up care. Continuity is sometimes achieved by ensuring that the client always sees the same primary care provider; in other situations, it is achieved by keeping accurate medical records so that a new provider knows the patient's history and can build upon and complement the diagnosis and treatment of previous providers. The absence of continuity can compromise effectiveness, decrease efficiency, and reduce the quality of interpersonal relations.

7. Safety

As a dimension of quality, safety means minimizing the risks of injury, infection, harmful side effects, or other dangers related to service delivery. Safety involves the provider as well as the patient. For example, safety is an important dimension of quality for blood transfusions, especially since the advent of AIDS. Patients must be protected from infection, and health workers who handle blood and needles must be protected by safety procedures. Additional safety issues related to blood transfusions include maintaining aseptic conditions and using proper techniques for transfusing blood. While safety may seem most important when complex clinical services are provided, there are safety concerns in the provision of basic health services as well. For example, health center waiting rooms can put clients at risk of infection from other patients if risk-reducing measures are not taken. If a health worker does not provide proper instruction on the preparation of oral rehydration solution (ORS), a mother may administer to her child (ORS) containing a dangerously high concentration of salt.

8. Amenities

Amenities refer to the features of health services that do not directly relate to clinical effectiveness but may enhance the client's satisfaction and willingness to return to the facility for subsequent health care needs. Amenities are also important because they may affect the client's expectations about and confidence in other aspects of the service or product. Where cost recovery is a consideration, amenities may enhance the client's willingness to pay for services. Amenities relate to the physical appearance of facilities, personnel, and materials; as well as to comfort, cleanliness, and privacy. Other amenities may include features that make the wait more pleasant such as music, educational or recreational videos, and reading materials. While some amenities—clean, accessible restrooms; and privacy curtains in examination rooms—are considered luxuries in most LDC health care settings, they are nevertheless important for attracting and retaining clients and for ensuring continuity and coverage.

B. Perspectives on the Meaning of Quality

The definitions and dimensions outlined above constitute a broad conceptual framework that includes almost every aspect of the health system performance. All these dimensions come into play as clients, health providers, and health care managers try to define quality of care from their unique perspectives. What does quality of health care mean for the communities and clients that depend on it, the clinicians who provide it, and the managers and administrators who oversee it?

The Client

For the clients and communities served by health care facilities, quality care meets their perceived needs, and is delivered courteously and on time. In sum, the client wants services that effectively relieve symptoms and prevent illness. The client's perspective is very important because satisfied clients often are more likely to comply with treatment and to continue to use primary health services. Thus, the dimensions of quality that relate to client satisfaction affect the health and well-being of the community.

Patients and communities often focus on effectiveness, accessibility, interpersonal relations, continuity, and amenities as the most important dimensions of quality. However, it is important to note that communities do not always fully understand their health service needs—especially for preventive services—and cannot adequately assess technical competence. Health providers must learn about their community's health status and health service needs, educate the community about basic health services, and involve it in defining how care is to be most effectively delivered. Which decisions should be made by health professionals and which should be made by the community? Where does the technical domain begin and end? This is a subjective and value-laden area that requires an ongoing dialogue between health workers and the community. Answering these questions requires a relationship of trust and two-way communication between the parties.

The Health Service Provider

From the provider's perspective, quality care implies that he or she has the skills, resources, and conditions necessary to improve the health status of the patient and the community, according to current technical standards and available resources. The provider's commitment and motivation depend on the ability to carry out his or her duties in an ideal or optimal way.

Providers tend to focus on technical competence, effectiveness, and safety. Key questions for providers may be: How many patients are providers expected to see per hour? What laboratory services are available to them, and how accurate, efficient, and reliable are they? What referral systems are in place when specialty services or higher technologies are needed? Are the physical working conditions adequate and sanitary, ensuring the privacy of patients and a professional environment? Does the pharmacy have a reliable supply of all the needed medicines? Are there opportunities for continuing medical education? Just as the health care system must respond to the patients' perspectives and demands, it must also respond to the needs and requirements of the health care provider. In this sense, health care providers can be thought of as the health care system's "internal clients." They need and expect effective and efficient technical, administrative, and support services in providing high-quality care.

The Health Care Manager

Quality care requires that managers are rarely involved in delivering patient care, although the quality of patient care is central to everything they do. The varied demands of supervision and financial and logistic management present many unexpected challenges and crises. This can leave a manager without a clear sense of priorities or purpose. Focusing on the various dimensions of quality can help to set administrative priorities. Health care managers must provide for the needs and demands of both providers and patients. Also, they must be responsible stewards of the resources entrusted to them by the government, private entities, and the community. Health care managers must consider the needs of multiple clients in addressing questions about resource allocation, fee schedules, staffing patterns, and management practices. The multidimensional concept of quality presented here is particularly helpful to managers who tend to feel that access, effectiveness, technical competence, and efficiency are the most important dimensions of quality.

IV. What is Quality Assurance?

As the QA field has evolved and developed, various definitions of quality assurance have emerged. Dr. Donabedian broadly defines it as "all the arrangements and activities that are meant to safeguard, maintain, and promote the quality of care."[4] Drs. Ruelas and Frenk, who have conducted extensive QA work in Mexico, define it as "a systematic process for closing the gap between actual performance and the desirable outcomes. . . ."[5] According to Dr. Heather Palmer, a QA expert in U.S. ambulatory care, it is a "process of measuring quality, analyzing the deficiencies discovered, and taking action to improve performance followed by measuring quality again to determine whether improvement has been achieved. It is a systematic, cyclic activity using standards of measurement."[6] Dr. Donald Berwick, a U.S.-based clinician, is working to apply principles of continuous quality improvement (CQI) to health services. This approach to QA is an integrated organizational approach for meeting client needs and expectations involving both management and staff while improving processes and services using quantitative techniques and analytical tools. According to Berwick, it is ". . . a systematic managerial transformation designed to address the needs and opportunities of all organizations as they try to cope with increasing change, complexity and tension within their environments."[7]

All these definitions of QA share several characteristics. Each, for example, refers to a systematic, ongoing process that is oriented toward improving performance and using data in the process, either implicitly or explicitly. In essence, quality assurance is that set of activities that are carried out to set standards and to monitor and improve performance so that the care provided is as effective and as safe as possible.

Quality assurance is not a new "magic bullet," but has been a part of health care for the past 100 years. It was introduced into modern medicine by a British nurse, Florence Nightingale, who assessed the quality of care in military hospitals during the Crimean War. She introduced the first standards in nursing care; these resulted in dramatic reductions of mortality rates in hospitals. Until recently, quality assurance was primarily used by hospitals in developed countries and relied heavily on standards of care developed by accrediting agencies. In the 1980s, quality assurance expanded to primary health care in the United States and Europe. Simultaneously, internationally accepted standards of care were introduced by diarrhea and acute respiratory infection (ARI) case management algorithms developed by WHO. After 1985, WHO and several projects such as PRICOR and CCCD began using systems analysis and facility assessments to assess the quality of care.

There has recently been a revolution in quality assurance approaches and an explosion of interest in developing national QA programs for several reasons:

- Democratization movements have led politicians to consider more carefully the demands of citizens for better quality care.
- Economic problems in all countries have limited their ability to improve quality by spending more. Countries have realized that improvements in quality must come by improving the efficiency and effectiveness of current resources.
- Managers see the need for more cost recovery, but realize that it will be difficult to charge for services unless the quality is improved.
- The success of quality management approaches employed by industry in Japan, and recently in the United States and Europe, has inspired health care organizations to apply these same methods to their quality assurance programs. After only five years, there are dramatic examples of the improvements in quality and efficiency that can be achieved.

Recent experience in applying quality management to health care systems suggests that four tenets should be adhered to in an ideal quality assurance program:

The Four Tenets of Quality Assurance

- Quality Assurance is oriented toward meeting the needs and expectations of the patient and the community.
- Quality assurance focuses on systems and processes.
- Quality assurance uses data to analyze service delivery processes.
- Quality assurance encourages a team approach to problem-solving and quality improvement.

Quality assurance is oriented toward meeting the needs and expectations of the patient and the community. Quality assurance requires a commitment to finding out what patients and the community need, want, and expect from the health services. The health team must work with communities to meet service demand and to promote acceptance of needed preventive services. Subsequent program planning and quality improvement efforts should be evaluated according to these needs and expectations. Quality assurance also requires that health workers' professional needs and expectations be met.

Quality assurance focuses on systems and processes. By focusing on the analysis of service delivery processes, activities, and tasks as well as outcomes, quality assurance approaches allow health care providers and managers to develop an in-depth understanding of a problem and to address its root causes. Rather than merely treating the symptoms of a quality-related problem, quality assurance seeks to find a cure. In the advanced stages of a QA program, the health center team can go even further by analyzing processes to prevent problems before they occur.

Quality assurance uses data to analyze service delivery processes. Simple quantitative approaches to problem analysis and monitoring are another important aspect of quality improvement. Data-oriented methods allow the QA team to test its theories about root causes; effective problem-solving should be based on facts, not assumptions.

Quality assurance encourages a team approach to problem-solving and quality improvement. Participatory approaches offer two advantages. First, the technical product is likely to be of higher quality because each team member brings unique perspective and insight to the quality improvement effort. Collaboration facilitates a thorough problem analysis and makes development of a feasible solution more likely. Second, staff members are more likely to accept and support changes that they helped to develop. Thus, participation in quality improvement builds consensus and reduces resistance to change.

It is important to note that the definition of QA can be extremely broad and can include all program management activities. QA can include everything from applied research to comprehensive management assessments and interventions. In practice, the scope of a QA effort depends on the needs and capacities of the health service organization. Usually, the QA effort will be developed as a limited activity that is integrated into the existing management system. However if an organization desires a comprehensive approach, a QA initiative can be developed as a component of a general management improvement effort or a total quality management system.

V. The Quality Assurance Process

The QA process is based on QAP's experience working with health services in developing countries. However, it also integrates lessons learned from earlier quality assurance methodologies. A.I.D.'s PRICOR Project developed a simple, practical approach to quality improvement that was applied in Africa, Asia, and Latin America. WHO has promoted a QA paradigm developed by Hannu Vuori that has been applied in selected international settings.

Some U.S. models include the quality assurance cycle used by Palmer in ambulatory care settings; the 10-step process developed by the Joint

Commission on Accreditation of Health Care Organizations; and CQI which applies total quality management to health services. The QAP quality improvement model attempts to integrate the strengths of the various models into a simple, logical process for planning and implementing QA activities. Consistent with earlier models, QAP's quality improvement model defines norms, conducts an assessment, works with health care providers in a participatory fashion, takes action based on the assessment, and monitors results. Perhaps most important, it puts forth a replicable process for improving the quality of health care service delivery. This process can, over time, be integrated into ongoing program management.

Many health center teams will find that they are already taking steps toward improving quality, although they might not use the term "quality assurance" to describe their activities. The time and effort required for each step will depend on which QA activities are already in place. For example, an organization that has an existing monitoring system will spend less time on Step 4—monitoring quality—than an organization that is monitoring quality for the first time. During Step 2—developing guidelines and setting standards—some organizations may review existing norms or practice guidelines; others may need to spend considerable time developing norms before a quality improvement effort can begin. It is important for an organization new to QA to go through all steps, at least in a cursory way. This will ensure that essential components will not be missed and all those involved in the process will receive essential information.

In practice, QA is a cyclical, iterative process that must be applied flexibly to meet the needs of a specific program. The process may begin with a comprehensive effort to define standards and norms as described in Steps 1-3, or it may start with small-scale quality improvement activities (Steps 5-10). Alternatively, the process may begin with monitoring (Step 4). Some teams may even choose to simultaneously begin in two places. For instance, comprehensive monitoring and focused problem-solving may start as a coordinated, parallel effort. The ten steps in the QA process are discussed in the following section.

1. Planning for Quality Assurance

This first step prepares an organization to carry out QA activities. Planning begins with a review of the organization's scope of care to determine which services should be addressed. For most organizations, it is impossible to improve quality in all areas at once. Instead, QA activities are initiated in a few critical areas. High-priority, high-volume, or problem-prone services are often selected for special attention at the start of a QA program. Once organizational leaders have decided where the QA effort will begin, they must select a quality improvement approach. They may focus on monitoring desired or adverse outcomes, or they may study service delivery and support processes to determine areas for improvement. Another component of planning is assigning responsibilities for the QA activities. This may entail forming a QA committee or an *ad hoc* team responsible for initial QA activities.

If the program mission is unclear or unresponsive to community needs, or if overall planning in an organization is weak, in-depth strategic planning might be required. Strategic planning begins with defining the organization's mission. The next step is to assess the opportunities and constraints in the external environment as well as the organization's internal strengths and weaknesses. Strategic planning produces a clear vision of what the organization must do to achieve its mission in the light of its environment. The organization can then determine QA priorities based on the program mission and vision.

2. Setting Standards and Specifications

To provide consistently high-quality services, an organization must translate its programmatic goals and objectives into operational procedures. In its widest sense, a "standard" is a statement of the quality that is expected. Under the broad rubric of standards there are practice guidelines or clinical protocols, administrative procedures or standard operating procedures, product specifications, and performance standards.

Practice guidelines, sometimes called clinical protocols or practice parameters, define how clinical processes such as antenatal care are carried out. Administrative procedures, sometimes called standard operating procedures, define routine non-clinical processes. Specifications usually pertain to product characteristics or material inputs such as drugs or technical equipment related to health service delivery.

Performance standards are specific criteria used to measure the outcome of service delivery and the activities that support it. They are also used to measure compliance with guidelines. These standards differ from guidelines or standard operating procedures; they are designed to evaluate practice rather than to assist practitioners and patients. Standards have been defined as "authoritative statements of: (1) minimum levels of acceptable performance or results, (2) excellent levels of performance or results, or (3) the range of acceptable performance or results."[9] Standards can be related to the care process by measuring health out- comes or guideline compliance. While health outcomes are sometimes difficult and costly to measure, it is often possible to monitor intermediate outcomes such as utilization or coverage in assessing program effectiveness. Performance standards form the core of the monitoring system, as discussed in Step 4.

Guidelines, standard operating procedures, and performance standards should be developed for both clinical and management areas. They should reflect the perspectives of their communities and health care specialists. Both perspectives are essential to ensure the effectiveness of planned activities and their accessibility and acceptability to the community. Program staff should periodically review and revise guidelines and standard procedures.

For some programs, setting standards and specifications involves a simple review of current guidelines and standard operating procedures to ensure that they are up-to-date. For others, it may be important to develop consensus among professionals to ensure support. Others may require creating new guidelines and standards. In such cases, some widely accepted resources are available. For example, WHO helps in defining service delivery protocols appropriate for health centers and small hospitals in developing countries. The PRICOR Project developed clinical guidelines for use in primary health care in developing countries. The PRICOR Thesaurus sets forth guidelines for seven child survival services: immunization, oral rehydration therapy, prenatal care, family planning, growth monitoring, treatment of acute respiratory infections, and malaria. The project also developed guidelines in seven management areas: planning, supervision, training, logistics, financial management, management information systems, and community organization. In sum, the Thesaurus is a useful reference for setting standards.[10]

Health workers at all levels should participate in developing guidelines and setting standards. Because health workers often understand local conditions better than high-level managers, the resulting guidelines are likely to be more appropriate and effective. Also, staff participation will generate commitment to quality because health workers are more likely to implement and support an effort that they have helped to develop. Finally, staff members are more likely to accept QA activities if they have been involved in defining quality. Their standards will become the measure for judging the quality of their services.

3. Communicating Guidelines and Standards

Once practice guidelines, standard operating procedures, and performance standards have been defined, it is essential that staff members communicate and promote their use. This will ensure that each health worker, supervisor, manager, and support person understands what is expected of him or her. This is particularly important if ongoing training and supervision have been weak or if guidelines and procedures have recently changed. Assessing quality before communicating expectations can lead to erroneously blaming individuals for poor performance when fault actually lies with systemic deficiencies. Additionally, QA efforts that begin with a surprise examination are likely to cause suspicion rather than support.

Managers and the health center team share a mutual responsibility for quality; the notion of this partnership should be communicated along with guidelines and standards. A dialogue about guidelines and standards can take place in the context of supervision, training, or other channels. Activities that communicate guidelines and standards include developing job descriptions, translating performance guidelines into job aids, developing and conducting training programs, holding formal conferences or informal presentations about new procedures, providing on-the-job training through supervisory activities, and informing providers of changes in protocols through administrative announcements.

4. Monitoring Quality

Monitoring is the routine collection and review of data that helps to assess whether program norms are being followed or whether outcomes are improved. By monitoring key indicators, managers and supervisors can determine whether the services delivered follow the prescribed practices and achieve the desired results. QA involves a new process orientation that has profound implications for monitoring and collecting data in LDCs. Outcome measures alone, or other service statistics that are generally part of LDC monitoring systems, offer limited guidance in problem-solving. Detailed assessment of processes through special comprehensive studies or routine assessments can provide useful information about specific service delivery problems.

The monitoring system is central to a QA program. Unfortunately, existing data collection systems in many developing countries can be difficult to use for QA. At some point, existing monitoring systems may require redesign. However, this is not recommended as an initial activity; it is likely to be very time consuming and to meet resistance. It is often better to involve program staff members in using data to solve problems (see Steps 5-11) and to work with them in redesigning their system.

Designing (or redesigning) a monitoring system requires translating statements about expected quality into measurable indicators. It also demands setting performance thresholds, selecting information sources, designing a system for collecting data and compiling results, and carrying out monitoring activities. (Each of these activities is briefly discussed below.) It is important to define which data are to be used at the various levels in the system. For example, a front-line supervisor may collect a great deal of information about service quality and delivery, but may summarize only some of this information for higher-level managers. Generally, all levels of staff should be involved in designing a monitoring system so that everyone receives all necessary information.

- *Selecting indicators*: An indicator is a measurable characteristic of actual system performance that determines the extent to which desired outcomes are achieved, or the degree to which guidelines and standard operating procedures are adhered. Indicators are used to monitor the quality or appropriateness of important clinical and management activities. It is unnecessary to choose an indicator for every standard or specification. The number of indicators should be minimized when assessing key processes and identifying potential problem areas.
- *Setting thresholds*: Thresholds define a program's acceptable performance levels, as measured by indicators, at a given point in time. They allow program staff to detect potential problems or areas for improvement. Performance thresholds can be based on clinical or medical knowledge of risks or on what is operationally feasible. For example, some immunization

programs set 80 percent coverage as a threshold. The acceptable level of performance is relative and should be revised as conditions and priorities change. The role of thresholds is to trigger action when the monitored indicators suggest inadequate program performance. Performance thresholds are not needed in all cases and should be set only after consultation with program staff. It is important to note the potential drawbacks of using thresholds in a quality improvement effort. Rather than encouraging continual improvement, using thresholds may give the mistaken impression that some errors are acceptable and that, once met, there is no need for further improvement. In spite of these potential drawbacks, performance thresholds, used correctly, can help teams to set priorities and can promote gradual improvement.

- *Selecting information sources*: Because many organizations already collect data, the first information source to examine is the existing information systems. Sometimes it is possible to make a minor change that would provide information without major efforts. Other information sources include suggestion boxes, complaint registers, clinical records, health center registers, interviews, facility review, and job performance observations. Because monitoring is a routine exercise, additional data collection should be kept to a minimum. It is especially important to minimize the burden of data collection on peripheral health workers. Generally, health workers should not be asked to collect data that they cannot use in their work. Data that are used at the local level and then compiled for higher-level managers are more likely to provide a basis for a constructive dialogue between health workers and managers about problems and priorities.
- *Designing a system for collecting and compiling data*: It is important to specify who will collect and compile the data, determine the frequency of collection and compilation, and develop a mechanism and schedule for disseminating the results. This system should be developed with staff participation at all levels, and it should be periodically reviewed. Over time, staff members should become adept at self-monitoring, relying less on district- and central-level managers.
- *Implementing the monitoring activities*: Once the system has been designed and responsibility has been assigned, data collection and compilation can begin. During the initial phase of a monitoring system, health workers will need assistance in collecting and using data. This support is essential if monitoring is to serve as a screening tool.

Rather than constantly monitoring all activities, monitoring systems might use an index of activities or tracer conditions that cover various program dimensions. For example, a program manager could monitor immunization, hypertension, and treatment of pneumonia. Together, these tracer conditions might cover preventive services and management of chronic and acute illness, encompassing both child and adult care. Eventually, the conditions monitored should be rotated or modified to meet the community's changing needs. They should also expand with the QA effort. It is important to limit the monitoring system by emphasizing the collection and use of only essential data.

Systems analysis is another assessment method that can be used to identify service delivery problems. The service quality assessment technique originally applied to LDC primary health care by PRICOR consists of a comprehensive assessment of standard procedures and health worker performance. It is based primarily on observing actual or simulated performance.

Such systems analyses can be carried out as a baseline in identifying and measuring major problems before a QA program is launched. They can also be carried out periodically, in whole or in part, to evaluate general improvement and to prove the validity of program institutionalization.

5. Identifying Problems and Selecting Opportunities for Improvement

Program managers can identify quality improvement opportunities by monitoring and evaluating activities. With effective monitoring systems, health programs can conduct special community or patient surveys or comprehensive assessments such as PRICOR II's systems analysis methodology.[11] These studies highlight specific service delivery problems requiring attention. Other means include soliciting suggestions from health workers, performing system process analyses, reviewing patient feedback or complaints, and generating ideas through brainstorming or other group techniques. Employing a participatory approach to problem identification offers several advantages. First, the quality of the assessment and preliminary analysis is likely to be superior because those who are directly involved with the processes are participating. Second, staff members are more likely to contribute and to cooperate if they are involved in identifying problems.

Once a health facility team has identified several problems, it should set quality improvement priorities by choosing one or two problem areas on which to focus. Selection criteria will vary from program to program. Two important principles should guide this process. The criteria should reflect team, not individual, priorities. They should also be explicit so that the decision-making process is as objective and as thorough as possible. Criteria might include the technical feasibility of addressing the problem, the potential impact of improving quality on the population's health, or the adequacy of the necessary available resources.

PRICOR II's quality improvement work in developing countries resulted in some noteworthy insights about priority setting. First, the problem must be within the scope of responsibility and authority of those carrying out the QA effort. Trying to change something that is outside local control is a frustrating experience that has little hope for success. In the same vein, it is often preferable to begin QA efforts by focusing on a smaller, manageable problem rather than on a large, complex one. Tackling a solvable problem encourages confidence in the QA process. Teams can select priorities using various group decision-making techniques such as ranking and voting exercises or decision matrices that consider several criteria in the priority-setting process.

6. Defining the Problem

Having selected a problem, the team must define it operationally—as a gap between actual performance and performance as prescribed by guidelines and standards. The problem statement should identify the problem and how it manifests itself. It should clearly state where the problem begins and ends, and how to recognize when the problem is solved. Developing a problem statement is a crucial step in the QA process, and its apparent simplicity is deceptive. Often, the initial formulation of a problem will include only the cause of a problem—"we don't have a laboratory"—or its premature solution—"we need more staff." Sometimes problems are too general to permit concrete, incremental action—"we don't work as a team." Problem statements also may err by focusing on blame rather than on the problem description—"nurses are not willing to be polite to patients." Problems should explicitly relate to the quality of services or the health of the population. They should refer to specific processes or activities so that the improvement effort is well focused and measurable.[12]

Problem definition is an iterative process: as team members attempt to define a problem, they will be forced to rethink many of their steps. They may decide to narrow the problem or choose to address one cause of a multifaceted problem. While defining a concrete operational problem, team members are likely to vacillate between large, unmanageable problems and the smaller one that they are trying to define. They may even feel that the discrete operational problem they are defining is not worth addressing because it is such a small part of the wider problem. It is important for a team to take the time to develop clarity about the problem and consensus about its importance. Without these ingredients, the QA effort will stall. The examples provided on the top of page 19 illustrate how problem statements can be reformulated to show the relation to service quality.

7. Choosing a Team

Once a health facility staff has employed a participatory approach to selecting and defining a problem, it should assign a small team to address the specific problem. The team will analyze the problem, develop a quality improvement plan, and implement and evaluate the quality improvement effort. The team should comprise those who are involved with, contribute inputs or resources to, and/or benefit from the activity or activities in which the problem occurs. This ensures the involvement of those most knowledgeable about the process.

Learning to work effectively as a team is a challenging and continuous process. Health center teams often will need training in basic skills related to planning and facilitating meetings, communicating effectively, making group decisions, and resolving conflict. Building a high-performance team takes time, requiring patience and persistence.[13]

8. Analyzing and Studying the Problem to Identify the Root Cause

Achieving a meaningful and sustainable quality improvement effort depends on understanding the problem and its root causes. Given the complexity of health service delivery, clearly identifying root causes requires systematic, in-depth analysis. Analytical tools such as system modeling, flow charting, and cause-and-effect diagrams can be used to analyze a process or problem.

Once several potential causes are identified, the team should determine which ones are the most damaging, since two or three causes may be responsible for up to 80 percent of quality problems. By addressing these critical causes, a problem-solving team can realize significant improvement with minimal effort. Analytical tools alone will not always provide enough information. A problem-solving team may need to conduct an in-depth examination. Such studies can be based on clinical record reviews, health center register data, staff or patient interviews, service delivery observations, or any combination of the above. These studies must go beyond documenting the problem; they should examine root causes.

At this stage, problem-solving teams often employ some basic statistical tools. These may include check sheets, histograms, scattergrams, pareto charts, run charts, and control charts. The check sheet is a data collection tool used in assessing variables related to a specific process. The resultant data can be presented in a histogram that assesses the extent of variation, in a distribution scattergram that indicate trends, or in a pareto chart that classifies problems according to cause in descending order of importance. Run charts make it easy to monitor change in a process over time. Control charts help to monitor variation and provide clues that can help to identify the type of variation. Some causes are inherent to the process, while others have their roots outside the process.

9. Developing Solutions and Actions for Quality Improvement

The problem-solving team should now be ready to develop and evaluate potential solutions. Unless the procedure in question is the sole responsibility of an individual, developing solutions should be a team effort. It may be necessary to involve personnel responsible for processes related to the root cause. Solutions to quality problems or quality improvement activities can take several forms. A solution may be very straightforward: it may be as simple as reminding staff about clinical guidelines through supervision or focused in-service training. Solutions may also take the form of job aids such as wall charts and checklists. They become part of the process that provides information and checks at the point of service delivery, thereby reducing error or variation. Often, solutions and improvements are rooted in management systems related to supervision, training, and logistics. Some problems, however, are more difficult to solve because they require procedural redesign. This should be considered if the team determines that there is no existing process in the problem area or that the defined process is not responsive to the clients' needs and expectations. In such cases, tools such as flowcharts and design matrices can be very helpful in designing solutions that build on the strengths of existing practices and take client requirements into account.

Problem-solving teams are encouraged to think creatively and to generate a variety of solution options. Choices among potential solutions should be based on an examination of the option's potential costs and effectiveness. Teams may employ techniques such as multiple criteria utility assessment or multi-voting to help them in evaluating solutions and making a decision. The team also should gauge potential opposition to change and develop a plan to minimize resistance.

10. Implementing and Evaluating Quality Improvement Efforts

Implementing quality improvement requires careful planning. The team must determine the necessary resources and time frame and decide who will be responsible for implementation. It must also decide whether implementation should begin with a pilot test in a limited area or should be launched on a larger scale. A pilot project is merited if the solution requires substantial resources or if there is considerable uncertainty about the solution's potential effectiveness. The team should select indicators to evaluate whether the solution was implemented correctly and whether it resolved the problem it was designed to address. In-depth monitoring should begin when the quality improvement plan is implemented. It should continue until either the solution is proven effective and sustainable, or the solution is proven ineffective and is abandoned or modified. When a solution is effective, the teams should continue limited monitoring. Teams should modify solutions as needed and should fully document results and lessons learned.

Once the solution has proved to be effective, program managers should codify and disseminate the new process so that others can learn from the experience. The QA team should also make plans to identify a new problem, either through a team process or through data generated by an existing monitoring system. The team may then repeat the quality improvement cycle.

VI. Building a Quality Assurance Program

A QA program is a comprehensive set of quality assessment and improvement activities that is incorporated into an organization's routine management functions. As health care organizations learn more about the

QA process, they are likely to discover that some of their current activities are related to quality improvement. In fact, most organizations already do some type of QA. These existing activities provide a foundation upon which to build a comprehensive QA program. The previous section describes how program managers and staff can conduct quality-related activities more thoroughly. The following section discusses how QA can be permanently integrated into health program management in developing countries. There are two distinct approaches to building a QA program. The first is the comprehensive QA strategy; the second is the problem-oriented strategy. The two approaches are contrasted here to provide an overview of the wide range of strategic options available to program managers. In practice, most organizations will want to combine these approaches as they introduce quality assurance.

In the comprehensive approach, QA policies, procedures, and processes are implemented simultaneously, starting at the top and moving down the organizational structure. A comprehensive approach typically begins with a thorough review of standards and specifications.

This may be followed by an assessment of health care and support services. This assessment may be conducted through an existing management information system or through a monitoring system specifically developed to measure service quality. Start-up also includes an extensive training effort to strengthen technical competencies and to impart quality improvement knowledge and skills.

Comprehensive service quality assessments are useful in countries where information systems are inadequate. Systems analysis allows managers to use interviews and observation to assess primary health care services and their associated support activities. Priority areas for quality improvement can be identified based on the results of comprehensive monitoring or systems analysis. The comprehensive approach works best when there is a commitment throughout the system to addressing quality of care and when organizations have the necessary resources to implement a QA program on a large scale.

The problem-oriented approach to QA emphasizes practical, small-scale, quality-related activities that produce incremental quality improvements. Rather than carrying out a comprehensive assessment, individuals or teams focus on a single problem that is important to them. In this model, comprehensive assessment and monitoring are de-emphasized in favour of immediate action. This is based on the assumption that monitoring systems and a more systematic approach can be developed over time once problem-solving has become part of the organizational culture. Often, the problem-oriented approach is introduced early at a few clinics rather than throughout the organization. This allows an organization to modify and adapt the problem-solving strategy before wider implementation.

With careful planning, problem-orientation can evolve into a more comprehensive approach. Eventually, all types of services can be covered by the QA effort and a simple monitoring system can be emplaced. It is also important to note that a comprehensive approach can benefit from some small-scale, problem-oriented activities. One danger of an exclusively comprehensive approach is that staff at all levels may grow impatient with the tedious process of setting up systems and of participating in training activities that do not yield immediate, concrete results. Potential resistance can be averted by conducting small-scale, quality improvement activities that demonstrate quick, short-term outcomes. Also, these results can be incorporated into training efforts, thus providing local examples of QA.

There is no recipe for developing a QA program. It is a creative process that requires flexibility in order to adapt to a given health program's unique features. This section describes key activities that are usually carried out in building a QA program. Most of the key activities described take place concurrently, and many must be continually renegotiated as the program evolves and conditions change.

Key Activities in the Development of a Quality Assurance Program

- Foster commitment to quality
- Conduct a preliminary review of QA-related activities
- Develop the purpose and vision for the QA effort
- Determine level and scope of initial QA activities
- Assign responsibility for QA
- Allocate resources for QA
- Develop a written QA plan
- Strengthen QA skills and critical management systems
- Disseminate QA activities
- Manage change

A QA program may be developed gradually through a carefully planned, phased process, or it may be implemented in one step as part of a fundamental organizational change. A gradual, phased approach is frequently appropriate for organizations with rudimentary management systems.

Foster Commitment to Quality

Building a permanent QA program requires the early support of top- and mid-level managers. Over time, this commitment to QA should be shared by all staff and reflected in the organization's mission, purpose, and procedures. The process of fostering and developing commitment is not an isolated activity; it must continue throughout the life of a project and at all levels of the organization.

Commitment is developed by raising awareness and by fostering a dialogue among top-level managers. This can be done through awareness-raising seminars, special planning meetings, or one-to-one discussions with an organization's leaders. During the awareness-raising process, basic concepts are introduced that relate to quality and quality assessment and improvement methods. Discussing the importance of quality and presenting empirical information about quality problems at the local level can also foster commitment.

Conduct a Preliminary Review of Quality-related Activities

Before introducing new QA activities, it is important to conduct an initial review of the organization and to develop a general description of the existing system. This review will allow the new QA effort to build on existing strengths. QA efforts will likely be sustained if they are built into the existing system in a logical way. For example, an existing supervisory system that monitors compliance with technical norms is a logical place to begin QA activities. Failing to recognize such an opportunity can result in turf battles between managers and in confusion among service providers. One important function of the initial assessment is to determine the best place in the organization to launch a QA initiative. This preliminary analysis can include the following:

- Review of the program's clinical and managerial standards or norms. Are they technically sound? Are they appropriate for local conditions? Are they complete? Are they up-to-date? Are they available to staff?
- Assessment of the quality of service currently provided, and patient and community satisfaction with the services.
- Review of the supervisory system and related management activities to determine which type of QA is already in place. What problems are faced by supervisors? Are they able to solve them?
- Examination of the management information system. Consider the scope, validity, sensitivity, specificity, and reliability of the indicators currently being monitored. Are data used for management and decision-making? Could the existing data be used to support a QA program?
- Review of existing training capacity. Could training be carried out by the organization or would outside help be needed? Do current training programs include skills that could be used in QA?
- Study of the organizational structure. Profile the organization's lines of communication and authority. Who is doing QA now? Who should be doing QA?
- Assessment of the adequacy of facilities, logistics, and equipment. Different approaches can be used to conduct a preliminary assessment. Depending on the resources available, the assessment can be a comprehensive study. It may include collecting new data or a rapid assessment based on available data and the expert opinion of key informants.

Develop the Purpose and Vision for the Quality Assurance Effort

Building commitment to QA within an organization requires that top managers and their staff share an overall vision of quality improvement. The purpose of a vision statement is to build consensus between managers and to set boundaries for the QA effort. The vision statement will help staff at all levels to understand how their day-to-day work relates to quality improvement. It can be developed through a variety of consensus-building techniques that can be employed by the senior management team. The vision statement should be developed at the QA effort's outset and revised periodically if there are strategic changes in the organization or if there is a significant staff turnover.

Determine Level and Scope of Initial Quality Assurance Activities

The level and scope of initial QA activities depend on the resources available, the implementation time frame, and the receptivity of management and program staff to the idea of QA. An organization must also consider external political factors.

A QA effort can be implemented at the national, regional, and district level or within a single health facility. Where services are organized as vertical programs, one program may be the focus of initial QA activities. An organization must also use a small-scale effort such as a pilot study or series of demonstration projects in testing QA strategies and in learning more about their local application. Small-scale efforts are often attractive to managers because they offer progress at little risk, and because successful programs can be replicated or expanded. Unfortunately, it is frequently difficult to replicate developed models, often because the demonstration sites have advantages over the rest of the organization.

Assign Responsibility for Quality Assurance

To ensure continuity, accountability for QA activities must be clear, and QA must be a prominent organizational emphasis. In some organizations a single person may be responsible for QA, while in others it may be the domain of quality committees. Occasionally, an existing committee or management body will take on responsibility for QA, integrating it into the general management structure. In others, a QA program will be established whose role is defined in relation to other departments. The titles of those responsible for QA should denote a facilitative rather than a directive role; they might be called quality coordinators, coaches, or advisors. QA coordinators and the QA committee are responsible for monitoring and supporting QA activities, providing technical assistance to teams, assigning staff to develop indicators, and facilitating communication about QA issues between top-level management and staff.

Allocate Resources for Quality Assurance

Local resources must be allocated to quality assurance in order for a

QA program to become a permanent part of a health care organization. Often, the initial QA effort may depend on outside technical and financial assistance. Over time, the organization should support its own QA program with minimal dependency on external resources. While QA efforts may not become self-financing immediately, organizations should weigh resource considerations in the design phase. Externally funded QA activities should be designed so that they can be replicated with local resources. It is important to note that even QA programs that are to be integrated into an existing management system often need initial resources to support training and miscellaneous costs. While the QA staff may be the same as the management staff, it will need resources earmarked for new activities. QA staff may travel more to health service facilities or may require additional materials for data collection maintenance.

Develop a Written Quality Assurance Plan

A QA plan is a written document that describes the program objectives and scope, defines lines of responsibility and authority, and puts forth implementation strategies. The plan should help staff members to relate quality goals and objectives to their routine activities. It should also be a living document that is regularly referred to and revised.

Strengthen Quality Assurance Skills and Critical Management Systems

QA activities are an important part of management and may occasionally be reformulated into a total quality management system. In general, however, QA efforts will focus more narrowly on three critical management systems: supervision, training, and management information systems. Special effort should be made to strengthen these systems as a QA program develops. Organizations should develop supervision systems that not only evaluate and manage activities, but also support health workers through a process of professional growth. In the long-term, this approach can lead to self-managed, self-directed individual and collective work. While this may seem difficult, it is necessary since many health providers in developing countries work at the periphery without daily supervision. Supervisors can take the lead in QA efforts by providing an example of participatory leadership and problem-solving skills; over time, health workers can initiate quality improvement activities. Methods for self-management and concurrent QA such as health worker and supervisor self-assessments and other job aids can be introduced by the supervisor to improve performance.

The training system should incorporate competency-based training for specific routine tasks, including service delivery, counseling, and health education, as well as for management support services. Besides improving training in skill areas essential for high-quality services, the training capacity should be developed and expanded to include such QA skills as problem-solving, evaluation, and teamwork. It is also important to revise the management information system so that it serves as an effective QA monitoring system. This can be done early or late in the QA process, when managers and staff have an idea of what information they need and how to use it more effectively. Resistance to change in this area may be easier to manage after the QA program has achieved some initial successes.

Disseminate QA Experiences

Early in the life of a QA program, a dissemination strategy should be devised to share experiences inside and outside the organization. Some dissemination programs use newsletters that contain educational articles and project progress reports. Newsletters also serve as an effective way to recognize the initiative of local individuals and groups. Conferences at the local regional, national, and international level can also be effective because they reinforce success, encourage dialogue and creativity, and generate political momentum for the program. Developing a Quality Assurance Resource Center is another effective dissemination strategy. Making information about QA methods and experiences available to staff will encourage initiative and will accelerate the learning rate. Resource centers are particularly important for program leaders and trainers because they offer valuable self-study programs.

Participation in professional societies such as local medical and nursing associations or the International Society for Quality Assurance is also an excellent way to disseminate QA-related experiences. Storytelling is a potent dissemination tool for documenting the quality improvement efforts of local teams. It is an accurate and appealing way to document quality improvement, employing graphic techniques that eliminate the need for laborious report writing.

Manage Change

Resistance is almost inevitable when trying to implement a QA program. Initially, some managers and staff fear criticism, loss of power, and change itself. Staff members who are new to leadership and decision-making roles may be fearful or nervous about their new responsibilities. Even healthy changes involve discomfort, uncertainty, and conflict.

SOURCES

1. Nicholas, David D., Heiby, James R., and Hatzell, Theresa A., "The Quality Assurance Project: Introducing Quality Improvement to Primary Health Care in Less Developed Countries," *Quality Assurance in Health Care,* 3:3, Great Britain, 1991, pp. 147-65.
2. Health Administration Press, 1980, pp. 5-6. Roemer, M.I., and Montoya-Aguilar, C., "Quality Assessment and Assurance in Primary Health Care," WHO Offset Publication No., 105, World Health Organization, Geneva, Switzerland, 1988. Donabedian, pp. 5-6.
3. Donabedian, Avedis, Explorations in Quality Assessment and Monitoring, Ann Arbor, Ruelas, Enrique and Frenk, Julio, "Framework for the Analysis of Quality in Transition: The Case of Mexico," *Australian Clinical Review,* 9, 1989, pp. 9-16.

4. Palmer, Heather, Ambulatory Health Care Evaluation Principles and Practice, Chicago: American Hospital Association, 1983, p. 139.
5. Berwick, Donald, Improving Health Care Quality, Boston: Institute for Health Care Improvement, 1991, p. II-3.
6. Field, Marilyn J., and Lohr, Kathleen N. (editors), Clinical Practice Guidelines - Directions for a New Program, Institute of Medicine, National Academy Press, Washington, D.C., 1990, p. 8.
7. *Ibid.*
8. Copies can be obtained by writing to Center for Human Services, 7200 Wisconsin Avenue, Suite 600, Bethesda, MD 20814, U.S.A.
9. The comparative analyses summarize the work of PRICOR II: Burns Jaeger, Janice, Franco, Lynne Miller, and Newman, Jeanne S., "Oral Rehydration Therapy in Diarrheal Disease Control: A Review of Experience in Eight Countries," September 1990.
10. DiPrete, Lori, "Acute Lower Respiratory Infection: A Review of Experience in Four Countries," September 1991.
11. Franco, Lynne Miller, "Malaria Treatment: A Review of Experience in Four Countries," June 1991.
12. Sonnemann, James C., McMeekin, Elizabeth, Bossert, Thomas, "Expanded Program on Immunization: A Review of Experience in Nine Countries," September 1991.
13. Stinson, Wayne and Sayer, Patricia, "Growth Monitoring and Promotion: A Review of Experience in Seven Countries," August 1991.

5

Health Care Systems in the Western World

"Health Care is claimed to be better in the western world as compared to communist countries as well as that of third world countries. Obviously, poverty breeds poor health and unmanaged health care. Even in the developed countries of the western world, there is no single health care model that the world follows. Each country's system is the product of its development status, economy, unique conditions, history, politics, and national character, and many are undergoing significant reforms. Under a single-payer health care system, the government pays for the health care of all citizens. It collects taxes, administers the supply of health care, and pays providers directly. Typically, the government establishes a budget, deciding how much of the nation's resources should be allocated to health care, and sets prices or reimbursement rates for providers. In some cases, providers may be salaried government employees. In others, they may remain independent and be reimbursed according to the services and procedures they provide. Single payer is the system advocated by Michael Moore, Paul Krugman, Dennis Kucinich, and Physicians for a National Health Program, among others. This is the ideal system, hence not achieved."

Cost-sharing is a Practical Option

Cost-sharing is well accepted concept/options in various countries of the developed as well as under-developed countries. Some countries, such as France and Japan, impose significant cost sharing on consumers in an effort to discourage over-utilization and to control costs. Other countries strictly limit the amount that consumers must pay out of pocket. Some countries permit free choice of providers, while others limit it. In some countries there is widespread purchase of alternative or supplemental private insurance, whereas in others, private insurance is prohibited or used very little. Resource allocation and prioritization vary greatly. Japan spends heavily on technology but limits reimbursement for surgery, while France has exceptionally high levels of prescription drug use. Outcomes also vary significantly. Canada, Great Britain, Norway, and Spain all heavily ration health care or have long waiting lists for care, while France and Switzerland have generally avoided waiting lists. At the same time, France, Italy, and Germany are struggling with rising health care costs and budget strain, compared with Canada and Great Britain, which have done better at containing growth in expenditures. And some countries such as Greece have fallen far short of claims of universal coverage.

France

Some people tout the French health care system as ideal. Jonathan Cohn of the New Republic has written that "the best showcase for what universal health care can achieve may be France." EzraKlein of the *American Prospect* calls France "the closest thing to a model structure out there." The French system ranks at or near the top of most cross-country comparisons and is ranked number one by the WHO. Although the French system is facing looming budgetary pressures, it does provide at least some level of universal coverage and manages to avoid many of the problems that afflict other national health care systems. However, it does so in large part by adopting market-oriented approaches, including consumer cost sharing. Other aspects of the system appear to reflect French customs and political attitudes in such a way that would make it difficult to import the system to the United States. France provides a basic level of universal health insurance through a series of mandatory, largely occupation-based, health insurance funds. These funds are ostensibly private entities but are heavily regulated and supervised by the French government. Premiums (funded primarily through payroll taxes), benefits, and provider reimbursement rates are all set by the government. The largest fund, the General National Health Insurance Scheme, covers most non-agricultural workers and their dependents, about 83 percent of French residents. Separate insurance plans cover agricultural workers, the self-employed, and certain special occupations like miners, transportation workers, artists, clergy, and notaries public. Another fund covers the unemployed. These larger insurance schemes are broken down into smaller pools based on geographic region. Overall, about 99 percent of French citizens are covered by national health insurance.

Third most expensive

The French health care system costs roughly 11 per cent of GDP, behind only the United States (17 percent) and Switzerland (11.5 percent). Employers must pay 12.8 percent of wages for every employee, while employees contribute an additional 0.75 percent of wages, for a total pay-roll tax of 13.55 percent. In addition, there is a 5.25 general social contribution tax on income (reduced to 3.95 percent on pension income and unemployment benefits). Thus, most French workers are effectively paying 18.8 percent of their income for health insurance. Finally, dedicated taxes are assessed on tobacco, alcohol, and pharmaceutical company revenues. The National Health Authority sets a global budget for national health care spending, but actual spending has consistently exceeded those targets. In 2006, the health care system ran a €€10.3 billion deficit. This actually shows improvement over 2005, when the system ran an €€11.6 billion deficit. The health care system is the largest single factor driving France's overall budget deficit, which has grown to €€49.6 billion, or 2.5 percent of GDP.

In general, the funds provide coverage for inpatient and outpatient care, physician and specialist services, diagnostic testing, prescription drugs, and home care services. Most services require substantial co-payments, ranging from 10 to 40 percent of the cost. As a result, French consumers pay for roughly 13 percent of health care out of pocket, roughly the same percentage as U.S. consumers. Moreover, because many health care services are not covered, and because many of the best providers refuse to accept the fee schedules imposed by the insurance funds, more than 92 percent of French residents purchase complementary private insurance. In fact, private insurance now makes up roughly 12.7 percent of all health care spending in France, a percentage exceeded only by the Netherlands (15.2 percent) and the United States (35 percent) among industrialized countries. The combination of out-of-pocket and insurance payments means that non-government sources account for roughly 20 percent of all health care spending, less than half the amount spent in the United States but still more than most countries with national health care systems. The private insurance market in France is in many ways less regulated than the U.S. market. In general, French patients pay up front for treatment and are then reimbursed by their government health insurance fund and/or private insurance. The amount of reimbursement, minus the copayment, is based on a fee schedule negotiated between health care providers and the national health insurance funds. These fee schedules operate similarly to the diagnostic-related groups (DRGs) under the U.S. system.

Physicians allowed to overcharge

The French system permits providers to charge more than the reimbursement schedule, and approximately one-third of French physicians do so. In some areas, such as Paris, the percentage of physicians who bill above reimbursement schedules runs as high as 80 percent. In general, however, competition prevents most physicians from billing too far outside negotiated rates; and physicians employed by hospitals, as opposed to those in private practice; do not have the same ability to charge more than the negotiated rate. In general, the quality of French health care is high, but there are problem areas. Until very recently, the French have generally had quick access to their primary care physician of choice. Now, a patient can't go from one doctor to another until it is driving up costs to the system. The government has responded by increasing co-payments and attempting to limit physician reimbursements. Much of the burden for cost containment in the French system appears to have fallen on physicians. The average French doctor earns just €€40,000 per year ($55,000), compared to $146,000 for primary care physicians and $271,000 for specialists in the United States.

"Under the new system, which operates very much like managed care in the United States, patients are encouraged to choose a "preferred doctor" and to follow the "pathway" suggested by that doctor. The effect is both to lock patients into a choice of primary care physician and to establish a "gatekeeper" who limits access to specialists, tests, and some advanced treatment options. But if costs continue to rise, the new system may be extended and made more rigorous. Strong disparities are also evident in the geographic distribution of health care resources, making access to care easier in some regions than others. Government regulation and bureaucracy have also been blamed for rigidity in the French system, preventing it from reacting quickly to changing circumstances. For example, mismanagement and the inability of the system to cope with emergencies were blamed in part for the deaths of 15,000 elderly individuals in the summer of 2003 during the European heat wave; and a shortage of hospital beds occurred in 2004 when a nationwide flu and bronchitis epidemic broke out. Slightly less than half consider the waiting time between diagnosis and treatment to be acceptable. Some French health professionals have suggested that waiting times for care have begun to lengthen. However, patients may ignore the "coordinated care pathway" and accept higher prices, paying more for immediate access. In essence, the French system avoids widespread rationing because, unlike true single-payer systems, it employs market forces. Waiting lists for elective surgery generally tend to be found in countries which combine public health insurance (with zero or low patient cost sharing) and constraints on surgical capacity.

Moral hazard

French system's innovative response to one of the trickier problems bedeviling health-policy experts: an economic concept called "moral hazard." Moral hazard describes people's tendency to overuse goods or services that offer more marginal benefit without a proportionate marginal cost. Means, you eat more at a buffet because the refills are free, and you use more health care because insurers generally make you pay up front in premiums, rather than at the point of care. The obvious solution is to shift more of the cost away from premiums and into co-pays or deductibles, thus increasing sensitivity of consumers to the real cost of each unit of care they purchase. A 2004 poll showed that the French had the highest level of satisfaction with their health care system among all European countries. This is partly because their hybrid system has avoided many of the biggest problems of other national health care systems. Yet it also stems from French social character. For example, by a three-to-one margin, the French believe the quality of care they receive is less important than everyone having equal access to that care. The new French government has made a crackdown on health care spending one of its top priorities. Thus, the French health care system clearly works better than most national health care systems. Despite some problems, France has generally avoided the rationing inherent in other systems. However, the program is threatened by increasing costs and may be forced to resort to rationing in the future.

Italy

Italy's national health care system is rated second in the world by the WHO. Yet a closer examination shows the system to be deeply troubled, plagued with crippling bureaucracy, mismanagement and general disorganization, spiraling costs, and long waiting lists. Generally, the Italian system is similar to the British National Health Service but enjoys more decentralization. The central government sets goals on how money should be spent, monitors the overall health status of the nation, and negotiates the labour contracts of medical staff. The Italian Constitution was changed in 2001 such that the national government now sets the "essential levels of care". Thus, while the national Ministry of Health continues to outline funding needs based on weighted capitation and past spending, recent reforms have shifted more and more power and responsibility to regional governments who set their own budgets. The regions establish one or more Local Health Authorities, which are responsible for the provision of care either through government-run hospitals and clinics or by contracting with private providers. It should be noted that governance in Italy is often as much art as science and regions frequently fail to implement rules, guidelines, reimbursement schedules, and budgets set by the central government.

Inpatient care and primary care are free at the point of treatment. However, copayments are required for diagnostic procedures, specialists, and prescription drugs. The size of such copayments has crept steadily upward over the past decade and now runs as high as 30 percent for some services. Several attempts have been made to impose copayments for a broad range of services, including primary care, but have collapsed in the face of public protests. In addition, nearly 40 percent of the population (the elderly, pregnant women, and children) are exempt from copayments. Italians have limited choice of physician. They must register with a general practitioner within their LHA. They may choose any GP in the LHA but may not go outside it. Except for emergency care, a referral from a GP is required for diagnostic services, hospitalization, and treatment by a specialist. Despite these limits, Italians enjoy more choice of physician than do the British or Spanish.

Most physicians are reimbursed on a capitated basis (i.e., according to the number of patients served over a given time period rather than the services actually provided), although some hospital physicians receive a monthly salary. Hospitals are generally reimbursed according to DRGs, with rates set by the central government—though regions sometimes disregard those rates and set their own. Private health insurance is available in Italy but is not widespread. Where offered, it is usually provided by employers. About 10 percent of Italians have private health insurance, below the percentage in most OECD countries. According to the insurance industry, this is partly because it is not possible to opt out of the National Health System and because health insurance premiums are not tax deductible. Private health insurance allows free choice of doctors, including specialists, and treatment in private hospitals. Even with-out private insurance, however, many Italians use private health resources (and presumably pay out of pocket). Estimates suggest that as much as 35 percent of the population uses at least some private health services. Although Italy spends a relatively low percentage of GDP on health care, expenditures have been rising rapidly in recent years and have consistently exceeded government forecasts. Between 1995 and 2003, total health care spending rose by 68 percent. The Italian government has taken various steps to try to control costs, such as reducing reimbursement rates, increasing copayments, reducing capital expenditures, contracting with private providers, limiting prescription drugs. All of these measures have met with protests, including physician strikes, and many have been repealed after only a short time. The Italian government does not provide official information on waiting lists, but numerous studies have shown them to be widespread and growing, particularly for diagnostic tests. For example, the average wait for a mammogram is 70 days; for endoscopy, 74 days; for a sonogram, 23 days. Undoubtedly, this is due in part to a shortage of modern medical technology. The United States has twice as many MRI units per million people and 25 percent more CT scanners. Ironically, the best-equipped hospitals in northern Italy have even longer waiting lists since they draw patients from the poorer southern regions as well. If delays become excessive, patients may seek permission from the regional government to obtain treatment from private doctors or hospitals at NHS expense. A recent court decision allows patients whose life would be endangered by delays under the NHS to seek treatment in private hospitals even without prior permission from the regional government.

Reducing the drug cost

Italy has imposed a relatively strict drug formulary as well as price controls, and has thereby succeeded in reducing pharmaceutical spending, long considered a problem for the Italian health care system. In 2006, Italian drug prices fell (or were pushed) 5 per cent, even as drug prices rose in the United States and much of the rest of the world. However, the savings came at a cost: the introduction of many of the newest and most innovative drugs was blocked. Conditions in public hospitals are considered substandard, particularly in the south. They lack not just modern technology, but basic goods and services; and overcrowding is widespread. Conditions are frequently unsanitary. For example, one of the largest public hospitals in

Rome was recently found to have garbage piled in the hallways, unguarded radioactive materials, abandoned medical records, and staff smoking next to patients. Private hospitals are considered much better and some regions have contracted with private hospitals to treat NHS patients. Dissatisfaction with the Italian health care system is extremely high, by some measures the highest in Europe. In polls, Italians say that their health care system is much worse than that of other countries and give it poor marks for meeting their needs. Roughly 60 percent of Italians believe that health care reform is "urgent," and another 24 percent believe it is "desirable." In general, Italians believe that such reform should incorporate market-based solutions. More than two-thirds (69 percent) believe that giving patients more control over health care spending will improve the system's quality. And 55 percent believe that it should be easier for patients to spend their own money on health care. However, given the general dysfunction of the Italian political system, and the entrenched opposition of special interest groups, substantial reform is not likely anytime soon.

Spain

The Spanish Constitution guarantees all citizens the "right" to health care, including equal access to preventive, curative, and rehabilitative services; but responsibility for implementing the country's universal system is being devolved to regional governments. The degree and speed of devolution is uneven, however, with some regions only recently achieving maximum autonomy. Coverage under the Spanish system is nearly universal, estimated at 98.7 percent of the population. The system provides primary health care, including general health and pediatric care, outpatient and inpatient surgery, emergency and acute care, long-term disease management, and prescription drugs (although some drugs may require a copayment). Many mental health services, particularly out-patient services, are excluded, as is cosmetic surgery. The federal government provides each region with a block grant. The money is not earmarked: the region decides how to use it. The block grant itself is based primarily on a region's population with some consideration given to other factors such as the population's demographics. Regions may use their own funds to supplement federal monies. Not surprisingly, health care spending varies widely from region to region. The differences in expenditures, as well as in spending priorities, lead to considerable variance in the availability of health resources. For example, Catalonia has more than 4.5 hospital beds per 1,000 residents, while Valencia has just 2.8. Spanish patients cannot choose their physicians, either primary care or specialists. Rather, they are assigned a primary care doctor from a list of physicians in their local community. If more specialized care is needed, the primary care physician refers patients to a network of specialists. Unlike U.S. managed care, it is not possible to go "out of network" unless the patient has private health insurance. This has sparked an interesting phenomenon whereby sick Spaniards move in order to change physicians or find networks with shorter waiting lists. Waiting lists vary from region to region but are a significant problem everywhere. On average, Spaniards wait 65 days to see a specialist, and in some regions the wait can be much longer. For instance, the wait for a specialist in the Canary Islands is 140 days. Even on the mainland, in Galacia, the wait can be as long as 81 days. For some specialties the problem is far worse, with a national average of 71 days for a gynecologist and 81 days for a neurologist. Waits for specific procedures are also lengthy. The mean waiting time for a prostectomy is 62 days; for hip replacement surgery, 123 days. Some health services that U.S. citizens take for granted are almost totally unavailable. For example, rehabilitation, convalescence, and care for those with terminal illness are usually left to the patient's relatives. About 12 percent of the population currently has private health insurance. (This amounts to double coverage since opting out of the government system is not allowed. In larger cities such as Madrid and Barcelona, the number of privately insured reaches as high as 25 percent. Overall, private insurance payments account for 21 percent of total health care expenditures. More commonly, Spaniards pay for care outside of the national health care system out of pocket. In fact, nearly 24 percent of health care spending in Spain is out of pocket, more than any European country except Greece and Switzerland, and even more than the United States. Here again, a two-tier system has developed, with the wealthy able to buy their way around the defects of the national health care system, and the poor consigned to substandard services.

Lacks behind in technology

There are also shortages of modern medical technologies. Spain has one-third as many MRI units per million people as the United States, just over one-third as many CT units, and fewer lithotripters. Again, there is wide variation by region. For example, two regions, Ceuta and Melilla, do not have a single MRI unit. The regional variation is important because Spaniards face bureaucratic barriers in trying to go to another region for treatment. All hospital-based physicians and approximately 75 percent of all other physicians are considered quasi-civil servants and are paid a salary rather than receiving payment based on services provided. Compensation is based on years of practice or the attainment of certain professional credentials, with across-the-board annual increases unrelated to merit, performance, or patient satisfaction. As a result, Spain has fewer physicians and fewer nurses per capita than most European countries and the United States. The lack of primary care physicians is particularly acute. Even so, Spaniards are generally happy with their system. Nearly 60 percent describe their system as good, the second highest favourability rating in Europe. (France was first.) Accordingly, health care reform does not rank high on the average Spaniard's political agenda. One observer described health care as "conspicuous by its absence as a major issue" in recent elections. Only about 46 percent of Spaniards describe the need for reform as "urgent," while 35 percent see reform as "desirable." And

Spaniards are less inclined toward market-based reforms than most other European countries. Only 42 percent of Spaniards believe that it should be easier for patients to spend their own money on health care, and only 58 percent believe that giving patients more control over spending will improve quality. However, Spaniards do want more choice of doctors and hospitals, and they want the government to do a better job of dealing with waiting lists.

Japan

Japan has a universal health insurance system centered primarily on mandatory, employment-based insurance. On the surface, Japan's national health insurance program defies easy description, comprising some 2,000 private insurers and more than 3,000 government units. However, in a broader sense, the system encompasses four principal insurance schemes. The Employee Health Insurance Program requires companies with 700 or more employees to provide workers with health insurance from among some 1,800 "society-managed insurance" plans. Nearly 85 percent of these plans cover a single company and can be thought of as similar to the self-insurance plans operated by many large U.S companies. Most of the rest are industry-based. About 26 percent of the population participates in these plans. Such plans are financed through mandatory employer and employee contributions, effectively a payroll tax. The total contribution averages around 8.5 percent of wages. It is generally split evenly between employer and employee, although some companies assume slightly more than half the contribution. As a result, workers contribute about 45 percent of payments overall. It should be noted that studies have found that the majority of the burden of the employer's contribution to health insurance is borne by the employees in the form of reduced wages. These contributions are frequently insufficient to operate the insurance plans. In 2003, more than half lost money. A number of companies have responded by dissolving their individual plans and entering larger industry-based plans. However, growing costs continue to pressure many businesses. Workers in businesses with fewer than 700 workers must enroll in the government-run, small-business national health insurance program. This plan covers about 30 per cent of the population and is funded primarily through mandatory contributions, around 8.2 percent of wages, and supplemented by government funds. The self-employed and retirees are covered under the Citizens Insurance Program administered by municipal governments. Funding comes primarily from a self-employment tax, but additional revenues come from an assessment on the society-managed insurance programs discussed above and the small business program. General revenue contributions from the national government are used to plug shortfalls.

Elderly do not pay

The elderly are covered through a fund financed by contributions from the other three schemes, as well as contributions from the central government. The elderly do not pay directly into this plan, known as the Roken, but contribute to the plan they were enrolled in while employed. The Roken is simply a cost-sharing mechanism. A number of small programs exist to handle special populations such as farmers, fisher-men, and government workers. The unemployed remain under their former employers' plan, although they are not required to continue contributing. Private supplemental insurance exists, but very few Japanese carry it. Private health insurance pays for less than 1 percent of total Japanese health care spending. Benefits under all four schemes are extremely generous, including hospital and physician care, as well as dental care, maternity care, prescription drugs, and even some transportation costs. There are no restrictions on hospital or physician choice and generally no preauthorization or gatekeeper requirements. Significant copayments accompany most services, ranging from 10 percent to, more commonly, 30 percent (capped at $677 per month for a middle-income family). As a result, the average Japanese household pays about $2,300 per year out of pocket.

It is not all free

Overall out-of-pocket expenditures amount to roughly 17 percent of total health care spending. The vast majority of hospitals and clinics in Japan are privately owned, but because the government sets all fee schedules, the distinction between privately and publicly owned is irrelevant for patients. Reimbursement for both hospitals and clinics is on a fee-for-service basis, with the government setting fees and prescription prices. The fee schedule is identical for inpatient and outpatient treatment. Because hospitals must absorb both physician and capital costs from the same level of reimbursement, the tendency has been to shift patients to outpatient services. Recently, some attempts have been made to introduce alternate reimbursement mechanisms for hospitals, including DRGs and Diagnosis and Procedure Combinations—classification systems that tie reimbursements more closely to the resources that a particular patient consumes. But the medical establishment has resisted, and only about 80 hospitals participate in the experiment. Hospital physicians are salaried employees. Non-hospital physicians' work in the private sector and the government sets their reimbursement schedules. Generally, reimbursement is on a fee-for-service basis, although recently some chronic conditions have been "price bundled" into a single fee. Reimbursement schedules are set within the context of an overall global budget on health spending, but the division of resources is the subject of extensive negotiation with providers. The fee schedule reflects both the Japanese style of medicine and attempts to contain costs. For example, because of a strong cultural bias against invasive procedures, surgery tends to be reimbursed at a much lower rate than non-surgical procedures. The fee-setting system has had serious corruption problems. Because the fees for each of more than 3,000 procedures or services are set individually and adjusted every two years on an individual basis, it is possible to manipulate particular fees without attracting much attention. In 2004, a group of dentists was indicted for bribing the fee-setting board. In addition, the reimbursement schedule for physicians creates an incentive for them to see as many patients as possible. The result is assembly line medicine. Two-thirds of patients spend less than 10 minutes with their doctor; 18 percent spend less than 3 minutes. On the other hand, the Japanese, like Americans, practice a very technology-intensive style of medicine. Capital investment in technology has been given high priority, and the Japanese have at least as much access to technology such as MRI units, CT scanners, and lithotripters as patients in the United States. Because the government imposes uniform fee schedules on hospitals, there is no price competition. Instead, hospitals attempt to lure patients by having the best technology. While this can benefit patients, it has also led to queues at the best hospitals and a black market with "under the table" payments for faster access. Some restrictions have been added in the last few years, capping the number of diagnostic imaging procedures that a hospital can perform in a calendar month, as well as reducing the fees for those services. These changes have not led to visible rationing yet but could in the future. To date, Japan has done a fairly good job of controlling costs without resorting to the rationing common in many universal care systems. This is due in part to factors outside the health care system, such as generally healthy lifestyles, low vehicle accident rates, low crime rates, low rates of drug abuse, and other cultural factors. One study estimated that 25 percent of the difference in health care spending between the United States and Japan is attributable to a lower incidence of disease and 15 percent to less aggressive practice styles. But rationing has also been avoided through the management of the health care system and the imposition of significant consumer cost sharing. Nonetheless, spending is beginning to escalate, especially in government-managed programs such as the Roken, where there has been less of an attempt at cost sharing and cost containment. As one observer explained : We Japanese have a tendency to go to the hospital even when we have only minor ailments such as the flu, headaches, or stomach aches. If medical expenses are not high and we do not feel well, then why not go see a doctor and get some medication. . . . The result, of course, is that waiting rooms of clinics and hospitals are full of people. Everyone is welcome and there are, in fact, regular customers. Sometimes elderly people come to see a friend and the hospital waiting room becomes a sort of salon. This problem is aggravated by the demographics of a rapidly aging society. By some estimates, the elderly are responsible for 90 per cent of the aggregate increase in Japan's health care costs. If current trends continue, Japan will almost triple its government spending on health care in the next 20 years. And the situation will only grow less stable with time. Japan is expected to lose 35 million workers by 2050, with 35 percent of its population in retirement. This raises questions of how a system that relies on payroll taxes for funding can continue to fund rising costs even as its payroll base shrinks.

Norway

Norway has a universal, tax-funded, single-payer, national health system. All Norwegian citizens, as well as anyone living or working in Norway, are covered under the National Insurance Scheme. Norwegians can, however, opt out of the government system by paying out of pocket. In addition, many Norwegians go abroad for treatment to avoid the waiting lists endemic under the government program. The system is financed through general tax revenues, with no earmarked or dedicated tax for health care. Thus, health care becomes one large contributor to a tax burden that consumes 45 percent of GDP. Among industrialized countries, only Sweden has a higher tax burden. Benefits are extensive and include inpatient and outpatient care, diagnostic services, specialist care, maternity services, preventive medicine, palliative care, and prescription drugs. At public hospitals, there are no charges for stays or treatment, including drugs. However, small copayments may be charged for outpatient treatment and for treatment by a general practitioner, psychologist, or psychiatrist. The program also provides "sick pay" and disability benefits. As Michael Moore has noted; the Norwegian system will even pay for "spa treatments" in some cases. Although the central government retains overall responsibility for and authority over the system, some management and funding responsibilities have devolved to regional and municipal governments. In general, municipal governments are responsible for primary health care, while four regional health authorities are responsible for specialist care. Prior to 2002, public hospitals were run by local or county governments. In the face of chronic problems, notably long waiting lists and rising costs, the central government took direct control of all public hospitals in January 2002. A small number of private hospitals do exist outside the public system. The government sets a global budget limiting overall health expenditures, and setting capital investment expenditures for hospitals. Most general practitioners and physician specialists outside hospitals receive a fixed salary, although some specialists working on a contract basis receive both an annual grant and fee-for-service payments. Reimbursement rates are set by the government and balance-billing is prohibited. Most other health care personnel are salaried government employees.

GP is the gate-keeper

Patient choice of physician is constrained. All Norwegian citizens must choose a general practitioner from a government list. The GP acts as a gatekeeper for other services and providers. Patients may switch GPs, but no more than twice per year and only if there is no waiting list for the requested GP. Specialists may only be seen with a referral from the GP. The Norwegian health care system has experienced serious problems with long and growing waiting lists. Approximately 280,000 Norwegians are estimated to be waiting for care on any given day (out of a population of just 4.6 million). The average wait for hip replacement surgery is more than four months; for a prostectomy, close to three months; and for a hysterectomy, more than two months. Approximately 23 percent of all patients referred for hospital admission have to wait longer than three months for admission. The Norwegian government has responded by repeatedly and unsuccessfully attempting to legislate waiting lists out of existence. For example, under the 1990 Patients' Rights Act, patients with a condition that would lead to "catastrophic or very serious consequences" have a right to treatment within six months, if the treatment is available. In 2001, after several government reports had documented repeated violations of this policy, the government passed a new mandate requiring that a patient's medical condition be at least "assessed" within 30 days. Despite these paper guarantees, waiting lists have not been substantially reduced. Moreover, such delays may represent only the tip of the iceberg when it comes to rationing care in Norway. In some cases, care may be denied altogether if it is judged not to be cost-effective. As Knut Erik Tranoy, Professor Emeritus at the Centre for Medical Ethics of the University of Oslo and an original member of the government's Health Care Priorities Commission, explains: It is important to see (a) that, in a public health service of the Nordic type, any given amount of resources always has alternative uses, and (b) it is neither medically nor morally defensible to put scarce resources to uses which will foreseeable yield less favourable outcomes than other uses-save fewer lives, cure fewer patients.

Tranoy differentiates between Norwegian-style systems of national health care and "a health care system where patients buy services in a market, and where justice means equality of opportunity to buy what you need. Decisions about alternative use are then (largely) patients' decisions." While Norwegians generally report that they are "fairly satisfied" with the way their health care system is run, there has been growing discontent over such issues as the ability to choose a health care provider, involvement in decisions regarding care or treatment, and waiting times—which has been an ongoing issue in Norwegian politics. However, at this time there doesn't appear to be any widespread movement for larger reform.

Portugal

The Portuguese health care system is a classic, universal, centrally run National Health System, a single-payer system funded through taxes with comprehensive benefits provided free or with little cost at the point of service. Also, a number of occupation-related health insurance schemes-originally intended to be integrated into the NHS-now coexist with it. The primary source of care is the NHS, which is funded primarily through general tax revenues, accounting for approximately 13 per cent of all government expenditures. In theory, the NHS operates within an annual global budget for health care spending. In reality, it regularly exceeds this budget by a wide margin, necessitating supplemental funding. Portugal is one of the few OECD countries where public health care spending has been rising as a proportion of total health spending, up more than four percentage points since 1997. Theoretically, benefits under the NHS include all necessary inpatient and outpatient health care services including specialists, diagnostic tests, mother and child care, and prescription drugs. On paper, no health-related expense is specifically excluded from coverage by the NHS, though in reality services such as dental care and rehabilitation therapy are seldom provided. Copayments are required for diagnostic tests, hospital admissions, consultations with specialists, and prescription drugs, where copayments can run to 40 per cent or higher. Primary care physicians and hospital-based physicians are public employees, paid directly by the NHS. However, NHS doctors are permitted to practice privately as well, and roughly half do so. Specialists are often in private practice and are reimbursed by the NHS on a contractual basis. About 25 percent of the population, mostly government workers, military, telecommunication workers, and their families, remain under a series of industry or occupation-based insurance schemes, known collectively as "sub-systems," which are a legacy of the country's pre-NHS health care system. These plans were originally intended to be incorporated into the NHS, but their powerful constituencies have prevented that from occurring. Participants in the subsystems pay a premium equal to approximately 1 percent of their salary. Benefits are generally superior to those offered through the NHS. Not surprisingly, premiums fall far short of what is needed to finance benefits. The resulting shortfall is shifted to the NHS. In addition, approximately 10 percent of the population has private insurance, usually through their employer. Private insurance generally pays for hospital and specialty care but not for primary care physicians. Policies are medically underwritten and have no requirement for renewability, meaning insurers can raise premiums or drop customers with extremely high claims. Choice of provider is heavily constrained under the NHS. Every citizen must choose a primary care physician from a list of those available within a specified geographic area. This area is usually based on the person's area of residence but may be based on the area of employment. The average general practitioner serves as many as 1,500 people, though some may have more than 2,000 patients, leading to long waits and difficulties in getting appointments. People may change GPs only by applying in writing to the NHS and explaining their reasons. Access to specialists or hospital care, except in emergencies, requires referral from the patient's GP. Since this is often difficult to secure in a timely manner, patients often seek care through hospital emergency rooms. By some estimates, at least 25 percent of emergency room patients do not need immediate treatment.

Waiting list are long

Despite guarantees of "universal coverage," access to care remains a serious problem. Waiting lists are so long and so prevalent that the European Observatory on Health Systems says that they veer toward "de facto rationing." Currently, more than 150,000 Portuguese are on waiting lists for surgery, out of a population of just 10.6 million. However, that may understate the problem in poorer and rural areas, which have fewer health resources and less access to care. Modern health technology is far less available than in the United States. The United States has almost seven times more MRI units per million people, and 20 percent more CT scanners. To avoid waiting lists, Portuguese patients frequently pay out of pocket to see physicians in private practice. In some cases, Portuguese patients have crossed the border to receive treatment in Spain. While there appears to be a consensus in Portugal that the system needs some kind of reform, weak governments and strong structural interest groups have combined to prevent the development of any consensus over the direction reform should take. For the moment, Portugal drifts.

Greece

Although ostensibly an employer-based system, the Greek system operates more like a single-payer system in that it is highly centralized and regulated. Virtually every aspect of health care financing and provision is strictly controlled by the Ministry of Social Health and Cohesion. Some attempts have been made to decentralize decision making, with 17 regional organizations having some responsibility for implementing policy and managing the delivery of health care, but most power remains with the central government. Greek employers must enrol their workers in one of 35 "social insurance funds," funded in part through a payroll tax and in part through general tax revenues. Unlike Germany, where employers have a choice among competing sickness funds, Greek social insurance funds are specific to industry sectors. The range of benefits offered by each fund, the contribution rates, and the types of providers that the insured can access are all determined by the Ministry of Social Health and Cohesion. Certain funds known as "noble funds," primarily used by government workers, the banking sector, and public utility workers, offer more extensive benefits and require smaller worker contributions. The powerful unions representing workers from these sectors have consistently blocked attempts to merge these funds with other social insurance funds or to allow buy-ins from other industry sectors. Social insurance funds reimburse doctors in two ways. Some providers are employed directly by the funds at fund-operated clinics and are effectively salaried employees. Others practice privately but contract with funds to provide care. Contract physicians are reimbursed on a fee-for-service basis, but reimbursement rates are extremely low. Balance-billing is prohibited. In theory, funds provide first-dollar coverage, with no deductibles and low copayments for only a few services.

Most physicians demand "informal" payments

In addition to the social insurance funds, the National Health Service employs physicians and operates hospitals. The NHS operates parallel to the social insurance funds, acting essentially as a back-up mechanism, although it may be the principal provider of health services in some rural areas. It also provides health care for the uninsured and the elderly. In addition to NHS hospitals, other public hospitals contract with the social insurance funds. In both cases, the Ministry of Social Health and Cohesion determines not only the hospital's budget, but the number of personnel, the specialties of the personnel, salary levels, number of beds, and the purchase of technology. Budgets are rigidly monitored and hospital administrators have little leeway. Hospitals are reimbursed on a per diem payment system, a type of a fixed charge. NHS hospitals in particular are considered substandard. Most suffer from severe staffing shortages caused by low pay and poor living conditions in rural areas. It has been estimated that less than half of authorized medical positions are actually filled. Low salaries have also led to personnel shortages in public hospitals associated with social insurance funds. A series of reforms implemented in 2005 imposed a referral requirement for hospital admissions. Patients seeking free treatment in a public NHS hospital must have a referral from a general practitioner, who acts as a gatekeeper. Private practice physicians may not make referrals to public or NHS hospitals. Unfortunately, general practitioners are in severely short supply. Greece needs an estimated 5,000 general practitioners to meet demand. In actuality it has only around 600. Despite overlapping health plans, the Greek system falls short of universal coverage. About 83 percent of the population is covered for primary care (on par with the United States), and about 97 percent for hospital care. In theory, the uninsured can always receive treatment by walking into an NHS clinic or hospital. Only about 8 percent of Greeks have private supplemental health insurance, although this percentage has risen substantially in the past few years and further growth is predicted.

Accurate information on waiting lists is difficult to come by. According to the WHO, "although 'patient registries' at the hospital level do exist, there is no systematic data processing available at any level of care," to provide adequate analysis. However, most observers agree that waiting lists are a severe problem at almost every level of care, and particularly bad at both NHS and public hospitals. An examination of waiting lists at Athens hospitals by the Ta Nea newspaper found the wait for surgery was as long as six months; for an outpatient appointment with either the hypertension or neurology departments, 150 days. Even simple blood tests required a month-long wait. The Greek system has developed a level of endemic corruption as patients have sought ways around the system's rationing, bureaucracy, and inefficiencies. For example, Greeks routinely provide physicians with "informal" payments for seeing a patient from a sickness fund that has not contracted with the doctor, for moving a patient up in the queue, or for providing treatment outside government guidelines. In addition, physicians actively attempt to persuade patients to move from a doctor's sickness fund contract to the doctor's private practice. Patients who switch pay out of pocket but receive faster and better care. Even NHS physicians see private patients on the side. (This practice was illegal until 2002 but went on despite the prohibition). Physicians also receive payments for referrals to private hospitals or diagnostic centers.

Such informal out-of-pocket payments made up 42 percent of total health expenditures in 2002, fully 4.5 per cent of GDP. Essentially, the Greek health care system is funded through payroll taxes, general tax revenue, and bribery. In addition, the health care bureaucracy has become highly politicized. Every staff appointment in the public health sector must be approved at the ministry level. All hospital administrators and other health officials are appointed on the basis of political affiliation with the governing party, often with little regard for relevant training or other qualifications. Not surprisingly, Greece has far less modern health care technology than the United States. The United States has more than twice as many MRI units per million people and 20 percent more CT scanners. Much of the state-of-the-art equipment that does exist is clustered in the country's small number of private clinics and hospitals. Indeed, the vast majority of high technology biomedical tests are performed by the private sector.

Problems with the Greek health care system

The Greek health system does not yet offer universal coverage and has fragmented funding and delivery. Funding is regressive, with a reliance on informal payments, and there are inequities in access, supply and quality of services. Inefficiencies arise from an over reliance on relatively expensive inputs, as evidenced by the oversupply of specialists and undersupply of nurses. Resource allocation mechanisms are historical and political with no relation to performance or output; therefore providers have little incentive to improve productivity.

Netherlands

Aside from Switzerland, the Netherlands has perhaps the most market-oriented national health care system in Europe. That was the case even before 2006, when a series of reforms introduced even more market mechanisms. The old pre-2006 Dutch system resembled Germany's. Dutch workers with incomes below €€32,600 were required to enrol in one of 30 government-controlled "sickness funds." Those with higher incomes had the option of enrolling in the funds if they wished, or opting out of the government system and purchasing private insurance. Sickness funds were financed through a payroll tax and a flat-rate, per-capita premium. The funds provided a uniform package of benefits including physician and hospital care, specialist care, diagnostic tests, prescription drugs, and dental care for children. While consumers could switch funds annually, there was little competition between funds and few consumers actually switched. The new Dutch system operates on the theory of managed competition like Switzerland. Both the social health insurance program and the alternative private health insurance option were replaced by a requirement that all Dutch citizens purchase a basic health insurance plan from one of 41 private insurance companies. Although a fine may be imposed for failure to comply, there is no comprehensive system for identifying citizens who do not meet the mandate. An estimated 1.5 to 2 percent of the population is currently uninsured. The required plan, which covers minimum benefits set by the government, includes general practitioner and specialist care, hospital stays, some dental care, prenatal care, some medicines, and travel expenses. In one interesting innovation, most of the required benefits are specified in terms of "functions of care" rather than by provider category. Thus, "rehabilitation care" is required, but no particular type of rehabilitation provider is mandated. This may mean that the benefits package will be less susceptible to manipulation by provider interest groups, but it is much too early to tell.

The Health Ministry sets premiums, which average around €€100 per month for an individual. Insurance companies can offer varying deductibles, ranging from €€150 to €€1,000 per year, allowing for a small level of price competition. Policies can also offer rebates of up to €€225 if a policy-holder uses no health services in a given year beyond seeing a primary care physician. About 90 percent of the population also buys supplemental insurance covering services over and above the required standard benefits package. Employers generally pay half of insurance premiums, with individual workers picking up the other half. Individual premiums are tax deductible. Subsidies, or care allowances, that help low- and middle-income workers purchase the basic insurance plan are extensive and reach well into the middle class. Currently, 5 million Dutch citizens qualify for some level of subsidy on a sliding scale based on income. Those subsidies are financed through a tax on salaried workers. Because of the high levels of subsidy, the Dutch government remains a large source of health spending, one area of significant difference with the Swiss system. Insurers negotiate quality, quantity, and price of services with providers. Notably, many insurers require providers to document the quality of the care they provide, frequently relying on evidence-based guidelines and performance metrics. Some insurers provide care directly, using their own staffs and their own facilities, such as primary care centers and pharmacies. Other insurers contract with a network of providers similar to U.S. preferred provider organizations (PPOs). Patients can go out of network but will receive only partial reimbursement. Most insurers require a referral from a primary care provider before a patient can see a specialist. Pharmaceutical prices are capped nationwide at the average price of medicines in a therapeutic class. Individuals may choose more expensive drugs but must pay the difference out of pocket. The new system has been in place for only two years, which is not enough time to permit a thorough evaluation. However, preliminary indications suggest that it is an improvement over the pre-2006 system.

Transparency is now visible

Dutch consumers appear to have embraced the reforms. Consumer organizations are participating in negotiations with providers, insurers, and law-makers. The system is becoming more transparent, with far greater information available regarding both price and quality. Consumers seem willing to make decisions and change insurers on the basis of price and quality. Price competition under the new system has increased significantly and at least 20 percent of Dutch consumers have switched insurers. When the system was initiated, the Dutch government predicted premiums would cost €€1,106 on average. However, competition has forced the average premium down to €€1,028, 097.6 percent below the prediction. Overall, the new system is estimated to have increased the purchasing power of Dutch households by as much as 1.5 percent. However, not everyone has been a winner. The community rating requirement has resulted in steep increases in premiums for younger workers who were more heavily subsidized under the old system.

Under the old system, waiting lists were widespread—for example, more than three months for a hip replacement and two months for a prostectomy or hysterectomy. One study estimated that at least 100 heart patients died each year while on waiting lists. Early evidence suggests that some improvement has come as a result of the 2006 reforms. Hospitals are beginning to compete by expanding services such as neurosurgery and radiation therapy. Although some experts have expressed concern that smaller hospitals offering these services may not have sufficient utilization rates to ensure quality and efficacy, the expanded availability of services will likely increase access to care and reduce queues. The new system may even be having a positive impact on health care costs. Since the new system took effect, health care costs have been growing at an annual rate of just 3 per cent, compared to more than 4.5 percent in the year before the reforms.

Great Britain

The NHS is a highly centralized version of a single-payer system. The government pays directly for health care and finances the system through general tax revenues. Except for small co-payments for prescription drugs, dental care, and optician services, there are no direct charges to patients. Unlike many other single-payer systems such as those in Canada and Norway, most physicians and nurses are government employees. For years, British health policy has focused on controlling spending and in general has been quite successful, with the system spending just 7.5 percent of GDP on health care. Yet the system continues to face serious financial strains. In fiscal year 2006, the NHS faced a deficit of £700 million, according to government figures, and as much as £1 billion, according to outside observers. This comes despite a £43 billion increase in the NHS annual budget over the past five years. By some estimates, NHS spending will have to nearly triple by 2025 just to maintain the current level of services. And that level of services leaves much to be desired. Waiting lists are a major problem. As many as 750,000 Britons are currently awaiting admission to NHS hospitals. These waits are not insubstantial and can impose significant risks on patients. For example, by some estimates, cancer patients can wait as long as eight months for treatment. Delays in receiving treatment are often so long that nearly 20 percent of colon cancer patients considered treatable when first diagnosed are incurable by the time treatment is finally offered. In some cases, to prevent hospitals from using their resources too quickly, mandatory minimum waiting times have been imposed. The fear is that patients will flock to the most efficient hospitals or those with smaller backlogs. Thus a top-flight hospital like Suffolk East was ordered to impose a minimum waiting time of at least 122 days before patients could be treated or the hospital would lose a portion of its funding. As the Daily Telegraph explained: In a real competitive market, increased demand can allow prices to rise, thus increasing profits, which allow the market to grow. Efficient producers can then reduce their unit costs and their prices, and so give a better deal to the consumer. The prevailing logic is that the more customers who are served—or products that are sold—in a given period of time, the better the business does.

The problem affects not only hospitals. There are also lengthy waits to see physicians, particularly specialists. In 2004, as a cost-cutting measure, the government negotiated low salaries for general practitioners in exchange for allowing them to cut back the hours they practice. Few are now available nights or weekends. Problems with specialists are even more acute. For example, roughly 40 percent of cancer patients never get to see an oncology specialist. The government's official target for diagnostic testing is a wait of no more than 18 weeks by 2008. In reality, it doesn't come close. The latest estimates suggest that for most specialties, only 30 to 50 percent of patients are treated within 18 weeks. For trauma and orthopedics patients, the figure is only 20 percent. Overall, more than half of British patients wait more than 18 weeks for care. Explicit rationing also exists for some types of care, notably kidney dialysis, open heart surgery, and some other expensive procedures and technologies. Patients judged too ill or aged for the procedures to be cost-effective may be denied treatment altogether.

Recently, the British government introduced some tiny steps toward market-based reforms. Under the experimental London Patient Choice Project, patients who have been waiting longer than six months for treatment are offered a choice of up to four alternate providers. This experiment has been extended nationwide for coronary heart patients who have been waiting longer than six months. Some proposed solutions are far more radical. David Cameron, leader of the Conservative Party, has proposed that the NHS be allowed to refuse treatment to individuals who don't practice healthy lifestyles, for example, who smoke or are overweight. Then again, he has also proposed that the government pay for gym memberships and subsidize the purchase of fresh fruit and vegetables. A small but growing private health care system has emerged in the UK. About 10 percent of Britons have private health insurance. Some receive it through their employer, while others purchase it individually. In general, the insurance replicates care provided through the NHS and is purchased to gain access to a wider choice of providers or to avoid waiting lists. Private health insurance is lightly regulated and risk-rating is allowed. The British government treats health insurance more or less the same as other types of insurance. Fully 60 percent of Britons believe that making it easier for patients to spend their own money on health care would improve quality. Yet Britons are also extremely proud of their health care system and wary of any reforms that would "Americanize" it.

Switzerland

Switzerland has one of the most market-oriented systems. Indeed, the Swiss government actually pays for a smaller amount of total health care expenditures than the U.S. government, 24.9 percent versus 44.7 percent. The Swiss system is based on the idea of managed competition, the same concept that underlay the 1993 Clinton health care plan and Mitt Romney's reforms in Massachusetts. Managed competition leaves the provision of health care and health insurance in private hands but creates a highly regulated artificial marketplace as a framework within which the health care industry operates. Swiss law requires all citizens to purchase a basic package of health insurance, an individual mandate. Coverage is close to universal, estimated at 99.5 percent. This level of compliance is due in part to the Swiss national character and may not be replicable in the United States where the record of complying with mandates is much more mixed (even if such a mandate were desirable). For example, nearly 100 percent of Swiss drivers comply with their country's mandate for automobile insurance, compared with only 83 percent of U.S. drivers. The term "basic benefits package" is somewhat misleading since the required benefits are quite extensive, including inpatient and outpatient care, care for the elderly and the physically and mentally handicapped, long-term nursing home care, diagnostic tests, prescription drugs, and even complementary and alternative therapies.

Insurance is generally purchased on an individual basis. Few employers contribute to the purchase or provide insurance. The policies are provided by private insurers. Currently, some 93 insurers operate in Switzerland, although not every insurer operates in every canton, or region. Originally, insurers were required to be nonprofit entities, but that restriction was eliminated in 2002. Insurers cannot reject an applicant on the basis of health status, and all policies are community rated within a geographic area, meaning that the healthier pay higher premiums to subsidize the less healthy. One exception to community rating is for non-smokers, who can receive premiums as much as 20 percent lower than smokers. A formula adjusts premiums based on sex and age.259 The geographic variation can be significant, with premiums differing as much as 50 percent between cantons. Unable to compete on the basis of managing and pricing risk, and required to offer nearly identical basic benefits packages, insurers compete primarily on price. Since they cannot reduce costs by risk management or benefit design, they generally manage prices by varying the level of deductibles and copayments. Individuals can purchase expensive policies with very low deductibles and copayments, or far less expensive policies with high deductibles or extensive copayments. Thus, premiums vary according to their cost-sharing attributes and plan type, running from $1,428 per year for a plan with a deductible of approximately $2,000 to $2,388 for a plan with a $250 deductible.

Swiss pay for their health insurance cover

Because employers do not pay for workers' health insurance, the Swiss are exposed to the full cost of their insurance purchases. As a result, many Swiss have opted for high-deductible insurance. Thus, with high deductibles and extensive copayments, the Swiss pay out of pocket for 31.5 percent of health care, twice as much as in the United States. Recently, there has also been a growing market in managed care plans that, like those in the United States, offer lower premiums in exchange for limitations on access to specialists and other services. Premiums for such plans run around $1,900 per year. The Swiss government offers subsidies to low-income citizens to help them purchase a policy. Subsidies are based on both income and assets, and the maximum available subsidy covers the cost of an average premium in the individual's canton. These subsidies are designed to prevent any individual from having to pay more than 10 percent of income on insurance. They do not, however, pay the entire cost of insurance because the Swiss do not want to create an incentive for subsidized individuals to choose the most expensive plan with the lowest deductibles and copayments. Roughly one-third of Swiss citizens receive some form of subsidy, and approximately 19 percent of all health insurance premiums are paid with government funds. Swiss insurers operate as cartels to negotiate provider reimbursements on a cantonal basis. Providers must accept the negotiated payment, and balance-billing is prohibited. If insurers and providers are unable to reach agreement on a fee schedule, canton governments are empowered to step in and impose an agreement. There are no restrictions on where physicians may set-up practice, so to some degree providers can vote with their feet, moving to cantons that offer higher reimbursements, a practice that has led to physician shortages in some areas. The system includes both public and private hospitals. Private hospitals negotiate reimbursement with insurance cartels and physicians in the same manner. Public hospitals are operated by cantons, which negotiate reimbursement rates with insurers and provide subsidies to the hospitals. In some cantons, individuals with only the basic insurance plan must use public hospitals; supplementary insurance is required for admission to private hospitals. Recently, some providers have begun operating outside the negotiated fee schedules. A separate supplemental insurance market is starting to develop to cover the cost of these providers, which are presumed to offer higher quality or more advanced services. Supplementary insurance also allows access to private hospitals in those cantons that do not permit access under the basic insurance plan.

Supplemental insurance

Even within public hospitals, supplementary insurance can be used to pay for services such as private rooms that are not covered under the basic plan. By some estimates as many as 40 percent of Swiss citizens have purchased supplemental insurance. The Swiss do not impose a global budget on their health care system and have therefore avoided the waiting lists common in other systems. In addition, the Swiss have a high degree of access to modern medical technology, but it has come at a cost. The Swiss spend 11.5 percent of GDP on health care, second only to the United States.

Since Swiss health care consumers are exposed to the cost consequences of their health care decisions, this trade-off between access and cost can be presumed to reflect the desires of Swiss patients. They have chosen high quality care even though it costs them more. Given that economists consider health care to be a "normal good"—that is, consumption rises along with income—and Switzerland is a wealthy nation, such a decision seems entirely reasonable. At the same time, it is notable that Swiss health care spending remains below that of the United States for nearly comparable care. Strong evidence suggests that the exposure of Swiss consumers to the cost consequences of their health care decisions has made them more conscious consumers and helped limit overall health care costs. As Regina Herzlinger and Ramin Parsa-Parsi of Harvard have concluded, "Cost control may be attributed to the Swiss consumer's significant role in health care payments and the resulting cost transparency." The transparency of the system also makes it responsive to consumer preferences. The WHO survey ranked Switzerland second only to the United States in terms of responsiveness to patients' needs for choice of provider, dignity, autonomy, timely care, and confidentiality. The Swiss generally seem pleased with their system. Earlier this year, Swiss voters over-whelmingly rejected a proposal to replace the current system with a single-payer plan; more than 71 percent of Swiss voters turned down the proposal in a nationwide referendum. Nonetheless, the Swiss system has its own problems, most of them predictable outgrowths of the individual mandate and the regulation inherent in managed competition. In most markets, consumers impose a certain discipline on prices because they can refuse to buy a product if it costs too much. The individual mandate removes this power since consumers must purchase the product (in this case, insurance) even if they believe the cost outweighs the value. Moreover, the establishment of a government- defined benefits package is an open-ended invitation to special interests representing various health care providers and disease constituencies, who can certainly be expected to lobby for the inclusion of additional services or coverage.

Basic benefits package

Public choice dynamics are such that providers (who would make money from the increased demand for their services) and disease constituencies (whose members naturally have an urgent desire for coverage of their illness or condition) will always have a strong incentive to lobby legislators for inclusion under any minimum benefits package. The public at large will likely be unaware of the debate or see resisting the small premium increase caused by any particular additional benefit as unworthy of a similar effort-a simple case of concentrated benefits and diffused costs. That is exactly what has happened in Switzerland, leading to a growing expansion of the basic benefits package. In particular, a powerful hospital and physician lobbying coalition known as the "Blue Front" was able to demand a significant expansion in covered benefits in exchange for a relaxation of "any willing provider" laws so as to permit managed-care contracts. The expansion of benefits has driven up the cost of insurance, a cost only partially off-set by larger deductibles. Although the proportion of health expenditures paid out of pocket remains high, it has decreased by roughly 10 percent in the past decade.

Moreover, the growth in covered benefits has helped drive up costs for the system as a whole, as the Swiss become more insulated from the costs of their health care purchasing decisions. If that trend continues, it could undermine the cost transparency that is at the heart of the Swiss system." "Over time, the growth in compulsory benefits has absorbed an increasing fraction of the consumers' payment, thus compromising the consumer-driven aspects of the Swiss system." Evidence shows that the community rating requirements are creating distortions within the Swiss market, leading to the over provision of care to the healthy and the under provision of care to the sick. In addition, the prohibition on risk management discourages the development of new and innovative products. Peter Zweifel of the University of Zurich, a member of the Swiss Competitive Committee which oversees insurance regulation, believes that a return to some degree of risk-rating is essential to the long-term success of the Swiss system. As Zweifel puts it, "Let competition work its magic. Let those who are bad risks get the message that they need to become better risks, if possible. If not possible, still get a subsidy which keeps their costs down to little more than 8-10 percent of taxable income."

Physicians can desert low paying zones

Third, the cartel structure for negotiating reimbursement schedules can create a number of distortions. Effectively monopsony purchasers, the cartels have enormous leverage when it comes to negotiations. Not surprisingly, physicians have tended to set-up practice in cantons with the highest levels of reimbursement, leading to shortages in other areas. Reimbursement rates have reportedly created wasteful incentives—for example, hospitals shifting patients from outpatient to inpatient care. And the combination of increased demand and low reimbursement has led to the first signs of queues for the most complex surgeries. In addition, the negotiations freeze in place a pricing structure that inhibits the development of innovative approaches that do not tie payments to specific benefits. This includes both managed care approaches and health services integration. Finally, Switzerland has some of Europe's strongest regulation of non-physician health care professionals. As a result, patients are often forced to use more expensive providers where a less expensive professional would do. All of the above combine to undermine the consumer-driven nature of Switzerland's health system. Despite these problems, the Swiss system provides a useful lesson for the United States about the value of consumer-directed health care. In particular, we can see that when the cost of insurance becomes more transparent, consumers shift their purchasing preferences toward true insurance (spreading catastrophic risk), rather than purchasing pre-payment for routine, low-cost services. That gives consumers an overall incentive to makecost *versus* value decisions when purchasing health care, resulting in reduced costs while maintaining individual choice and quality care.

Germany

Germany has been ranked 25th in the WHO ratings. Despite that low ranking, however, the country is worth examining because it is frequently cited as a model by advocates of national health care. National health insurance in Germany is part of a social insurance system that dates back to Bismarck. All German citizens with incomes under €€46,300 (roughly $60,000) are required to enroll in one of approximately 250 statutory "sickness funds." Those with higher incomes may enrol in the funds if they wish, or may opt out of the government system and purchase private insurance. About three-quarters of workers with incomes above the statutory limit choose to remain in the sickness funds, which currently cover approximately 90 percent of the population. Overall, insurance coverage is nearly universal. However, the number of uninsured has been rising, roughly tripling in the last 10 years to 300,000 people. About 9 percent of the population purchases supplemental insurance to cover items that are not included in the standard benefits package. Sickness funds are financed through a pay-roll tax split equally between the employer and employee. The size of the tax varies depending on which fund the worker has chosen, but averages around 15 percent of wages. Sickness funds are supposed to be solvent and self-supporting, but in reality the system ran a €€7 billion deficit in 2006. The German government has proposed a 1 percent increase in the payroll tax, split evenly between employer and employee, starting next year. In addition, general tax revenues finance capital costs for acute care hospitals and many rehabilitative services, especially for retirees.

Sickness fund provide insurance

Benefits are extensive, covering physicians, hospital and chronic care, diagnostic tests, preventive care, prescription drugs, and part of dental care. In addition to the medical benefits, sickness funds provide sick pay to those who cannot work due to illness, ranging from 70 to 90 percent of the patient's last gross salary, for up to 78 weeks. The central government and state governments split the regulation of the health care system. The central government establishes the national global budget for health care spending, defines any new medical procedures to be included in benefit packages, and sets reimbursement rates for physicians. Some of this is accomplished through legislation, while the rest is handled through negotiations between the National Association of Sickness Funds and the National Association of Physicians. At the state level, state associations of sickness funds and physicians negotiate overall health budgets, reimbursement contracts for physicians, procedures for monitoring physicians, and reference standards for prescription drugs. The bargaining power in these negotiations clearly lies with the sickness funds backed by the government, allowing them to effectively impose fee schedules and other restrictions on providers. The purchasing power of a German physician's wages is now about 20 percent that of a U.S. physician.

Although Germany spends less on health care than the United States, both as a percentage of GDP and per capita, expenditures have been rising at an alarming rate in recent years. Friedrich Breyer, an economist from Konstanz University, estimates that health care spending could reach 30 percent of GDP by 2020 unless significant changes are made. Germans now pay €€10 per quarter to see a general practitioner, €€10 per day of hospital stay, €€10 per prescription, and for certain specialty services. The highest copayments are 10 percent for prescription drugs. Overall, Germans pay out of pocket for about 13 percent of total health care spending, only slightly less than Americans. Preliminary evidence suggests that the introduction of cost sharing has slightly reduced utilization and spending. In 2006, Chancellor Angela Merkel proposed a sweeping set of health care reforms that included creating a centralized health fund, shifting financing in part from payroll taxes to general revenues, trimming benefits, imposing greater cost sharing, and making the system more transparent. She was forced to abandon the package in the face of public and political opposition. The degree of health care rationing in Germany is the subject of considerable debate. Unlike many OECD countries, the German government does not compile data on waiting lists. One frequently cited study suggests that Germans are no more likely than Americans to wait more than four weeks to see a specialist. The WHO says, "Waiting lists and explicit rationing decisions are virtually unknown." However, at least one study concludes that rationing is occurring for the elderly and those with terminal illness, and concludes that "the question remains as to whether lives at advanced ages could be saved if age rationing were discontinued and maximum medical treatment were to be applied to everyone, irrespective of their age." In addition, a survey of German hospitals reported that "waiting times were prolonged" due to both a lack of capacity and hospital target budgets that make the treatment of sickness fund patients with serious conditions financially unattractive. Also, Germans have less access to modern medical technology than Americans. The United States has four times as many MRI units per million people and twice as many CT scanners.

Some analysts blame price restrictions and reimbursement rates for increasing bureaucratic interference in how German physicians practice medicine. Physicians trying to work within the maze of reimbursement caps and budget restrictions have no financial incentive to provide more than the minimally necessary care. That has led to questions of quality assurance, and the government has responded with ever greater micromanagement of practice standards. The result has been a huge increase in red tape for physicians and a general loss of innovation. Germans seem aware of the need to reform their health care system. In a 2004 poll, 76 percent of Germans thought health care reform was "urgent," while an additional 14 percent thought it was "desirable."

Equal access preferred over best care

However, Germans are split nearly down the middle about what that reform should be. Roughly 47 percent would like to see an increase in private health care spending, whereas 49 percent would not. Similarly, 45 percent of Germans believe that more patient choice would improve health care quality, whereas 50 percent do not. The reluctance to fully embrace market reforms undoubtedly stems from a long-standing German belief in social solidarity. By a margin of 81 to 18 percent, Germans believe that equal access to the same quality of care for everyone is more important than their own access to the best possible care.

Canada

Canada is another country that did not make the top 20 health care systems in the WHO rankings (it finished 30th), and yet few serious advocates of universal health care look to it as a model. Although Canada is frequently referred to as having a "national health system," the system is actually decentralized with considerable responsibility devolved to Canada's 10 provinces and 2 territories. It is financed jointly by the provinces and the federal government, similar to the U.S. Medicaid program. In order to qualify for federal funds, each provincial program must meet five criteria: (1) universality-available to all provincial residents on uniform terms and conditions; (2) comprehensiveness-covering all medically necessary hospital and physician services; (3) portability-allowing residents to remain covered when moving from province to province; (4) accessibility-having no financial barriers to access such as deductibles or copayments; and (5) public administration—administered by a non-profit authority accountable to the provincial government. Federal financing comes from general tax revenue. The federal government provides a block grant to each province which amounts to around 16 percent of health care spending. However, most funding comes from provincial taxes, primarily personal and corporate income taxes. Some provinces also use funds from other financial sources like sales taxes and lottery proceeds. And some (British Columbia, Alberta, and Ontario) charge premiums, although health services cannot be denied because of inability to pay. The health care system is an enormous part of the Canadian welfare state. On the provincial level, the health care system amounts to between one-third and one-half of all social welfare spending. Provinces must provide certain benefits, including primary care doctors, specialists, hospitals, and dental surgery. Other benefits, such as routine dental care, physiotherapy, and prescription drugs, are optional. Some provinces offer substantial coverage for these services, some cover them only partially, and some do not cover them at all. Except for emergencies, treatment by specialists or hospital admission requires a referral from a primary care physician.

Provider reimbursement is set by each province, and some provinces restrict overall physician income. In general, however, reimbursement is on a fee-for-service basis. Hospitals are paid a specific pre-set amount to cover all non-capital costs. Capital expenditures must be approved on a case-by-case basis. An increasing number of Canadians also carry private insurance, most often provided through their employer. Originally this insurance was designed to cover those few services not covered by the national health care system. At one time, all provinces prohibited private insurance from covering any service or procedure provided under the government program. But in 2005, the Canadian Supreme Court struck down Quebec's prohibition on private insurance contracting. Litigation to permit private contracting is now pending in several other provinces. In addition to the public hospitals covered by the government, many private clinics now operate, offering specialized services. Although private clinics are legally barred from providing services covered by the Canada Health Act, many do offer such services in a black market. The biggest advantage of private clinics is that they typically offer services with reduced wait times compared to the public health care system. Obtaining an MRI scan in a hospital could require a wait of months, whereas it could be obtained much faster in a private clinic. Waiting lists are a major problem under the Canadian system. No accurate government data exists, but provincial reports do show at least moderate waiting lists. The best information may come from a survey of Canadian physicians by the Fraser Institute, which suggests that as many as 800,000 Canadians are waiting for treatment at any given time. According to this survey, treatment time from initial referral by a GP through consultation with a specialist, to final treatment, across all specialties and all procedures (emergency, non-urgent, and elective), averaged 17.7 weeks in 2005. And that doesn't include waiting to see the GP in the first place.

NHS defended by 70% Canadians

Defenders of national health care have attempted to discount these waiting lists, suggesting that the waits are shorter than commonly portrayed or that most of those on the waiting list are seeking elective surgery. A look at specialties with especially long waits shows that the longest waits are for procedures such as hip or knee replacement and cataract surgery, which could arguably be considered elective. However, fields that could have significant impact on a patient's health, such as neurosurgery, also have significant waiting times. In such cases, the delays could be life threatening. A study in the *Canadian Medical Association Journal* found that at least 50 patients in Ontario alone have died while on the waiting list for cardiac catheterization. Data from the Joint Canada-United States Survey of Health (a project of Statistics Canada and the National Center for Health Statistics) revealed that "thirty-three percent of Canadians who say they have an unmet medical need reported being in pain that limits their daily activities." In a 2005 decision striking down part of Quebec's universal care law, Canadian Supreme Court Chief Justice Beverly McLachlin wrote that it was undisputed that many Canadians waiting for treatment suffer chronic pain and that "patients die while on the waiting list." Clearly there is limited access to modern medical technology in Canada. The United States has five times as many MRI units per million people and three times as many CT scanners. Indeed, there are more CT scanners in the city of Seattle than in the entire province of British Columbia. Physicians are also in short supply. Canada has roughly 2.1 practicing physicians per 1,000 people, far less than the OECD average. Worse, the number of physicians per 1,000 people has not grown at all since 1990. And while the number of nurses per 1,000 people remains near the OECD average, that number has been declining since 1990. In addition, although national health care systems are frequently touted as doing a better job of providing preventive care, U.S. patients are actually more likely than Canadians to receive preventive care for chronic or serious health conditions. In particular, Americans are more likely to get screened for common cancers, including cancers of the breast, cervix, prostate, and colon. Canada has been relatively effective at controlling spending. The country spends about 9 percent of GDP on health care, a percentage that has risen only slightly over the last decade. Relative to average OECD expenditures, Canadian health expenditures have declined by 4 percent since 1997. The cost control, however, has clearly come at the expense of access to care. Canadians' dissatisfaction with the problems in their system has been growing for some time. One survey showed that some 59 percent of Canadians believe that their system requires "fundamental changes," and another 18 percent believe the system needs to be scrapped and totally rebuilt. Still, Canadians are reluctant to embrace market reforms that are associated with the U.S. health care system—a system that Canadians disdainfully reject. As one observer put it: Anxiety about Americanization and the constantly reinforced strain of national pride in Canadian health care coexist[s] with considerable uneasiness about the actual state of that care. It is as if, when Canadians look south across the border they swell with pride, but when they look within they shrink back, seeing many problems and feeling uncertainty about the future. Canadians may jealously guard their system and resist "Americanizing" it.

However, a closer look shows that nearly all health care systems worldwide are wrestling with problems of rising costs and lack of access to care. There is no single international model for national health care, of course. Countries vary dramatically in the degree of central control, regulation, and cost sharing they impose, and in the role of private insurance.

Experts suggest the following:

- o Health insurance does not mean universal access to health care. In practice, many countries promise universal coverage but ration care or have long waiting lists for treatment.
- o Rising health care costs are not a uniquely American phenomenon. Although other countries spend considerably less than the United States on health care, both as a percentage of GDP and per capita, costs are rising almost everywhere, leading to budget deficits, tax increases, and benefit reductions.
- o In countries weighted heavily toward government control, people are most likely to face waiting lists, rationing, restrictions on physician choice, and other obstacles to care.
- o Countries with more effective national health care systems are successful to the degree that they incorporate market mechanisms such as competition, cost sharing, market prices, and consumer choice, and eschew centralized government control. Although no country with a national health care system is contemplating abandoning universal coverage, the broad and growing trend is to move away from centralized government control and to introduce more market-oriented features.

A comparison

Michael Moore and Krugman explore problems with the U.S. health care system and advocate the adoption of a government-run, single-payer system. Moore compares the U.S. system unfavourably with those of Canada, Great Britain, and France. These and other critics of the U.S. health care system note that countries with such systems spend far less per capita on health care than the United States does and, by some measures, seem to have better health outcomes. Krugman says, "The obvious way to make the U.S. health care system more efficient is to make it more like the systems of other advanced countries." United States now spends close to 16 percent of GDP on health care, nearly 6.1 percent more than the average for other industrialized countries. Overall health care costs are rising faster than GDP growth and now total more than $1.8 trillion, more than Americans spend on housing, food, national defense, or automobiles. Economists consider health care a "normal good," meaning that spending is positively correlated with income. As incomes rise, people want more of that good. On average, health insurance now costs $4,479 for an individual and $12,106 for a family per year. Health insurance premiums rose by a little more than 6 percent in 2007, faster on average than wages. Moreover, government health care programs, particularly Medicare and Medicaid, are piling up enormous burdens of debt for future generations. Medicare's unfunded liabilities now top $50 trillion. Unchecked, Medicaid spending will increase four-fold as a percentage of federal outlays over the next century.

Many Americans lack of health cover

At the same time, too many Americans remain uninsured. Although the number of uninsured Americans is often exaggerated by critics of the system, approximately 47 million Americans are without health insurance at any given time. Many are already eligible for government programs; many are young and healthy; many are uninsured for only a short-time. Yet there is no denying that a lack of insurance can pose a hardship for many Americans. The Institute of Medicine estimates that some 44,000-90,000 annual deaths are due to medical errors. Many critics of U.S. health care suggest that the answers to these problems lie in a single-payer, national health care system. Under such a system, health care would be financed through taxes rather than consumer payments or private insurance. Direct charges to patients would be prohibited or severely restricted. Private insurance, if allowed at all, would be limited to a few supplemental services not covered by the government plan.

Quality of Health Care across Countries

A World Health Organization study ranks the U.S. health care system 37th in the world, "slightly better than Slovenia." The United States is actually penalized for low fairness and adopting Health Savings Accounts and because, according to the WHO, patients pay too much out of pocket. Such Judgments clearly reflect a particular political point of view, rather than a neutral measure of health care quality. Notably, the WHO report ranks the United States number one in the world in responsiveness to patients' needs in choice of provider, dignity, autonomy, timely care, and confidentiality.

Life expectancies are affected by exogenous factors such as violent crime, poverty, obesity, tobacco and drug use, and other issues unrelated to health care. As the Organization for Economic Co-operation and Development explains, "It is difficult to estimate the relative contribution of the numerous nonmedical and medical factors that might affect variations in life expectancy across countries and over time." Consider the nearly three-year disparity in life expectancy between Utah (78.7 years) and Nevada (75.9 years), despite the fact that the two states have essentially the same health care systems. In fact, a study by Robert Ohsfeldt and John Schneider for the American Enterprise Institute found that those exogenous factors are so distorting that if you correct for homicides and accidents, the United States rises to the top of the list for life expectancy. Similarly, infant mortality, a common measure in cross-country comparisons, is highly problematic. In the United States, very low birth-weight infants have a much greater chance of being brought to term with the latest medical technologies. Some of those low birth-weight babies die soon after birth, which boosts our infant mortality rate, but in many other Western countries, those high-risk, low birth-weight infants are not included when infant mortality is calculated. In addition, many countries use abortion to eliminate problem pregnancies. For example, Michael Moore cites low infant mortality rates in Cuba, yet that country has one of the world's highest abortion rates, meaning that many babies with health problems that could lead to early deaths are never brought to term.

When you compare the outcomes for specific diseases, the United States clearly outperforms the rest of the world. Whether the disease is cancer, pneumonia, heart disease, or AIDS, the chances of a patient surviving are far higher in the United States than in other countries. For example, according to a study published in the *British medical journal* The *Lancet*, the United States is at the top of the charts when it comes to surviving cancer. Among men, roughly 62.9 percent of those diagnosed with cancer survive for at least five years. The news is even better for women: the five year-survival rate is 66.3 percent, or two-thirds. The countries with the next best results are Iceland for men (61.8 percent) and Sweden for women (60.3 percent). Most countries with national health care fare far worse. For example, in Italy, 59.7 percent of men and 49.8 percent of women survive five years. In Spain, just 59 percent of men and 49.5 percent of women do. And in Great Britain, a dismal 44.8 percent of men and only a slightly better 52.7 percent of women live for five years after diagnosis. One U.S. hospital alone, the Mayo Clinic, treats roughly 7,200 foreigners every year. Johns Hopkins University Medical Center treats more than 6,000, and the Cleveland Clinic more than 5,000. One out of every three Canadian physicians sends a patient to the Unites States for treatment each year, and those patients along with the Canadian government spend more than $1 billion annually on health care in this country.

Eighteen of the last 25 winners of the Nobel Prize in Medicine are either U.S. citizens or individuals working here. U.S. companies have developed half of all new major medicines introduced worldwide over the past 20 years. In fact, Americans played a key role in 80 percent of the most important medical advances of the past 30 years. There is no dispute that more health care technology is invented and produced in the United States than anywhere else. Even when the original research is done in other countries, the work necessary to convert the idea into viable commercial products is most often done in the United States. Its costs are rising and are distributed in a way that makes it difficult for some people to afford the care they want or need. And while the U.S. provides the world's highest quality health care, that quality is uneven, and too often Americans don't receive the standard of care that they should. But the experiences of other countries with national health care systems show that the answer to these problems lies with more pro-market reform, not more government control. Of course, there is no single model for national health care systems in other countries. Those systems range from the managed competition approach of the Netherlands and Switzerland to the more rigid single-payer systems of

Great Britain, Canada and Norway, with many variations in between. Some require consumers to share a significant portion of health care costs through either high deductibles or high copayments. Others subsidize virtually first-dollar coverage. Some allow unfettered choice of physicians. Others allow a choice of primary care physicians but require referrals for specialists. Still others restrict even the choice of primary care doctors.

No premium, unlimited health cover?

In fact, about the only system one cannot find is the type of system described by Michael Moore, Physicians for a National Health Program, and other national health care advocates—a system that provides unlimited care with no premiums, deductibles, or copayments, from the physician of one's choice. Likewise, advocates for national health care tap into the anger many patients (and doctors) feel for the gatekeepers and prior approval required under American managed care. But many if not most foreign systems require similar gatekeepers. Moreover, copayments and other forms of cost sharing are commonplace. Americans are unlikely to accept the rationing or restrictions on care and technology that many countries use to control costs. Nor are U.S. physicians likely to accept a cut in income to the levels seen in countries like France or Germany. American attitudes are quite different. Even so, some important lessons can be drawn from the experiences of other countries:

- Universal health insurance does not mean universal access to health care. In practice, many countries promise universal coverage but ration care or have extremely long waiting lists for treatment. Nor does a national health care system necessarily mean universal coverage. Some countries with ostensibly universal systems actually fall far short of universal coverage, and most leave at least a small remnant (1-2 percent of the population) uncovered. Although this is certainly wider coverage than the United States provides, it shows the difficulty of achieving either truly universal coverage or universal access to care.
- Rising health care spending is not a uniquely American phenomenon. Other countries spend considerably less than the United States on health care, both as a percentage of GDP and per capita, often because they begin with a lower base of expenditures. Nonetheless, their costs are still rising, leading to budget deficits, tax increases, and/or benefit cuts. In 2004, the last year for which data is available, the average annual increase for per capita health spending in the countries discussed in this study was 5.55 percent, only slightly lower than the United States' 6.21 percent. As the Wall Street Journal notes, "Europeans . . . face steeper medical bills in the future in their cash-strapped governments." In short, there is no free lunch.

- o Those countries that have single-payer systems or systems heavily weighted toward government control are the most likely to face waiting lists, rationing, restrictions on the choice of physician, and other barriers to care. Those countries with national health care systems that work better, such as France, the Netherlands, and Switzerland, are successful to the degree that they incorporate market mechanisms such as competition, cost-consciousness, market prices, and consumer choice, and eschew centralized government control.
- o Dissatisfaction and discontent with a nation's health care system seems to be universal. Undoubtedly, Americans are unhappy with the current state of our health care system. According to the most recent Commonwealth Fund survey, an astounding 82 percent of Americans believe that our system either requires fundamental change or needs to be completely rebuilt. Not surprisingly, polls suggest health care reform is the top domestic policy issue in the upcoming presidential election. Yet, that same Commonwealth Fund study shows large majorities in every country, ranging from 58 percent in the Netherlands to 78 percent in Germany calling for fundamental reform or complete rebuilding of their health care systems. Earlier polling by the Stockholm Network found similar levels of unhappiness. Not as bad as in the United States, perhaps, but certainly no ringing endorsement of their systems.
- o Although no country with universal coverage is contemplating abandoning a universal system, the broad and growing trend in countries with national health care systems is to move away from centralized government control and introduce more market-oriented features. As Richard Saltman and Josep Figueras of the World Health Organization put it, "The presumption of public primacy is being reassessed." Alan Jacobs of Harvard points out that despite significant differences in goals, content, and strategies, European nations are generally converging toward market practices in health care. Thus, even as Americans debate adopting a government-run system, countries with those systems are debating how to make their systems look more like that of the United States.

In most cases, national health care systems have successfully expanded insurance coverage to the vast majority, if not quite all, of the population. But they have not solved the universal and seemingly intractable problem of rising health care costs. In many cases, attempts to control costs through governmental fiat have led to problems with access to care, either delays in receiving care or outright rationing.

Value for money

In wrestling with this dilemma, many countries are loosening government controls and injecting market mechanisms, particularly cost sharing by patients, market pricing of goods and services, and increased competition among insurers and providers. As Pat Cox, former president of the European Parliament put it in a report to the European Commission, "We should start to explore the power of the market as a way of achieving much better value for money." Moreover, the growth of the government share of health care spending, which had increased steadily from the end of World War II until the mid-1980s, has stopped, and in many countries the private share has begun to increase, in some cases substantially. Some evidence shows a growing shift from public to private provision of health care. If the trend in the United States over the last several years has been toward a more European-style system, the trend in Europe is toward a system that looks more like America's. Therefore, if U.S. policy-makers can take one lesson from national health care systems around the world, it is not to follow the road to government-run national health care, but to increase consumer incentives and control. The United States can increase coverage and access to care, improve quality, and control costs without importing the problems of national health care. In doing so, we should learn from the successes-and the failures-of systems in other countries.

Sources

Alain Enthoven, "The History and Principles of Managed Competition," *Health Affairs*, 12, suppl. 1 (1993): 24-48.

Michael Tanner, "No Miracle in Massachusetts: Why Governor Romney's Health Care Reform Won't Work," Cato Institute Briefing Paper No. 97, June 6, 2006.

Ezra Klein, "Health Care Wrap Up," www.ezralein. com, April 25, 2005; Philippe Manière *et al.*, "Perspectives on the European Health Care Systems: Some Lessons for America," Heritage Foundation Lecture No. 711, July 9, 2001.

"French Health Insurance System to Post 10.3-Billion-Euro Deficit," *EU Business*, August 6, 2006.

"Deficit-Saddled France under Fire over Budget," Reuters, July 5, 2007. Members of the Eurozone are required to keep budget deficits below 3 percent of GDP.

"French Health Care Is Badly Run," *BBC News*, August 8, 2006.

Martine Bellanger, Veneta Cherilova, and Valerie Paris, "The Health Benefit Package in France," *European Journal of Health Economics*, 6, suppl. 1 (2005): 24-29.

Buchmueller and Couffinhal, "Private Health Insurance in France." It is important to note, however, that this deregulated insurance is supplemental coverage. No one can be disqualified for health reasons from basic coverage.

Alexander Dorozynski, "French Health Staff Strike over Budget Cuts," *British Medical Journal*, 320 (February 2000): 333; Alexander Dorozynski, "French Medical System Beset by Strikes," *British Medical Journal* 324 (February 2002): 258.

Norman Ho, "A Long, Hot Summer," Harvard International Review 26 (Summer 2004); "French Health Care Is Badly Run," *BBC News*, January 23, 2004.

Valentin Petkantchin, "Bureaucratic Drug De-listing: The French Example," EU Reporter, January-February 2007.

"French Health Care Is Badly Run," *BBC News*, January 23, 2004.

Helen Disney *et al.*, Impatient for Change: European Attitudes to Health Care Reform (London: Stockholm Network, 2004), pp. 69-86.

Hurst and Luigi Siciliani, "Tackling Excessive Waiting Times for Elective Surgery: A Comparison of Policies in Twelve OECD Countries," *OECD Health Working Paper* No. 6, July 2003.

Ezra Klein, "The Health of Nations-Here's How Canada, France, Britain, Germany, and our Own Veterans Health Administration Manage to Cover Everybody at Less Cost and with Better Care than We Do," *American Prospect*, April 24, 2007.

E. van Doorslaer *et al.*, "Income-Related Inequality in the Use of Medical Care in 21 OECD Countries," in Towards High Performing Health Systems: Policy Studies from the OECD Health Project (Paris: OECD, 2004).

"Budget 2008: Tighter Controls on Health Care Spending as French Conservatives Crack Down on Social Security Deficit," *Global Insight*, 2007

Alexandra Bibbee and Benoît Bellone, "Economic Survey of Italy, 2007" (Paris: OECD, 2007).

Franco Reviglio, "Health Care and Its Financing in Italy: Issues and Reform Options," *IMF Working Paper 00-166*, October 2000.

Daniel Callahan and Angela Wasunna, Medicine and the Market: Equity v. Choice (Baltimore: Johns Hopkins University Press, 2006), p. 98.

George France, Francesco Taroni, and Andrea Donatini, "The Italian Health Care System," *Health Economics*, 14 (September 2005): 185-202.

Alberto Mingardi, "A Drug Price Path to Avoid," *Washington Post*, November 12, 2006.

Ariel David, "Italian Police Units Inspect Hospitals," *Washington Post*, January 8, 2007.

Vittorio Maio and Lamberto Manzoli, "The Italian Health Care System: WHO Ranking *versus* Public Perception," *PLoS Medicine*, 6 (June 2002): 301-03.

Guillem Lopez-Casasnovas, Joan Coasta-Font, and Ivan Planas, "Diversity and Regional Inequalities: Assessing the Outcomes of the Spanish System of Health Care Services," *UPF Working Paper No. 745*, April 2004.

Emilio Cerda, Laura de Pablos, and Maria Rodriguez, "Waiting Lists for Surgery," in Patient Flow: Reducing Delay in Health Care Delivery (Hoboken, NJ: Springer, 2006).

Xavier Bosch, "Spain: The Old Frequently Live with Their Families," *British Medical Journal*, 324 (June 29, 2002): 1543.

Luis Rajmil *et al.*, "The Quality of Care and Influence of Double Health Care Coverage in Catalonia (Spain)," *Archive of Disease in Childhood*, 83 (September 2000): 211-14.

Tetsuo Fukawa, "Public Health Insurance in Japan," *World Bank Institute Working Paper No. 37201* (2002).

Kohei Komamura and Atsuhiro Yamada, "Who Bears the Burden of Social Insurance? Evidence from Japanese Health and Long-Term Care Insurance Data," *Journal of Japanese and International Economics*, 18 (December 2004): 565-81.

"Japanese Health Insurance Industry Faces Winnowing Out," Medical Insurance News, March 21, 2004.

Noriyuki Takayama, "Japan's Never-Ending Social Security Reforms," *International Social Security Review*, 55 (2002): 11-22.

M. Ryan Baker, "Japan and Massachusetts: A Comparison of Universal Health Care Systems," *Missouri Foundation for Health*, Spring 2006.

Naoki Ikagami and John Campbell, "Japan's Health Care System: Containing Costs and Attempting Reform," *Health Affairs*, 23 (2004): 29-34.

Naoki Ikagami and John Campbell, "Health Care Reform in Japan: The Virtues of Muddling Through," *Health Affairs*, 18 (Fall 1999): 56-75.

OECD, "OECD Health Data 2007: Statistics and Indicators for 30 Countries."

Rihito Kimura, "Bioethics and Japanese Health Care," *Washington-Japan Journal*, 3 (1994): 2.

Jan Roth Johnsen, Health Systems in Transition: Norway 8, No. 1 (Copenhagen: European Observatory on Health Systems and Policies, 2006).

Michael Moore, Remarks before the Washington, D.C., *Premiere of SiCKO*, June 20, 2007.

Paul van den Noord, Terje Hagen, and Tolversen, "The Norwegian Health Care System," *OECD Economics Department Working Paper No. 198*, 1998.

H. Piene, P. Nyen, and H. Hauge, "Waiting Lists and Hospital Capacity-Analyses Based on Theoretical Queue Models and Empirical Data," Paper presented to the Annual Meeting of the International Society for Technological Assessment of Health Care, Unimed, Norway, 1997.

Christine Furuholmen and Jon Magnussen, Health Care Systems in Transition: Norway (Copenhagen: European Observatory on Health Care Systems, 2000).

Luigi Siciliani and Jeremy Hurst, "Explaining Waiting Times Variations for Elective Surgery across OECD Countries," *OECD Health Working Paper* No. 7, October 2003.

M. Hoel and E. Saether, "Private Health Care as a Supplement to a Public Health System with Waiting Time for Treatment," *Ragnar Frisch Center for Economic Research*, Oslo, 2000.

Hagen and Kaarboe, "The Norwegian Hospital Reform of 2002: Central Government Takes Over Ownership of Public Hospitals." Directorate-General of Health, "National Health Plan, 2004-2010" (Lisbon: Ministry of Health, July 2004).

OECD, "Health at a Glance: OECD Indicators, 2005" (Paris: OECD, 2005).

Catarina Diogo, "The Reform of the NHS in Portugal," University of York, Department of Management, *Working Paper No. 5*, 2005.

Monica Duarte Oliveira and Gwyn Bevan, "Measuring Geographic Inequalities in the Portuguese Health Care System: An Estimation of Hospital Care Needs," *Health Policy*, 66 (March 2003): 277-93.

Konstantina Davaki and Elias Mossialos, "Plus Ca Change: Health Sector Reforms in Greece," *Journal of Health Politics, Policy, and Law*, 30 (February- April 2005): 143-67.

Elias Mossialos, Sara Allin, and Konstantina Davaki, "Analyzing the Greek Health System: A Tale of Fragmentation and Inertia," *Health Economics*, S1 (2005): S151.

Andre den Exter *et al.*, Health Care Systems in Transition: Netherlands (Copenhagen: European Observatory on Health Systems and Policies, 2004).

G.P. Westert and H. Verkleij, eds., Dutch Health Care Performance Report 2006 (Bilthoven, The Netherlands: Center for Prevention and Health Services Research, National Institute for Public Health and the Environment, 2006.)

Alain Enthoven and Wynand van den Ven, "Going Dutch-Managed-Competition Health Insurance in the Netherlands," *New England Journal of Medicine*, 357 (2007): 2421-23.

Stefan Greb, Maral Manougian, and Jurgen Wasem, "Health Insurance in the Netherlands," *CESifo DICE Report*, January 2007.

"Health Insurance System," Ministry of Health, Welfare and Sport, The Royal Netherlands Embassy, 2006,

J. Andre Knottnerus and Gabriel ten Velden, "Dutch Doctors and Patients-Effects of Health Care Reform in the Netherlands," *New England Journal of Medicine*, 357 (2007): 2424-26.

Gautam Naik, "Dutch Treatment: In Holland, Some See Model for U.S. Health care System," *Wall Street Journal*, September 6, 2007.

Rudolf Klein, "The Troubled Transformation of Britain's National Health Service," *New England Journal of Medicine*, 355 (2006): 409-15.

Ulla Schmidt, "Health Policy and Health Economics in Germany," Speech given at the conference, The American Model and Europe: Past-Present-Future, Washington, January 27, 2006.

Dennis Nowak, "Doctors on Strike-The Crisis in German Health Care Delivery," *New England Journal of Medicine*, 355, No. 15 (2006): 1520-22.

World Health Organization, "Highlights on Health, Germany, 2004, Dieter Braeuninger, "Health Policy in Germany: Health Reforms Need a Dose of Market Medicine," Deutsche Bank Research, June 13, 2006.

———2005: "Measuring the Sustainability of Provincial Public Health Expenditure in Canada," Fraser Institute, October 2005.

Nadeem Esmail, Michael Walker, and Dominika Wrona, "Waiting Our Turn, 16th Edition: Hospital Waiting Lists in Canada," Fraser Institute, 2006.

Madhu Natarajan *et al.*, "The Risks of Waiting for Cardiac Catheterization: A Prospective Study," Canadian Medical Association Journal, November 26, 2002.

"Edwards Campaign Unveils New 'Underdog' Television Ad in New Hampshire," John Edwards 08, news release, January 6, 2008,

Cathy Schoen *et al.*, "Toward Higher- Performance Health Systems: Adults' Health Care Experiences in Seven Countries, 2007," *Health Affairs*, October 31, 2007.

Richard Saltman and Josep Figueras, "Analyzing the Evidence on European Health Care Reforms," *Health Affairs*, March-April 1998.

Hans Maarse, "The Privatization of Health Care in Europe: An Eight Country Analysis," *Journal of Health Politics, Policy, and Law 3He1* (2006): 981-1014.

Paul Krugman, "The Waiting Game," *New York Times*, July 16, 2007.

Physicians for a National Health Program, "Insurance CEOs Fattened on the Suffering of Many," Paul Krugman and Robin Wells, "The Health Care Crisis and What to Do about It," *New York Review of Books*, March 23, 2006.

Organisation for Economic Co-operation andDevelopment, "OECD Health Data 2007: Statistics and Indicators for 30 Countries" (Paris:OECD, 2007).

Christine Borger *et al.*, "Health Spending Projections through 2015: Changes on the Horizon," *Health Affairs*, 25, No. 2 (2006): w61-w73

Kaiser Family Foundation, "Employer Health Benefits 2007 Annual Survey," *Kaiser Family Foundation*, September 11, 2007.

———2007: Annual Report of the Board of Trustees of the Federal Hospital Insurance and Federal Supplemental Medical Insurance Trust Funds (Washington: Government Printing Office, 2007).

Jagadeesh Gokhale, "Medicaid's Soaring Costs: Time to Step on the Brakes," Cato Institute Policy Analysis No. 597, July 19, 2007.

Carmen DeNavas-Walt *et al.*, "Income, Poverty and Health Insurance in the United States: 2005," Current Population Reports (Washington: U.S. Census Bureau, 2006).

Elizabeth McGlynn *et al.*, "The Quality of Health Care Delivered to Adults in the United States," *New England Journal of Medicine*, 348 (2003): 2635-45.

Rita Mangione-Smith *et al.*, "The Quality of Ambulatory Care Delivered to Children in the United States," *New England Journal of Medicine*, 357 (2007): 1515-23.

Robert L. Ohsfeldt and John E. Schneider, The Business of Health: The Role of Competition, Markets, and Regulation (Washington: American Enterprise Institute Press, 2006).

"World Briefing: Berlusconi Has Heart Surgery in US," *New York Times*, December 19, 2006.

Steve Findlay, "U.S. Hospitals Attracting Patients from Abroad," *USA Today*, July 22, 1997.

John Goodman, "Moore's SiCKO Could Put Lives at Risk," The Michael Moore Chronicles, National Center for Policy Analysis, 2007

"Nobel Prize in Physiology or Medicine Winners 2007-1901," The Nobel Prize Internet Archive, Pharmaceutical Research and Manufacturing of America, "R&D Spending by U.S. Bio-pharmaceutical Companies Reaches a Record $55.2 Billion in 2006," February 12, 2007.

Economic Report of the President (Washington: Government Printing Office, 2004), p. 192.

Gerard Anderson *et al.*, "It's the Prices Stupid: Why the United States Is So Different from Other Countries," *Health Affairs*, 22, No. 3 (2003): 99.

Cowen, "Poor U.S. Scores in Health Care Don't Measure Nobels or Innovation."

"The Novartis Warning," *Wall Street Journal*, May 8, 2002.

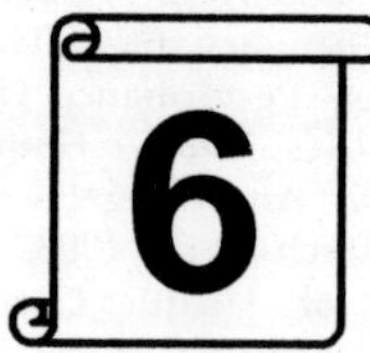

United States' Health Care System

'Health care facilities in USA are largely owned and operated by the private sector. Health insurance is primarily provided by the private sector, with the exception of programs such as Medicare, Medicaid, the Children's Health Insurance Program and the Veterans Health Administration. US is the world leader in biomedical and technology research and development as well as the introduction of new biomedical products. Pharmaceutical trade organizations also maintain that the high cost of health care in the US has encouraged substantial reinvestment in such research and development. US has world's best hospitals and highly skilled manpower. Yet, its health care system has been ranked at 37 by WHO. It is widely known that nearly 50 million US citizens do not have any health care cover. Many more have only limited medical-insurance. The private insurance companies are fattening themselves at the cost of the doctors as well the citizens. The passage of health care bill 2009 in the senate may bring cheer to 31 million uninsured citizens of US.'

There are many slips between cup and lips!

The Uninsured and Under-insured

At least 15% of the American population is completely uninsured, and a substantial additional portion of the population is "underinsured", or less than fully insured for medical costs they might incur. More money per person is spent on health care in the United States than in any other nation in the world, and a greater percentage of total income in the nation is spent on health care in the U.S. than in any United Nations member state except for East Timor. Medical debt is the principal cause of personal bankruptcy in the United States. The US pays twice as much yet lags behind other wealthy nations in such measures as infant mortality and life expectancy. Currently the U.S. has a higher infant mortality rate than most of the world's industrialized nations. The USA's life expectancy lags 42nd in the world, after most rich nations, lagging last of the G5 (Japan, France, Germany, UK, USA) and just after Chile (35th) and Cuba (37th). The USA's life expectancy is ranked 50th in the world after the European Union (40th).

Populations Over-utilize Health Care

It has been found that the 1% of the population with the highest spending accounted for 27% of aggregate health care spending. The highest-spending 5% of the population accounted for more than half of all spending. In 2004, private insurance paid for 36% of personal health expenditures, private out-of-pocket 15%, federal government 34%, state and local governments 11%, and other private funds 4%. Most Americans (59.3%) receive their health insurance coverage through an employer (which includes both private as well as civilian public-sector employees) under group coverage, although this percentage is declining. Workers with employer-sponsored insurance also contribute; in 2007, the average percentage of premium paid by covered workers was 16% for single coverage and 28% for family coverage. In addition to their premium contributions, most covered workers face additional payments when they use health care services, in the form of deductibles and co-payments. Some Americans do not qualify for government-provided health insurance, are not provided health insurance by an employer, and are unable to afford, cannot qualify for, or choose not to purchase, private health insurance. When charity or "uncompensated" care is not available, they sometimes simply go without needed medical treatment. This problem has become a source of considerable political controversy on the national level.

No Universal Health Care

The United States is a developed nation but without any universal health care system. Health care in the U.S, has some publicly funded components viz. Medicare covers the elderly and disabled, Medicaid is available for some of the poor, and the State Children's Health Insurance Program covers children of low-income families. The Veterans Health Administration directly provides health care to U.S. military veterans through government hospitals; while active duty service members, retired service members and their dependents are eligible for benefits through TRICARE. Together, these tax-financed programs cover 27.8% of the population. Roughly two-thirds of urban hospitals in the U.S. are non-profit hospitals and the balance evenly divided between for-profit hospitals and public hospitals. Care in the U.S. is generally provided by physicians in private practice and private hospitals.

Consumer driven health care is a scheme put forth by the National Center for Policy Analysis. It refers to a method of financing health care being the combination of a savings plan with a health insurance policy that pays only for the most catastrophic health care needs. This type of arrangements relieves the insurance company for paying for all but the most catastrophic of medical expenses. This reduces the monthly premium paid by the insured but the consumer is then expected to put aside money into Health Savings Accounts (HSAs), Health Reimbursement Arrangements (HRAs), or similar medical payment products, from which the majority of routine health care expenses and the first large slice of any catastrophic insurance claim would be used to pay health care providers and prescription medicines. The advantage of this system is that the consumer is expected to play a higher role in ensuring value for money.

The Plight of Uninsured

Uninsured live every day just one accident or illness away from bankruptcy. These are middle class Americans. Some can't get insurance on the job. Others are self-employed and can't afford it since buying insurance on your own costs you three times as much as the coverage you get from your employer. Many other Americans who are willing and able to pay are still denied insurance due to previous illnesses or conditions that insurance companies decide are too risky or too expensive to cover. One man from Illinois lost his coverage in the middle of chemotherapy because his insurer found that he hadn't reported gallstones. They delayed his treatment, and he died because of it. Then there's the problem of rising costs. This is one of the reasons that insurance premiums have gone up three times faster than wages. Finally, American health care system is placing an unsustainable burden on taxpayers. When health care costs grow at the rate they have, it puts greater pressure on programs like Medicare and Medicaid.

Views on New Comprehensive Health Insurance Plan: President Speaks

Some believe that the only way to fix the system is through a single-payer system like Canada's;—where we would severely restrict the private insurance market and have the government provide coverage for everybody. It's a plan that asks everyone to take responsibility for meeting this challenge—not just government, not just insurance companies, but everybody, including employers and individuals.

First, if you are among the hundreds of millions of Americans who already have health insurance, nothing in this plan will require you or your employer to change the coverage or the doctor you have. Under this plan, it will be against the law for insurance companies to deny you coverage because of a pre-existing condition. They will no longer be able to place some arbitrary cap on the amount of coverage you can receive in a given year or in a lifetime. We will place a limit on how much you can be charged for out-of-pocket expenses, because in the United States of America, no one should go broke because they get sick. And insurance companies will be required to cover, with no extra charge, routine checkups and preventive care, like mammograms and colonoscopies.

If you're one of the tens of millions of Americans who don't currently have health insurance, the second part of this plan will finally offer you quality, affordable choices. If you lose your job or you change your job, you'll be able to get coverage. If you strike out on your own and start a small business, you'll be able to get coverage. We'll do this by creating a new insurance exchange, a marketplace where individuals and small businesses will be able to shop for health insurance at competitive prices. As one big group, these customers will have greater leverage to bargain with the insurance companies for better prices and quality coverage. This is how large companies and government employees get affordable insurance. Now, for those individuals and small businesses who still can't afford the lower-priced insurance available in the exchange, we'll provide tax credits, the size of which will be based on your need.

In the meantime, for those Americans who can't get insurance today because they have pre-existing medical conditions, we will immediately offer low-cost coverage that will protect you against financial ruin if you become seriously ill.

Now, even if we provide these affordable options, there may be those, and especially the young and the healthy, who still want to take the risk and go without coverage. There may still be companies that refuse to do right by their workers by giving them coverage. If some businesses don't provide workers health care, it forces the rest of us to pick up the tab when their workers get sick, and gives those businesses an unfair advantage over their competitors. And unless everybody does their part, many of the insurance reforms we seek, especially requiring insurance companies to cover pre-existing conditions, just can't be achieved. That's why under my plan, individuals will be required to carry basic health insurance—just as most states require you to carry auto insurance. There will be a hardship waiver for those individuals who still can't afford coverage, and 95 percent of all small businesses, because of their size and narrow profit margin, would be exempt from these requirements.

... I believe a broad consensus exists for the aspects of the plan I just outlined: consumer protections for those with insurance; an exchange that allows individuals and small businesses to purchase affordable coverage; and a requirement that people who can afford insurance get insurance.— I realize that many Americans have grown nervous about reform.

Insurance Companies are the Villains

Unfortunately, in 34 states, 75 percent of the insurance market is controlled by five or fewer companies. In Alabama, almost 90 percent is controlled by just one company. And without competition, the price of insurance goes up and quality goes down. And it makes it easier for insurance companies to treat their customers badly—by cherry-picking the healthiest individuals and trying to drop the sickest; by overcharging small businesses who have no leverage; and by jacking up rates. They do it because it's profitable. As one former insurance executive testified before Congress, insurance companies are not only encouraged to find reasons to drop the seriously ill, they are rewarded for it.

Despite all this, the insurance companies and their allies don't like this idea. They argue that these private companies can't fairly compete with the government, and they'd be right if taxpayers were subsidizing this public insurance option, but they won't be. I've insisted that, like any private insurance company, the public insurance option would have to be self-sufficient and rely on the premiums its collects. But by avoiding some of the overhead that gets eaten up at private companies by profits and excessive administrative costs and executive salaries, it could provide a good deal for consumers and would also keep pressure on private insurers to keep their policies affordable and treat their customers better, the same way public colleges and universities provide additional choice and competition to students without in any way inhibiting a vibrant system of private colleges and universities.

The public option—the public option is only a means to that end, and we should remain open to other ideas that accomplish our ultimate goal. But I will not back down on the basic principle that, if Americans can't find affordable coverage, we will provide you with a choice.

Existing System is Currently Full of Waste and Abuse

Right now, too much of the hard-earned savings and tax dollars we spend on health care don't make us any healthier. That's not my judgment. It's the judgment of medical professionals across this country. And this is also true when it comes to Medicare and Medicaid. In fact, I want to speak directly to seniors for a moment, because Medicare is another issue that's been subjected to demagoguery and distortion during the course of this debate. More than four decades ago, this nation stood up for the principle that after a lifetime of hard work, our seniors should not be left to struggle with a pile of medical bills in their later years. That's how Medicare was born. And it remains a sacred trust that must be passed down from one generation to the next. That is why not a dollar of the Medicare trust fund will be used to pay for this plan.

The only thing this plan would eliminate is the hundreds of billions of dollars in waste and fraud, as well as unwarranted subsidies in Medicare that go to insurance companies... And we will also create an independent commission of doctors and medical experts charged with identifying more waste in the years ahead. Now, these steps will ensure that you—America's seniors—get the benefits you've been promised. They will ensure that Medicare is there for future generations. And we can use some of the savings to fill the gap in coverage that forces too many seniors to pay thousands of dollars a year out of their own pockets for prescription drugs. Now, because Medicare is such a big part of the health care system, making the program more efficient can help usher in changes in the way we deliver health care that can reduce costs for everybody. Reducing the waste and inefficiency in Medicare and Medicaid will pay for most of this plan. Much of the rest would be paid for with revenues from the very same drug and insurance companies that stand to benefit from tens of millions of new customers. And this reform will charge insurance companies a fee for their most expensive policies, which will encourage them to provide greater value for the money—an idea which has the support of Democratic and Republican experts. And according to these same experts, this modest change could help hold down the cost of health care for all of us in the long-run.

Defensive Medicine may be Contributing to Unnecessary Costs

So we move forward on a range of ideas about how to put patient safety first and let doctors focus on practicing medicine. ... ... Now, add it all up and the plan I'm proposing will cost around $900 billion over 10 years, less than we have spent on the Iraq and Afghanistan wars and less than the tax cuts for the wealthiest few Americans that Congress passed at the beginning of the previous administration. Now, most of these costs will be paid for with money already being spent—but spent badly—in the existing health care system. The plan will not add to our deficit. The middle class will realize greater security, not higher taxes. And if we are able to slow the growth of health care costs by just one-tenth of 1% each year—one-tenth of 1%—it will actually reduce the deficit by $4 trillion over the long-term. I will not waste time with those who have made the calculation that it's better politics to kill this plan than to improve it. And I will not accept the status quo as a solution. Not this time; not now. Our deficit will grow. More families will go bankrupt. More businesses will close. More Americans will lose their coverage when they are sick and need it the most. And more will die as a result.

Ted Kennedy's passion was born not of some rigid ideology, but of his own experience—the experience of having two children stricken with cancer. He never forgot the sheer terror and helplessness that any parent feels when a child is badly sick. And he was able to imagine what it must be like for those without insurance, what it'd be like to have to say to a wife or a child or an aging parent, "There is something that could make you better, but I just can't afford it." That large-heartedness, that concern and regard for the plight of others is not a partisan feeling. It's not a Republican or a Democratic feeling. It, too, is part of the American character.

History of Our Progress

In 1935, when over half of our seniors could not support themselves and millions had seen their savings wiped away, there were those who argued that Social Security would lead to socialism. But the men and women of Congress stood fast, and we are all the better for it. In 1965, when some argued that Medicare represented a government takeover of health care, members of Congress, Democrats and Republicans, did not back down. They joined together so that all of us could enter our golden years with some basic peace of mind. You see, our predecessors understood that government could not, and should not, solve every problem. They understood that there are instances when the gains in security from government action are not worth the added constraints on our freedom. But they also understood that the danger of too much government is matched by the perils of too little; that without the leavening hand of wise policy, markets can crash, monopolies can stifle competition, the vulnerable can be exploited.

And they knew that when any government measure, no matter how carefully crafted or beneficial, is subject to scorn; when any efforts to help people in need are attacked as un-American; when facts and reason are thrown overboard and only timidity passes for wisdom, and we can no longer even engage in a civil conversation with each other over the things that truly matter—that at that point we don't merely lose our capacity to solve big challenges. We lose something essential about ourselves.

. . . I still believe that we can act when it's hard. I still believe we can replace acrimony with civility and gridlock with progress. I still believe we can do great things and that here and now we will meet history's test.

Most Pressing Issue is Universality

Universality of access to health insurance is the most pressing issue. Universal health care simply means coverage for all eligible residents of a political area. The United States is the only industrialized country that has not implemented a universal system for citizens under age 65. Universal health care can be implemented in several ways. In some countries the government directly manages the health care system. This is usually called socialized medicine. In most countries universal coverage is achieved by a mix of public and private funding. Taxation is the primary source of funding but is supplemented by private payor arrangements. In 2000 the World Health Organization (WHO) produced a report which ranked all the health insurance systems used by its member-countries. The is the report usually quoted when discussing both the good and bad features of a health insurance system. It should be noted that the WHO has indicated it will no longer produce a ranking table because of the complexity of the task. The criteria for ranking the health care systems was based on a wide variety of findings, including but not limited to, life expectancy, infant mortality and cost. But do you know what the top 10 best health care system in the world are?

The top 10 in the order determined by the World Health Organization:

1. France
2. Italy
3. San Marino
4. Andorra
5. Malta
6. Singapore
7. Spain
8. Oman
9. Austria
10. Japan

The Beveridge Model

This model is named after William Beveridge, the social reformer who designed Britain's National Health Service. In this system, health care is provided and financed by the government through tax payments, just like the police force or the public library. Many, but not all, hospitals and clinics are owned by the government; some doctors are government employees, but there are also private doctors who collect their fees from the government. In Britain, you never get a doctor bill. These systems tend to have low costs per capita, because the government, as the sole payer, controls what doctors can do and what they can charge. Countries using the Beveridge plan or variations on it include its birthplace Great Britain, Spain, most of Scandinavia and New Zealand. Hong Kong still has its own Beveridge-style health care, because the populace simply refused to give it up when the Chinese took over that former British colony in 1997. Cuba represents the extreme application of the Beveridge approach; it is probably the world's purest example of total government control.

The Bismarck Model

It is named after Prussian Chancellor Otto von Bismarck, who invented the welfare state as part of the unification of Germany in the 19th century. Despite its European heritage, this system of providing health care would look fairly familiar to Americans. It uses an insurance system—the insurers are called "sickness funds"—usually financed jointly by employers and employees through payroll deduction. Unlike the U.S. insurance industry, though, Bismarck-type health insurance plans have to cover everybody, and they don't make a profit. Doctors and hospitals tend to be private in Bismarck countries; Japan has more private hospitals than the U.S. Although this is a multi-payer model—Germany has about 240 different funds—tight regulation gives government much of the cost-control clout that the single-payer Beveridge Model provides. The Bismarck model is found in Germany, of course, and France, Belgium, the Netherlands, Japan, Switzerland, and, to a degree, in Latin America.

The National Health Insurance Model

This system has elements of both Beveridge and Bismarck. It uses private-sector providers, but payment comes from a government-run insurance program that every citizen pays into. Since there's no need for marketing, no financial motive to deny claims and no profit, these universal insurance programs tend to be cheaper and much simpler administratively than American-style for-profit insurance.

The single payer tends to have considerable market power to negotiate for lower prices; Canada's system, for example, has negotiated such low prices from pharmaceutical companies that Americans have spurned their own drug stores to buy pills north of the border. National Health Insurance plans also control costs by limiting the medical services they will pay for, or by making patients wait to be treated. The classic NHI system is found in Canada, but some newly industrialized countries—Taiwan and South Korea, for example—have also adopted the NHI model.

The Out-of-Pocket Model

Only the developed, industrialized countries—perhaps 40 of the world's 200 countries—have established health care systems. Most of the nations on the planet are too poor and too disorganized to provide any kind of mass medical care. The basic rule in such countries is that the rich get medical care; the poor stay sick or die. In rural regions of Africa, India, China and South America, hundreds of millions of people go their whole lives without ever seeing a doctor. They may have access, though, to a village healer using home-brewed remedies that may or not be effective against disease. In the poor world, patients can sometimes scratch together enough money to pay a doctor bill; otherwise, they pay in potatoes or goat's milk or child care or whatever else they may have to give. If they have nothing, they don't get medical care.

These four models should be fairly easy for Americans to understand because they have elements of all of them in their fragmented national health care apparatus. When it comes to treating veterans, we're Britain or Cuba. For Americans over the age of 65 on Medicare, we're Canada. For working Americans who get insurance on the job, we're Germany.

For the 15 percent of the population who have no health insurance, the United States is rural India (or Cambodia or Burkina Faso), with access to a doctor available if you can pay the bill out-of-pocket at the time of treatment or if you're sick enough to be admitted to the emergency ward at the public hospital. The United States is unlike every other country because it maintains so many separate systems for separate classes of people. All the other countries have settled on one model for everybody.

Let us look at some democracies—the United Kingdom, Japan, Germany, Taiwan, Switzerland, Canada and India—how they deliver health care.

U.K.

Every single person who's born in the U.K. will use the NHS and none of them will be presented a bill at any point during that time. NHS is now trying some free-market tactics like "pay-for-performance," where doctors are paid more if they get good results controlling chronic diseases like diabetes. And now patients can choose where they go for medical procedures, forcing hospitals to compete head to head.

The British system is "socialized medicine" because the government both provides and pays for health care. Britons pay taxes for health care, and the government-run National Health Service (NHS) distributes those funds to health care providers. Hospital doctors are paid salaries. General practitioners (GPs), who run private practices, are paid based on the number of patients they see. A small number of specialists work outside the NHS and see private-paying patients. Because the system is funded through taxes, administrative costs are low; there are no bills to collect or claims to review. Patients have a "medical home" in their GP, who also serves as a gatekeeper to the rest of the system; patients must see their GP before going to a specialist. GPs, who are paid extra for keeping their patients healthy, are instrumental in preventive care, an area in which Britain is a world leader.

The stereotype of socialized medicine—long waits and limited choice—still has some truth. In response, the British government has instituted reforms to help make care more competitive and give patients more choice. Hospitals now compete for NHS funds distributed by local Primary Care Trusts, and starting in April 2008 patients are able to choose where they want to be treated for many procedures.

Japan

The Japanese go to the doctor three times as often as Americans, have more than twice as many MRI scans, use more drugs, and spend more days in the hospital. Yet Japan spends about half as much on health care per capita as the United States. One secret to Japan's success? By law, everyone must buy health insurance—either through an employer or a community plan—and, unlike in the U.S., insurers cannot turn down a patient for a pre-existing illness, nor are they allowed to make a profit.

Japan uses a "social insurance" system in which all citizens are required to have health insurance, either through their work or purchased from a non-profit, community-based plan. Those who can't afford the premiums receive public assistance. Most health insurance is private; doctors and almost all hospitals are in the private sector. Japan boasts some of the best health statistics in the world, no doubt due in part to the Japanese diet and lifestyle. Unlike the U.K., there are no gatekeepers; the Japanese can go to any specialist when and as often as they like. Every two years the Ministry of Health negotiates with physicians to set the price for every procedure. This helps keeps costs down.

In fact, Japan has been so successful at keeping costs down that Japan now spends too little on health care; half of the hospitals in Japan are operating in the red. Having no gate-keepers means there's no check on how often the Japanese use health care, and patients may lack a medical home.

Germany

For its 80 million people, Germany offers universal health care, including medical, dental, mental health, homeopathy and spa treatment. It is a system where the rich pay for the poor and where all are covered. As they do in Japan, medical providers must charge standard prices. This keeps costs down, but it also means physicians in Germany earn between half and two-thirds as much as their U.S. counterparts.

Germany, like Japan, uses a social insurance model. In fact, Germany is the birthplace of social insurance. But unlike the Japanese, who get insurance from work or are assigned to a community fund, Germans are free to buy their insurance from one of more than 200 private, non-profit "sickness funds." As in Japan, the poor receive public assistance to pay their premiums. Sickness funds are non-profit and cannot deny coverage based on preexisting conditions; they compete with each other for members, and fund managers are paid based on the size of their enrollments. Like Japan, Germany is a single-payment system, but instead of the government negotiating the prices, the sickness funds bargain with doctors as a group. Germans can go straight to a specialist without first seeing a gatekeeper doctor, but they may pay higher co-pay if they do.

The single-payment system leaves some German doctors feeling underpaid. A family doctor in Germany makes about half to two-thirds as much as he or she would in America. (Then again, German doctors pay much less for malpractice insurance, and many attend medical school for free.) Germany also lets the richest 10 percent opt out of the sickness funds in favour of U.S.-style for-profit insurance. These patients are generally seen more quickly by doctors, because the for-profit insurers pay doctors more than the sickness funds.

Taiwan

It has health care system where the government collects the money and pays providers. But the delivery of health care is left to the market. Every person in Taiwan has a "smart card" containing all of his or her relevant health information, and bills are paid automatically. But the Taiwanese are spending too little to sustain their health care system. Taiwan adopted a "National Health Insurance" model in 1995 after studying other countries' systems. Like Japan and Germany, all citizens must have insurance, but there is only one, government-run insurer. Working people pay premiums split with their employers; others pay flat rates with government help; and some groups, like the poor and veterans, are fully subsidized. The resulting system is similar to Canada's—and the U.S. Medicare program.

Taiwan's new health system extended insurance to the 40 percent of the population that lacked it while actually decreasing the growth of health care spending. The Taiwanese can see any doctor without a referral. Every citizen has a smart card, which is used to store his or her medical history and bill the national insurer. The system also helps public health officials monitor standards and effect policy changes nationwide. Thanks to this use of technology and the country's single insurer, Taiwan's health care system has the lowest administrative costs in the world. Like Japan, Taiwan's system is not taking in enough money to cover the medical care it provides. The problem is compounded by politics, because it is up to Taiwan's parliament to approve an increase in insurance premiums, which it has only done once since the program was enacted.

Switzerland

In 1994, a national referendum approved a law called LAMal ("the sickness"), which set-up a universal health care system, that among other things, restricted insurance companies from making a profit on basic medical care. "Everybody has a right to health care," says Pascal Couchepin, the current president of Switzerland. "It is a profound need for people to be sure that if they are struck by destiny ... they can have a good health system."

The Swiss system is social insurance like in Japan and Germany, voted in by a national referendum in 1994. Switzerland didn't have far to go to achieve universal coverage; 95 percent of the population already had voluntary insurance when the law was passed. All citizens are required to have coverage; those not covered were automatically assigned to a company. The government provides assistance to those who can't afford the premiums. The Swiss example shows that universal coverage is possible, even in a highly capitalist nation with powerful insurance and pharmaceutical industries. Insurance companies are not allowed to make a profit on basic care and are prohibited from cherry-picking only young and healthy applicants. They can make money on supplemental insurance, however. As in Germany, the insurers negotiate with providers to set standard prices for services, but drug prices are set by the government.

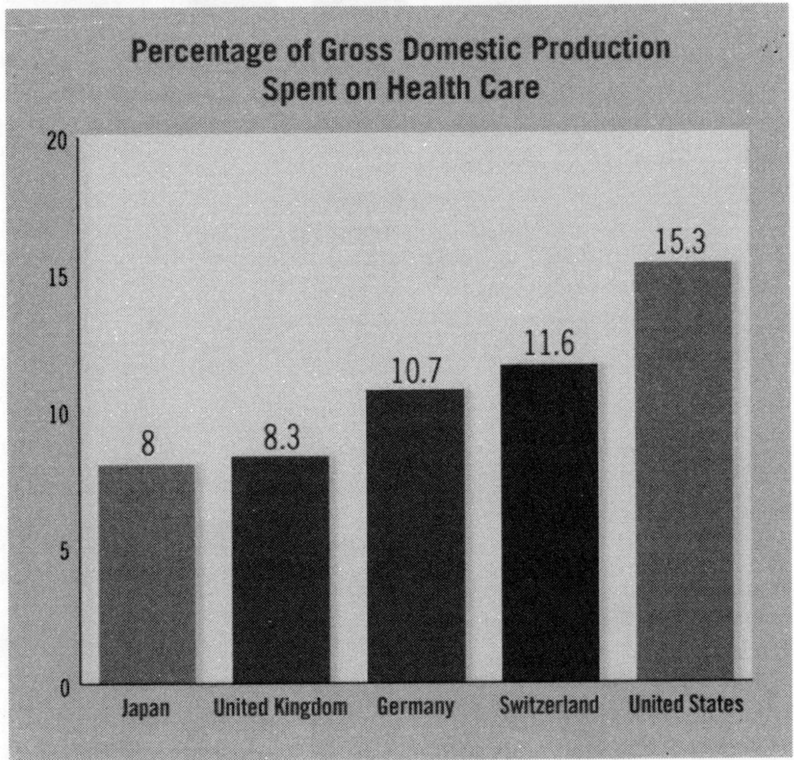

The Swiss system is the second most expensive in the world—but it's still far cheaper than U.S. health care. Drug prices are still slightly higher

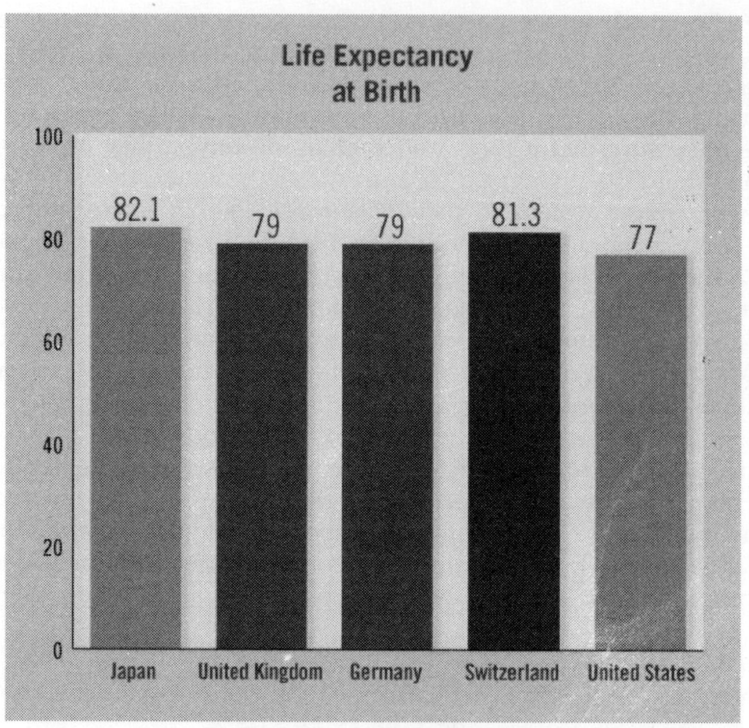
Life Expectancy
at Birth
100
80
60
40
20
0
82.1
79
79
81.3
77
Japan
United Kingdom
Germany
Switzerland
United States

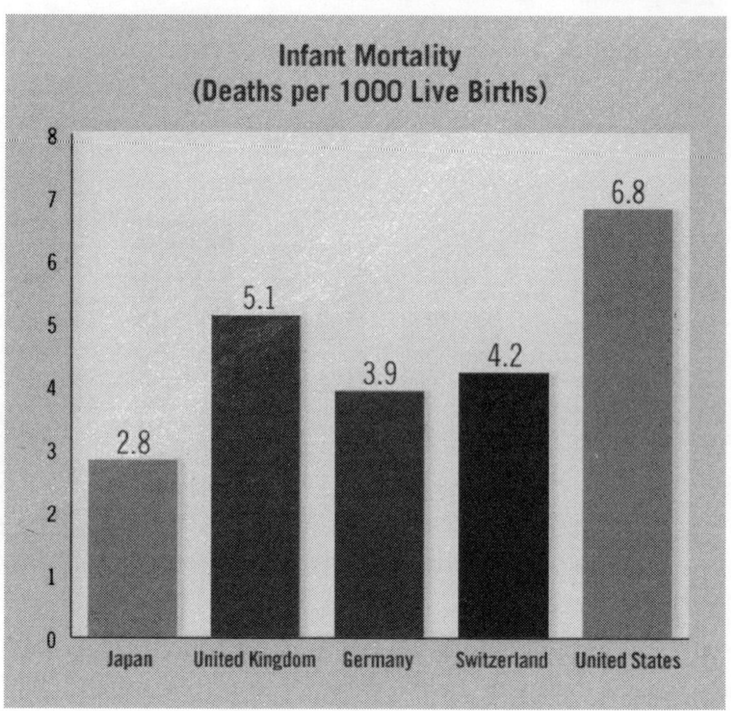
Infant Mortality
(Deaths per 1000 Live Births)
8
7
6
5
4
3
2
1
0
2.8
5.1
3.9
4.2
6.8
Japan
United Kingdom
Germany
Switzerland
United States

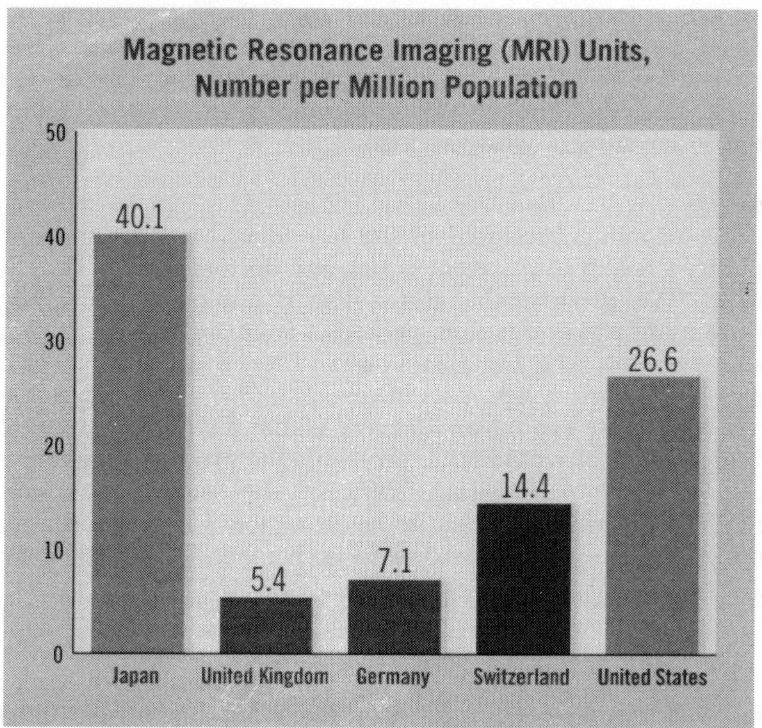
Magnetic Resonance Imaging (MRI) Units,
Number per Million Population
50
40
30
20
10
0
40.1
5.4
7.1
14.4
26.6
Japan
United Kingdom
Germany
Switzerland
United States

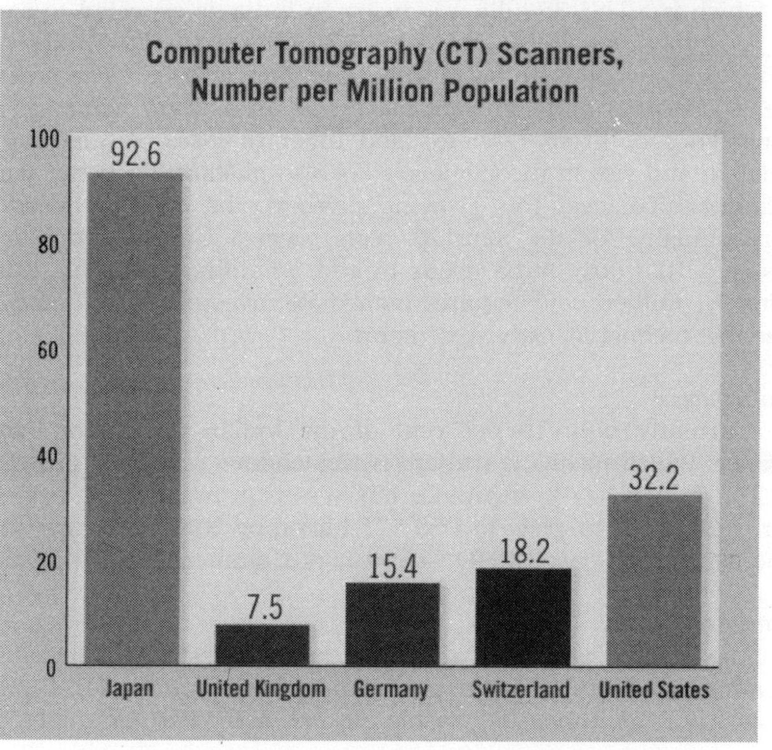
Computer Tomography (CT) Scanners,
Number per Million Population
100
80
60
40
20
0
92.6
7.5
15.4
18.2
32.2
Japan
United Kingdom
Germany
Switzerland
United States

than in other European nations, and even then the discounts may be subsidized by the more expensive U.S. market, where some Swiss drug companies make one-third of their profits. In general, the Swiss do not have gatekeeper doctors, although some insurance plans require them or give a discount to consumers who use them.

Canada

The incoming president of the Canadian Medical Association says this country's health care system is sick and doctors need to develop a plan to cure it. "We all agree that the system is imploding, we all agree that things are more precarious than perhaps Canadians realize," Doing said in an interview with The Canadian Press. There's a critical need to make Canada's health care system patient-centered. Ouellette believes there could be a role for private health care delivery within the public system. "A short-term achievable goal would be to accelerate the process of getting electronic medical records into physicians' offices," she said. "That's one I think ought to be a priority and ought to be achievable." A long-term goal would be getting health systems "talking to each other," so information can be quickly shared to help patients.

India

India is a third world country and its health care system is not working well. But we need to focus on India, for comparison. Indian health care, which is a US$ 35 billion industry in India, is expected to reach over US$ 75 billion by 2012 and US$ 150 billion by 2017, according to Technopak Advisors—'India Health Care Trends 2008'. The sector offers immense potential to health care players as the country witnesses a rise in the incidence of lifestyle-related and other diseases. A growing elderly population and rise in income levels are also pushing for better facilities in the country. To meet this growing demand, the country needs US$ 50 billion annually for the next 20 years, says a Confederation of Indian Industry (CII) study. India needs to add 3.1 million beds by 2018 to the existing 1.1 million, and requires immediate investments of US$ 82 billion, as per the Technopak Advisors report.

Health Insurance

Currently only 10 per cent of the Indian population has health insurance, which means that there is tremendous scope for growth in this area. The Indian health insurance business is growing at 50 per cent. The sector is projected to grow to US$ 5.75 billion by 2010, according to a study by the New Delhi-based PHD Chamber of Commerce and Industry.

Investments in Health Care

The sector has been attracting huge investments from domestic players as well as financial investors and private equity (PE) firms. Funds such as ICICI Ventures, IFC, Ashmore and Apax Partners invested about

US$ 450 million in the first six months of 2008-09 compared with US$ 125 million in the same period a year ago, according to an analysis carried out by Feedback Ventures. Feedback Ventures expects PE funds to invest at least US$ 1 billion in the health care sector in the next five years. Religare Venture Capital has entered into a 50:50 joint venture with PE player Milestone Capital to manage a US$ 120.09 million PE fund and tap the huge potential in health care and education sectors. GE Health Care has invested US$ 50 million in its Bangalore facility and will be investing an additional US$ 25 million soon. Philips plans to make India one of its global production hubs for medical equipment by investing substantially on upgrading of its two acquired manufacturing facilities in the country and increasing their capacity. The government, along with participation from the private sector, is planning to invest US$ 1 billion to US$ 2 billion in an effort to make India one of the top five global pharmaceutical innovation hubs by 2020.

Medical Tourism

In 2007 India treated 450,000 foreign patients ranking it second in medical tourism. The key selling points of the medical tourism industry are its cost effectiveness and its combination with the attractions of tourism. Treatment cost is lowest in India—10 to 20 per cent of the average cost incurred in the US, Singapore, Thailand and South Africa. Besides world class medical facilities, India is also trying to promote its traditional medicine such as ayurveda.

The fast growth in the Indian health care sector has created various pockets of opportunities for investors. A recent FICCI-Ernst and Young (E&Y) report highlights several such areas within the health care sector.

- Medical infrastructure forms the largest portion of the health care pie. Beds in excess of 1 million need to be added to reach a ratio of 1.85 per thousand at an investment of US$ 77.9 billion.
- The medical equipment industry is around US$ 2.17 billion and is growing at 15 per cent per year. It is estimated to reach US$ 4.97 billion by 2012.
- The medical textiles industry is projected to double to reach US$ 753 million by 2012.
- Clinical trials have the potential to become a US$ 1 billion industry by 2010 and the health services outsourcing sector has the potential to grow to US$ 7.4 billion by 2012, from US$ 3.7 billion in 2006.

In the face of intense Republican opposition, the White House signaled over the weekend it was not wedded to a public insurance option as long as the final health care measure increases choices for consumers and competition for insurers. "A public option is the best option to lower costs, improve the quality of health care, ensure choice and expand coverage," House of Representatives Speaker Nancy Pelosi said in a statement that cited strong House support for a government-run plan.

Republicans say a public plan, which has become the focus of their warnings about a government health care takeover, would unfairly compete with private plans and cripple the insurance industry. Six members of the Senate Finance Committee—three from each party—have been negotiating a reform package that would feature member-controlled non-profit cooperatives instead of the government-run plan. Members of the cooperatives would join together and purchase insurance for them.

What is a Single Payer Health Care System?

A single payer health care system is exactly what it sounds like—health care is paid for by only one entity. In all cases across the world where a single payer system has been implemented, that payer is the government. People often confuse a single payer system with universal health care, which instead refers to the fact that every citizen in that system has access to basic health care. Universal systems may be a combination of private and publicly funded care. Examples of single payer systems are found in the United Kingdom and Canada. Some consider these systems to be "socialized health care" because all funding comes from the government.

In the United States, Medicare is a single payer system for people age 65 and older. Those who favour a single payer system suggest it would look like Medicare for everyone. They also cite the fact that the total administrative cost for Medicare services is only 3%, whereas private insurance administrative costs may amount to 25% or more. Most Americans are surprised to learn that many physicians in the United States support a single payer system. In fact, more than 15,000 doctors support an organization called Physicians for a National Health Plan (PNHP) which has actively pursued a single payer system for many years. The biggest reason these physicians support a single payer system is because the billing aspects of their practices often cost more than the rest of their practice. It's not unusual for a doctor to devote more staff, therefore more expense, to billing than to patient care.

Most opposition to a single-payer system comes from the health insurance companies that would no longer provide the services they now offer, which means to them a reduction in revenue streams and profits.

Difference between Universal Health Care and a Single Payer System

Universal health care simply refers to making sure everyone has access to basic health care needs without regard to whether people can pay for care or not.

Many experts will tell you that even prior to any reform of the health care system, the United States has universal health care?:

- Some people have private insurance to cover their basic health care needs.

- The federal government covers the health care needs of everyone age 65 and older.
- Many (but not all) state governments provide health care coverage to the poor, especially children and some elderly residents.

For those with no formal coverage:

- Some pay for care out of their pockets.
- Some seek care in emergency rooms or free clinics, neither of which turn away patients, and most of which is then paid for by taxpayers.

Single-payer health care simply means everyone in a specific geography has universal care, and those services are paid for by one entity. While single payer by definition would not have to refer to a government as a single payer, in reality any country around the world that has a single payer system, uses a government-payer system.

Mr. Obama has been pressing for a government-run scheme to extend health care insurance to some 46 million people in the US. Health Care costs represent 16% of GDP, almost twice OECD average. Reform plans would require all Americans to get insurance

Some propose public insurance option to compete with private insurers:

More than $1.2 trillion spent on health care each year is a waste of money. Members of the medical community identify the leading causes

$ 1.2 trillion, That's half of the $2.2 trillion the United States spends on health care each year, according to the most recent data from accounting firm Price water house Coopers' Health Research Institute. The report identified 16 different areas in which health care dollars are squandered. But in talking to doctors, nurses, hospital groups and patient advocacy groups, six areas totaling nearly $500 billion stood out as issues to be dealt with in the health care reform debate.

1. Too Many Tests

Doctors ordering tests or procedures not based on need but concern over liability or increasing their income is the biggest waste of health care dollars, costing the system at least $210 billion a year, according to the report. The problem is called "defensive medicine." "Sometimes the motivation is to avoid malpractice suits, or to make more money because they are compensated more for doing more," said Dr. Arthur Garson, provost of the University of Virginia and former dean of its medical school. "Many are also convinced that doing more tests is the right thing to do." "But any money that is spent on a patient that doesn't improve the outcome is a waste," said Garson.

President Obama doesn't agree; instead, his reform proposal encourages doctors to practice "evidence-based" guidelines as a way to scale back on unnecessary tests.

2. Annoying Claim Forms

Inefficient claims processing is the second-biggest area of wasteful expenditure, costing as much as $210 billion annually, the PricewaterhouseCoopers report said, "We spend a lot of time and money trying to get paid by insurers," said Dr. Terry McGenney, a Kansas City, Mo.-based family physician. "Some practices spend 40% of their revenue filling out paperwork that has nothing to do with patient care."

"That adds to our administrative fees, extends the payment cycle and hurts our cash flow," he said. They also spend a lot of time getting "pre-certification" from insurers to approve higher-priced procedures such as MRIs. "We're already operating on paper-thin margins and this takes times away from our patients," he said. "Hundreds of billions" of dollars can be saved by standardizing procedures and using technology—something the White House has mentioned as a key to health care reform.

3. Using the ER as a Regular Clinic

More insured and uninsured consumers are getting their primary care in emergency rooms, wasting $14 billion every year in health care spending. "This is an inappropriate use of the ER," said the president of the American Academy of Nurse Practitioners. "You don't go to the ER for strep throat." Since emergency rooms are legally obligated to treat all patients, providers ultimately find ways to pass on the cost for treating the uninsured to other patients, such as to those who pay out-of-pocket for their medical care. "Going to the doctor for strep throat would cost $65-$70. In the ER, it's $600 to $800," he said. The $787 billion stimulus bill signed passed by President Obama earlier this year includes allocates $1 billion for a wellness and prevention fund, including $300 million for immunizations and $650 million for prevention programs to combat the rapid growth in chronic diseases such as obesity and diabetes.

4. Medical Errors

Medical errors are costing the industry $17 billion a year in wasted expenses, something that makes patient advocacy groups irate processes such as computerized order entry for drugs and use of electronic health records (EHR) could help ensure that patients get the correct dosage of medications in hospitals. The stimulus bill calls for the government to take a leading role in developing standards by 2010 to facilitate the adoption of health information exchanges across the system, including patient electronic health records by 2014. Obama has repeatedly said that the use of technology in the health sector will help boost savings, enhance the coordination of care and reduce medical errors and unnecessary procedures.

5. Going back to the Hospital

Discharging patients too soon is a "huge waste of money," said Swanson. "This happens a lot with elderly patients who are discharged prematurely because of insurance, bed unavailability or ageism," she said. Many times, patients also don't follow instructions for care after discharge. "So complications arise and they are readmitted in a week," Swanson said. PricewaterhouseCoopers estimates the cost of preventable hospital readmissions at $25 billion annually. Among the reform plans, one proposal being considered is for Medicare to potentially penalize hospitals who readmit patients within 30 days of discharge.

6. You Forgot to Wash Your Hands!

PricewaterhouseCoopers estimates that about $3 billion is wasted every year as a result of infections acquired during hospital stays. "The general belief is that hospitals are getting much better in managing this than they have in the past," said Richard Clarke, CEO of Health Care Financial Management Association, whose members include hospitals and managed care organizations. Something as simple as hand-washing often can reduce the problem. "The challenge here is that patients sometimes come in with infections which then spread in the hospital." The stimulus bill signed by Obama earlier this year includes $50 million for reducing health care-associated infections.

Other areas of waste identified in the PricewaterhouseCoopers report included up to $493 billion related to risky behaviour such as smoking, obesity and alcohol abuse, $21 billion in staffing turnover, $4 billion in prescriptions written on paper, and $1 billion in the over-prescribing of antibiotics.

US Health Care Reform Bill, 2009

The bill, which passed with 60 to 39 votes in senate, aims to cover 31 million uninsured Americans. "This will be the most important piece of social legislation since Social Security passed in the 1930s," President said.

It must still be reconciled with similar legislation passed by the House of Representatives.

Mr. Obama said: "We are now finally poised to deliver on the promise of real, meaningful health insurance reform that will bring additional security and stability to the American people."

He described the measures as "the toughest measures ever taken to hold the insurance industry accountable".

Among various reforms, Mr Obama said the insurance companies will no longer be able to deny coverage with a pre-existing condition nor end coverage when a person becomes ill.

"With today's vote, we are now incredibly close to making health insurance reform a reality in this country," the president said.

But he said it would be a challenge to "finish the job" of reform.

"For the sake of our citizens, our economy and our future, let's make

2010 the year we finally reform health care in the United States of America."

The process of reconciling the two bills is expected to begin in January and will require further tough negotiations.

Once that has been done—and the process could still be derailed by last-minute changes of heart among senators—Mr Obama will be able to sign the measure into law.

The bill's passage in an early morning vote on Christmas Eve follows months of political wrangling and 24 days of debate in the Senate chamber.

Opposition Republicans say the legislation is expensive, authoritarian and a threat to civil liberties, and accuse the Democrats of rushing it through.

Republican Senate leader Mitch McConnell said the bill's difficult history highlighted its failings.

"The most obvious problem with the bill before us is that it doesn't do what it was supposed to do. The one test for any bill was whether it would lower costs. This bill fails that test.

"It's also clear that even many of the people on this side who are going to support this bill don't like it—otherwise Democratic leaders wouldn't have had such a tough time rounding up the votes."

The non-partisan Congressional Budget Office estimates that efficiency savings made as a result of the Senate health care reform bill will cut the federal deficit by $132bn (£83bn) over 10 years, but critics say the predicted savings may never materialize.

As a nation, the US spent some $2.2tn (£1.36tn) on health care in 2007. That amounts to 16.2% of GDP, nearly twice the average of other rich, industrialized countries.

As costs have spiraled, millions of Americans have found themselves unable to afford health insurance and the cost to the government of providing care for the poor and elderly has risen hugely.

BILLS: KEY DIFFERENCES

Public option: House yes, Senate no.

Abortion: House bill has stricter restrictions on federal funding.

How to pay for reform: House relies heavily on income tax increase for high-earning Americans; Senate bill taxes high-cost health insurance plans

President Obama's Risks on Health Care Bill

Before Obama can sign a measure into law, differences must be resolved between the Senate bill and one passed last month by the U.S. House of Representatives. Democratic leaders have voiced confidence that Obama will get a final bill next month. "Democrats must produce a bill," said Ethan Siegal of the Washington Exchange, a private firm that tracks legislation and politics for institutional investors. "If they don't, they'd be seen as unable to govern." A victory on health care is critical for Obama, whose political standing and legislative agenda could hinge on its success.

Obama's approval rating has dropped to just under 50% from more than 60% earlier this year, due largely to the double-digit US unemployment rate. A signed bill would give Obama a boost—provided it proves to be popular and, as advertised, brings down costs, ends what are seen as insurance industry abuses and provides coverage to millions of uninsured Americans. No Republicans voted for the Senate bill and just one voted for the House bill. So Republican law-makers will likely rise or fall together on this issue, depending on the success or failure of the overhaul.

Republicans rallied their conservative base in recent weeks by denouncing the legislation as too expensive in televised speeches on the Senate floor. But the debate is now over. If the legislation proves to be effective, Democrats may be able to count on a new legion of supporters: the estimated 30 million Americans who would secure insurance coverage. But this centerpiece of the bill isn't due to kick in until 2014—after the next two congressional elections and after voters decide on whether to give Obama a second term.

Other provisions will take effect in 2010. They include making it illegal for insurance companies to drop coverage for Americans who get sick and providing grants for states to create ombudsmen to act as consumer advocates regarding health insurance coverage. Democrats are certain to promote these provisions as they head toward next year's election, when all 435 seats in the House and 38 of 100 in the Senate are up for election.

Sources

"Income, Poverty, and Health Insurance Coverage in the United States: 2007." U.S. Census Bureau. Issued August 2008.

Families USA (2009) press release summarizing a Lewin Group study: "New Report Finds 86.7 Million Americans were Uninsured at Some Point in 2007-08"[2].

"Underinsured Americans: Cost to you", Parija B. Kavilanz, CNNMoney.com, March 5, 2009.

Kaiser Commission on Medicaid and the uninsured, "Underinsured in America: Is Health Coverage Adequate?" July, 2002.

Two myths about the U.S. health care system". Montreal Economic Institute. June 2005. http://www.iedm.org/uploaded/pdf/juin05_en.pdf. Retrieved 2009-08-25.

WHO (May 2009). "World Health Statistics 2009". World Health Organization. http://www.who.int/whosis/whostat/2009/en/index.html. Retrieved 2009-08-02.

Medical Debt Huge Bankruptcy Culprit—Study: It's Behind Six-In-Ten Personal Filings". CBS. 2009-06-05. http://www.cbsnews.com/stories/2009/06/05/earlyshow/health/main5064981.shtml. Retrieved 2009-06-22.

Marian F MacDorman, Ph.D., and T.J. Mathews, M.S.. "Recent Trends in Infant Mortality in the United States" (pdf). National Center for Health Statistics, Centers for Disease Control.

Life Expectancy 2005-10 UN WPP 2006. PNG using: United Nations World Population Prospects: 2006 revision—Table A.17[3]. Life expectancy at birth (years) 2005-10. All data from the ranking is included, except for Martinique and Guadeloupe (due to imaging difficulties).

Stephen Ohlemacher, "US Slipping in Life Expectancy Rankings" *Washington Post*, August 12, 2007.

United Nations Department of Economic and Social Affairs, "World Population Prospects: The 2006 Revision", Life expectancy at p. 80ff, infant mortality at p. 85ff.

Factbook, Infant mortality rate by country.

World Health Organization assess the world's health system. Press Release WHO/44 21 June, 2000.

Health system attainment and performance in all Member States, ranked by eight measures, estimates for 1997.

Roehr, Bob (2008), "Health care in US ranks lowest among developed countries", BMJ 337 (jul21 1): a889, doi:10.1136/bmj.a889, PMID 18644774.

Insuring America's Health: Principles and Recommendations, Institute of Medicine of the National Academies of Science, 2004-01-14. Retrieved 2007-10-22.

The Case For Single Payer, Universal Health Care For The United States. *American Journal of Public Health*, December 2009, Vol. 99, No. 12.

State-by-state breakout of excess deaths from lack of insurance.

A 1997 study carried out by Professors David Himmelstein and Steffie Woolhandler (New England Journal of Medicine 336, No. 11 [1997]) "concluded that almost 100,000 people died in the United States each year because of lack of needed care-three times the number of people who died of AIDs." The Inhuman State of U.S. Health Care, *Monthly Review*, Vicente Navarro, September 2003. Retrieved 2009-09-10.

The Indian Health Service Fact Sheets.

EMRC WHITE PAPER: Present Status and Future Strategy for Medical Research in Europe Medical Research Spending Doubled Over Past Decade, Neil Osterweil, *MedPage Today*, September 20, 2005.

"National Health Expenditure Data: NHE Fact Sheet," Centers for Medicare and Medicaid Services, referenced February 26, 2008.

Sean Keehan, Andrea Sisko, Christopher Truffer, Sheila Smith, Cathy Cowan, John Poisal, M. Kent Clemens, and the National Health Expenditure Accounts Projections Team, "Health Spending Projections Through 2017: The Baby-Boom Generation Is Coming To Medicare", *Health Affairs* Web Exclusive, February 26, 2008. Retrieved February 27, 2008.

"National Health Expenditure Data: Overview," Centers for Medicare and Medicaid Services.

"National Health Expenditures, Forecast summary and selected tables", Office of the Actuary in the Centers for Medicare and Medicaid Services, 2008. Retrieved March 20, 2008 by David U. Himmelstein, Elizabeth Warren, Deborah Thorne, and Steffie Woolhandler, published at *Health Affairs Journal* in 2005, Accessed 10 May 2006.

U.S. Congressional Budget Office, "Technological Change and the Growth of Health Care Spending," January 2008.

"Health Care Costs 101", 2007 Edition. Katherine B. Wilson. April 2007.

Emily Cox, Doug Mager, Ed Weisbart, "Geographic Variation Trends in Prescription Use: 2000 to 2006" [dead link], Express Scripts, January 2008.

Gerard F. Anderson, Uwe E. Reinhardt, Peter S. Hussey and Varduhi Petrosyan, "It's The Prices, Stupid: Why The United States Is So Different From Other Countries", *Health Affairs*, Volume 22, Number 3, May/June 2003. Retrieved February 27, 2008.

Marc L. Berk and Alan, C. Monheit, "The Concentration Of Health Care Expenditures, Revisited", *Health Affairs*, Volume 20, Number 2, March/April 2001. Retrieved February 27, 2008.

Marc L. Berk and Alan C. Monheit, "Datawatch: The Concentration Of Health Expenditures: An Update", *Health Affairs*, Winter 1992. Retrieved February 27, 2008.

Steven B. Cohen and William Yu, "The Persistence in the Level of Health Expenditures over Time: Estimates for the U.S. Population, 2002-03," MEPS Statistical Brief #124, Agency for Health Care Research and Quality, May 2006.

Micah Hartman, Aaron Catlin, David Lassman, Jonathan Cylus and Stephen Heffler, "U.S. Health Spending By Age, Selected Years Through 2004", *Health Affairs*, web exclusive, November 6, 2007. Retrieved February 27, 2008.

John E. Wennberg, Elliott S. Fisher, David C. Goodman, and Jonathan S. Skinner, "Tracking the Care of Patients with Severe Chronic Illness: the Dartmouth Atlas of Health Care 2008." The Dartmouth Institute for Health Policy and Clinical Practice, May 2008, ISBN 978-0-9815862-0-5 (Executive Summary).

Coverage and Access | More Aggressive Hospital Care Does Not Lead to Improved Patient Outcomes in All Cases, Study Finds," *Kaiser Daily Health Policy Report*, Kaiser Family Foundation, May 30, 2008.

David Brown, "In the Balance: Some Candidates Disagree, but Studies Show It's Often Cheaper To Let People Get Sick," The Washington Post, April 8, 2008.

Vanessa Fuhrmans, "Consumers Cut Health Spending, As Economic Downturn Takes Toll," *The Wall Street Journal*, September 22, 2008

Health, United States, 2007. U.S. Department of Health and Human Services, Centers for Disease Control and Prevention, National Center for Health Statistics.

Kaiser Family Foundation (2007-09-11). "Health Insurance Premiums Rise 6.1 Percent In 2007, Less Rapidly Than In Recent Years But Still Faster Than Wages And Inflation".

OECD Health Data 2009 (pdf). How Does the United States Compare. OECD. http://www.oecd.org/dataoecd/43/23/40905066.pdf. Retrieved 2009-10-02.

Managed Care: Integrating the Delivery and Financing of Health Care—Part A, Health Insurance Association of America, 1995, p. 9 ISBN 1-879143-26-1

The Value of Provider Networks and the Role of Out-of-Network Charges in Rising Health Care Costs: A Survey of Changes Billed by Out-of-Network Physicians, America's Health Insurance Plans, August 2009.

Gina Kolata, "Survey Finds High Fees Common in Medical Care ," *The New York Times*, August 11, 2009.

Hurley, R.E., Strunk, B.C., White, J.S. (2004). "The puzzling popularity of the PPO". Health Aff (Millwood) 23 (2): 56-68. doi:10.1377/hlthaff.23.2.56. PMID 15046131. http://content.healthaffairs.org/cgi/pmidlookup?view=long&pmid=15046131.

Thomas M. Selden and Merrile Sing, "The Distribution Of Public Spending For Health Care In The United States, 2002," *Health Affairs*, 27, No. 5 (2008): w349-w359 (published online 29 July 2008).

Core Health Indicators: Per capita government expenditure on health at average exchange rate World Health Organization. Retrieved 2007-10-05.

Centers for Medicare and Medicaid Services: Medicare.

How the Tax Code Distorts Health Care Cato Institute?

"The Health Care Crisis and What to Do About It" By Paul Krugman, Robin Wells, *New York Review of Books*, March 23, 2006.

Employer-Sponsored Health Insurance: Past, Present and Future, *Journal of Forensic Economics*.

Verbal evidence of Robert Greenstein to 3rd Senate Finance Committee Meeting on Health Care Reform Financing, 2009.

Latest Enrolment Data Still Fail to Dispel Concerns about Health Savings Accounts: The Center on Budget and Policy Priorities.

Unsettling Scores: A Ranking of State Medicaid Programs, p. 15.

"Health and Human Services Statistics 2006" (PDF). U.S. Department of Health and Human Services. http://www.cms.hhs.gov/CapMarketUpdates/Downloads/2006CMSstat.pdf. Retrieved 2007-07-03.[dead link]

Cunningham, P., May, J. "Medicaid patients increasingly concentrated among physicians." Track Rep. 2006 Aug; (16):1-5. PMID 16918046.

"SCHIP Overview". U.S. Department of Health and Human Services, Centers for Medicare and Medicaid Services. http://www.cms.hhs.gov/LowCostHealthInsFamChild/. Retrieved 2007-07-03.

"SCHIP Ever Enrolled in Year" (PDF). U.S. Centers for Medicare and Medicaid Services. http://www.cms.hhs.gov/NationalSCHIPPolicy/downloads/SCHIPEverEnrolledYearGraph.pdf. Retrieved 2007-09-02.

"President's FY 2008 Budget and the State Children's Health Insurance Program (SCHIP)" (PDF). Henry J. Kaiser Family Foundation. http://www.kff.org/medicaid/upload/7635.pdf. Retrieved 2007-07-03.

Centers for Medicare and Medicaid Services: Emergency Medical Treatment and Active Labour Act.

Rowes, Jeffrey (2000). "EMTALA: OIG/HCFA Special Advisory Bulletin Clarifies EMTALA, American College of Emergency Physicians Criticizes It". *Journal of Law, Medicine and Ethics,* 28(1): 9092. http://www.aslme.org/news/jlme/28.1e.html. Retrieved 2008-01-02.[dead link]

Dubay, L., Holahan, J. and Cook, A., The Uninsured and the Affordability of Health Insurance Coverage, *Health Affairs* (Web Exclusive), November 2006. Retrieved February 4, 2007.

Characteristics of the Uninsured: Who is Eligible for Public Coverage and Who Needs Help Affording Coverage?" (PDF). Kaiser Commission on Medicaid and the Uninsured. http://www.kff.org/uninsured/upload/7613.pdf. Retrieved 2007-07-19.

Jack Hadley and John Holahan, How Much Medical Care Do the Uninsured Use and Who Pays for It?, *Health Affairs* Web Exclusive, 2003-02-13. Retrieved 2007-10-05.

Jack Hadley and John Holahan, Covering The Uninsured: How Much Would It Cost?, *Health Affairs Web Exclusive*, 2003-06-04. Retrieved 2007-10-05.

Wilhelmine Miller, Elizabeth Richardson Vigdor, and Willard G. Manning, Covering The Uninsured: What Is It Worth?, *Health Affairs Web Exclusive*, 2004-03-31. Retrieved 2007-10-05.

Centers for Medicare and Medicaid Services. CMS Programs and Information.. Retrieved August 30, 2006.

Centers for Medicare and Medicaid Services. Emergency Medical Treatment and Labour Act.. Retrieved August 30, 2006.

Anderson, Gerard F.; Uwe E. Reinhardt, Peter S. Hussey, Varduhi Petrosyan (2009). "It's the prices Stupid: Why the United States is so different from other countries" (pdf). *Health Affairs,* Volume 22, Number 3. http://content.healthaffairs.org/cgi/reprint/22/3/89.pdf. Retrieved 2009-10-02.

Organisation for Economic Co-operation and Development (pdf), OECD Health Data 2008: How Does Canada Compare, http://www.oecd.org/dataoecd/46/33/38979719.pdf, retrieved 2009-01-09.

Wangsness, Lisa (June 21, 2009). "Health debate shifting to public *vs.* private". Boston Globe. Retrieved September 21, 2009.

Fahrenthold, D.A. "Mass. Bill Requires Health Coverage."

Kaiser Daily Health Policy Report, Kaiser Family Foundation, April 23, 2008

Sidney M. Wolfe and Kate Resnevic, "Public Citizen's Health Research Group Ranking of the Rate of State Medical Boards' Serious Disciplinary Actions, 2005-07," Public Citizen, April 22, 2008.

Nursing Home Compare, Centers for Medicare and Medicaid Services (accessed 4/24/2008).

Special Focus Facility ("SFF") Initiative, Centers for Medicare and Medicaid Services (accessed 4/24/2008).

Kaiser Daily Health Policy Report, Kaiser Family Foundation, April 24, 2008.

United States Government Accountability Office, "NURSING HOMES: Federal Monitoring Surveys Demonstrate Continued Understatement of Serious Care Problems and CMS Oversight Weaknesses," GAO-08-517, May 2008 (GAO Summary).

Kaiser Daily Health Policy Report, Kaiser Family Foundation, May 15, 2008.

Victoria Craig Bunce and J.P. Wieske, "Health Insurance Mandates in the States 2008", The Council for Affordable Health Insurance, 2008.

Michael J. New, "The Effect of State Regulations on Health Insurance Premiums: A Preliminary Analysis," The Heritage Center for Data Analysis, October 27, 2005.

David Gratzer, Why Isn't Government Health Care The Answer?, Free Market Cure, 16 July 2007.

Robert J. Blendon, Minah Kim and John M. Benson, "The Public *Versus* The World Health Organization On Health System Performance," *Health Affairs*, May/June 2001.

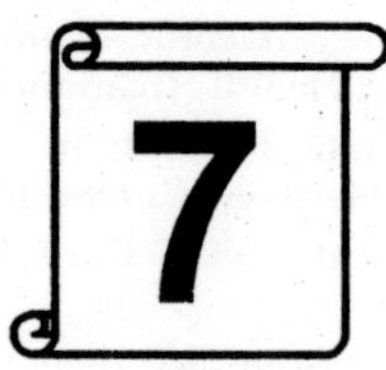

Universal Health Care Systems in the World

"Universal health care refers to access of health services by every citizen of a country. It could be by a combination of public and private systems. In U.K and Canada Government pay for the health care of its citizens and no citizen is presented a medical bill for payment. In Germany the payments are made by the insurance companies but it is cashless for the citizens. In USA the health care system is broken with over 47 millions of Americans not enjoying any health cover and many more have a limited cover. In India more than 80% citizens pay out of pocket, though they were entitled to seek health care from the Government-run institutions. Medical insurance cover is available to less than 10% of its citizens. Those who get insured abuse the system with impunity. The corporate hospitals also exploit the cashless facility offered to such insured patients. But the system has collapsed for all practical purposes. The situation is no better in many other third world countries."

Many countries claim to provide universal coverage but universal coverage is still a mirage for majority of the world population. Germany has universal coverage, and social insurance plans cover the majority of people. Government only subsidizes 15 per cent of the costs of the funds. There are also 42 private insurers that cover 9 per cent of the total population, viz. those in upper income brackets who are excluded from the public social-insurance programs. Netherlands, which has a similar system, has deemed that 35 per cent of its population is ineligible for the social insurance programs due to high income.

Even Multiple Payer Systems may not be Universal Health Care

USA is an example of multiple payer private insurance(for profit)-

based systems. Under this model, health care is paid for by premiums for insurance policies plus additional cost-sharing. In this system, there is less bargaining power over the price and quality of care. Currently, about one-third of Americans with private insurance are in self-insured plans. Complexity and fragmentation of the US health care system, particularly the payment system, results in higher prices. More is spent on administrative costs. USA health care is also far from satisfactory. It is one of the important political issues in the United States, under Obama administration. It is estimated that more than 47 million Americans are without health insurance, and 6.6 million of them reside in California alone. The skyrocketing costs of health care and the number of uninsured in the United States show no sign of slowing. Ironically, Americans spend more than 16% of the gross domestic product (GDP) on health care, yet health outcomes in the United States consistently rank on the lower rungs compared to other Western industrialized countries with developed economies. Further details about the US health care are described in a separate chapter. However, America is in the state of transformation with the health care bill 2009 having been passed by the congress as well as senate.

India and China Story: Far from Universal

In India universal health coverage is at the fore of Pep talk, though far from its realization. Barring a few islands of excellence in the form of corporate hospitals, which cater to the needs of the elite, health and medical services have more or less collapsed in this country. More than 80% expenditure on medical treatment is born by the citizens from their own pockets, despite poverty and indebtedness. In fact, increasing health care costs are quickly becoming a problem worldwide. Health care expenditures are mounting worldwide, in part because of aging populations, the prevalence of chronic disease, and increasing pharmaceutical costs. Coping with the rising cost of health care requires reconciling the oft-competing goals of health services; namely, the social goal of providing equal access, the medical goal of providing the highest quality care, the economic goal of cost containment, and the political goal of guaranteeing patient choice and getting input from medical professionals.

In case of China, the government supported or run hospitals provide most of the health care services and are currently making progress in health care insurance enterprises. In most cases government will pay a limited amount of the health care cost for city people. However, most people will pay the majority of the health care cost on their own, in addition to the health care insurances. In the countryside, there is a "rural health insurance system" consisting of some limited national and local support. Patients pay the cost for some kind of diseases. As a developing or transitional country China's health care expenditure is lower compared with the western countries ($261 per capita, per year),

OVERVIEW OF UNIVERSAL HEALTH CARE IN SOME COUNTRIES

CANADA

Canada provides universal access to health care to the 33.2 million people who reside there through a mixture of public, mixed, and private health care systems. The country's ten provinces are primarily responsible for health care in Canada, collectively called the Medicare systems. The provinces also govern their respective single-payer systems for universal hospital and medical services, paying for hospitals either directly or through global funding for regional health authorities. In addition, the provincial governments negotiate physician fee schedules with the provincial medical associations. The federal government does retain jurisdiction over certain aspects of the health care system, notably regulating prescription drugs and financing and administering health benefits for indigenous peoples, the armed forces and the Royal Canadian Mounted Police, veterans, and inmates in federal penitentiaries. In order to qualify for federal funding, each province must meet the following criteria:

1. *Universality*: Available to all provincial residents on uniform terms;
2. *Comprehensiveness*: Covering all necessary hospital and physician services;
3. *Portability*: Allowing residents to remain covered when moving from province;
4. *Accessibility*: Having no financial barriers to access such as deductibles; and
5. *Public administration*: Administered by a non-profit authority of government.

Who Pays for the Health Care?

Canada provides universal, medically necessary care for its residents free of charge, but its essentially single-payer system has created a bottleneck for timely access to services. Tax revenues at the provincial, territorial and federal governments account for nearly 70% of total health expenditures. Patients' out-of-pocket co-payments and private insurance reimbursements cover much of the remainder at 15% and 12%, respectively. Funding is provided jointly by the federal and state governments. The federal government uses funds from general revenue to provide a block grant to each of the provinces. The block grant finances only about 16% of each province's health care expenditures. The remainder is funded by provincial taxes: mostly personal and corporate income tax. Health care spending makes up between one-third to one-half of provincial social welfare spending. For the nation as a whole, health care costs only 9% of GDP. Physicians work in private practice and are paid on a fee-for-service basis. Since these fees are set by a centralized agency, wages are fairly low which has lead to a physician shortage. There are only 2.1 physicians per

1,000 people. In 2004, the C$130 billion spent on health care went to:

- o 43% on hospital (30%) and physician (13%) services,
- o 23% on provincial social service programs,
- o 30% on private health care services, and
- o 4% to direct federal services.

Canada spent approximately C$4548 per capita on health care in 2006. The regional health authorities have become the primary payer of health care services. Regional authorities have great freedom in allocating funds to best serve the particular needs of their population. Private health insurance mostly covers goods and services not covered by Medicare. Private insurance covered 33.8% of all prescription drugs, 21.7% of all vision care, and 53.6% of all dental care. Six of the provinces—British Columbia, Alberta, Manitoba, Ontario, Québec, and Prince Edward Island—go so far as to outlaw insurance that attempts to provide alternative or faster access to health care already covered by Medicare. Most private health insurance is group-based, sponsored by employers, unions, or other like organizations. Although employer-based insurance is part of the benefits package, this insurance is mandatory and thus most provinces do not tax those benefits.

Most of Canada's 1.5 million general practitioners and specialists work under fee-for-service arrangements. Fee-for-service payments account for 79.5% of physician income. Providers are discouraged from performing services in both the public and private spheres, although it is not illegal to do so. Although hospitals historically have been private, not-for-profit institutions, hospitalization has created a substantially integrated relationship between hospitals and provincial governments. Insured services include virtually all hospital, physician, and diagnostic services as well as primary care services covered under the provincial Medicare plans. Although financial barriers to care have essentially disappeared with the elimination of most Medicare user fees, access to timely care is a problem with which the provincial and territorial governments continue to struggle. The country as a whole also must address the rising costs of health care to ensure the sustainability of its programs.

DENMARK

All permanent residents of Denmark are entitled to coverage under the health system, including primary and hospital care, which are free at the point of service; however, many also choose to purchase private insurance supplements. All of Denmark's approximately 5.5 million residents are entitled to health insurance coverage. Denmark has a long history of providing social welfare services. Taxes levied at all levels of government paid for the services. The Health Act of 2005 reorganized the administration of the Danish health care system along three administrative levels. Implemented in 2007, the Ministry of Health and Prevention now oversees all health policy and sets goals for health care delivery. The regional authorities administer and deliver hospital services, while the local authorities purchase those services using state block grants.

Unlike the Canadian county-based system, the new regional authorities have no power to levy taxes. National health care tax revenues make up 81% of the funding for the Danish health care system. The government funds the regional authorities through state block grants. Copayments make up the remaining 19% of the overall health care budget. These payments cover mainly pharmaceutical products, dentistry, and physiotherapy for the majority of residents. About one-third of Danish residents purchase complementary insurance to cover these services. The popularity of supplementary insurance is increasing due to tax incentives for employer-based coverage.

The overwhelming majority of hospitals in Denmark (98%) are publicly funded and operated. There are about 3400 general practitioners in Denmark, and each cares for approximately 1600 patients. The distribution of general practitioners is regulated according to population size in a narrow geographic area to ensure an even distribution across the country. Entry is tightly restricted-not only must general practitioners complete sixty months of training, but they can only enter practice by purchasing the goodwill of a retiring physician or obtaining permission from the regional authorities. One-third of general practitioners have a private solo practice, while the others work in some form of group practice.

Health care providers at public health care facilities are salaried civil servants. General practitioners and private specialists are self-employed but bargain collectively through the Association of Private Specialists to contract for services with the regional authorities. General practitioners are paid on a mixed capitation and fee-for-service basis. The same fee schedule applies to all patients in both systems; however, as providers do not receive a capitation payment for the smaller of the two Danish health insurance plans, they are allowed to charge these patients a reasonable fee. The approximately 1200 specialists also negotiate a fee schedule but receive no capitation payments.

Insurance is a Must

Danish residents must choose between one of two health insurance plans. Ninety-eight percent of residents choose Group 1 insurance. These patients have open access to their general practitioner but must get a referral from their general practitioner to access specialist or hospital care (except to see an Ear, Nose and Throat doctor, an ophthalmology specialist, or to seek emergency care). Group 2 patients can access specialist care without a referral but must pay a copayment for all non-hospital-based services. Both groups must obtain a referral to access hospital services. Generally, patients are free to choose the hospital where they would like to receive care. In the event that a patient must wait longer than one month for public hospital care, the government will finance treatment at a private or foreign hospital. Patients may choose a new general practitioner every six months. Children under 16 years of age are covered under the same insurance as their parents. At 16, they are enrolled automatically in Group 1 unless they opt for Group 2 coverage. Reimbursement for pharmaceutical products is based on individual needs and also depends on the patient's prior consumption in the previous year. About 30% of residents purchase private insurance to cover statutory copayments.

The country spends 30.7% of its GDP on social protection programs. Welfare programs for the aging and vulnerable, disadvantaged, or socially excluded groups are key targets. Local government authorities provide long-term care services, financed through local taxes and state block grants.

FRANCE

France has universal health care, with few waiting lists. France has the highest level of satisfaction with their health care among all European countries. France provides a basic, universal health insurance through large occupation-based funds. The General National Health Insurance Scheme covers 83% of French workers, while other occupational specific (e.g.: for agricultural workers, for the self-employed, for miners, etc.) cover the remainder. About 99% of individuals are covered by this universal health insurance system. Copayment rates for most services are 10%-40%. About 92% of French residents have complementary private health insurance. "Proportion of the population with private health insurance" and the degree of cost sharing are key determinants of how severe waiting lists will be. France is the third most expensive health care system (~11% of GDP). While the system has generally been well funded, in 2005 the health care system ran a €11.6 billion deficit and in 2006 the health care system had a €10.3 billion deficit.

The French government provides health care for all 64 million residents under its jurisdiction. The vast majority of health insurance revenue, 88.1% in 2000, came from the general social contribution tax and the contributions of employers and employees. Each resident pays a general social contribution based on total income. The health insurance rate for earned income, capital gains, and gambling winnings is 5.25%, while benefits such as pensions or social allowances are taxed at a rate of 3.95%. Earnings-based contributions are levied at 0.75% of gross earnings. The remaining funds are provided through state subsidies and specifically earmarked taxes, such as car usage and alcohol and tobacco consumption. Pharmaceutical companies also contribute, mainly via a tax on advertising.

Three insurance funds make up the French health care system:

(1) the national health insurance fund for salaried workers (85.6% of the population),
(2) the agricultural scheme (7.2% of the population), and
(3) the national health insurance fund for independent professionals.

Under the statutory health insurance plan, the reimbursement of health care costs accounts for 84.9% of total expenditures. The remaining 15.1% is paid out as cash allowances for maternity, illness, work-related injuries, or disability. Reimbursements are made either to the patient, who paid out-of-pocket, or to the provider. To cover the cost of "copayments", i.e. the cost of coverage that is not reimbursed under the statutory health insurance scheme, 86% of the population purchased voluntary health insurance in 2000.

Approximately 4000 hospitals operate in France. Public hospitals account for about 25% of all hospitals. Non-profit private hospitals number 1400, about one-third of all French hospitals. Private for-profit hospitals are most numerous at 1750, but tend to specialize in particular medical, surgical, or obstetric procedures.

The number of general practitioners and specialists in France is almost evenly split-of the 194,000 physicians in France in 2000, 51% were specialists and 49% provided primary care. One-half of specialists and 29% of general practitioners are salaried, both working mostly in the hospital setting. Notably, private general practitioners in France still make home visits, which account for about 25% of their care activities. Providers receive payment from patients at the time of service; thus, providers negotiate with insurance schemes over the unit value to apply to the fee schedule to determine the rate of each procedure. Single residents whose taxable income falls below a certain amount per year (€8774 for 2008-09) are entitled to free coverage. The system is quite liberal in that patients may choose to see any licensed practitioner at any time without limit. The French average 4.7 contacts with a general practitioner, and not necessarily the same one, each year.

To make consumers price sensitive at the time the service is provided, most patients pay the full cost of services out-of-pocket and request reimbursement from the statutory plan, with the exception of those requiring hospitalization and low-income beneficiaries under the Universal Health Care Act. Typically, patients receive only partial reimbursement and thus pay the equivalent of a copayment for services. Patients without supplementary insurance typically receive a reimbursement rate of 70% for physician and dentist services and 60% for auxiliary and laboratory services. There are exemptions for patients with a certain chronic or debilitating health status, those receiving a certain type of care, or due to the status of the patient (such as pregnant women or those injured in the workplace). Out-of-pocket payments accounted for 11.1% of total health care expenditures in 2000.

Physician Compensation

French doctors are paid by the national health insurance system based on a centrally planned fee schedule, but doctors can charge whatever price they want. The fees are based on an up-front treatment lump sum, which is similar to DRGs in the U.S. The patient—or their private insurance—must make up the difference between the fee charged by the doctor and the amount paid for by the universal health care system. The average French doctor earns only €40,000, although medical school is free for them and the French legal system is fairly tort-averse. However, the program is threatened by increasing costs and may be forced to resort to rationing in the future." The French have a fair amount of choice in which doctors they choose. However, recently the French have moved towards a more "managed care" practice style where patients have a "preferred doctors" who acts as a gatekeeper for specialists.

The WHO has ranked France as the best health care system in the world. Yet even France must address challenges relating to sustainable financing and meeting growing demand due to aging populations.

ITALY

While France may have the highest rated health care system in the world, Italy is second according to the WHO. The Italian health care system is a decentralized version of the British NHS. Despite the high rankings by the WHO, Italians are dissatisfied with the quality of their care. Italians believe more patient choice will improve quality. Funding is based on a regressive payroll tax. The tax starts at 10.6% of income for the first €20,660 and drops to 4.6% of income between €20,51 and €77,480. The rest of the funding comes from federal and regional general taxation. The regions are responsible for health care provision. The Ministry of Health funds these regions according to a formula based on weighted capitation and past spending.

Private health insurance in Italy is uncommon, but is occasionally offered by employers. It is not possible to opt out of the National Health Insurance system and insurance premiums are not tax deductible. Many Italians do pay for private health care. It is estimated that about 35% of Italians use at least some private health services, but the public sector certainly dominates the private in terms if its relative importance.

Italians have limited choice of their physician but more than in the UK or in Spain. They must register with a general practitioner (GP). For any specialist services, patients must get a referral from their GP. Inpatient and primary care are free. For tests, diagnostic procedures and prescription drugs, copayments are as high as 30%. However, 40% of the population (e.g.: the elderly, pregnant women, kids) are exempt from these copayments. There is a shortage of medical technology in Italy. The U.S. has twice as may MRI units per million than Italy and 25% more CT scanners.

Waiting times are fairly long for diagnostic tests. The average wait for a mammogram is 70 days, for endoscopy 74 days. Tanner notes that: "Ironically, the best-equipped hospitals in northern Italy have even longer waiting lists since they draw patients from the poorer southern regions as well."

GERMANY

The most significant difference between Germany's health care system and that of other countries is its use of sickness funds. All Germans with incomes under €46,300 are required to enrol in one of the sickness funds. Those with higher incomes can either join a sickness fund themselves or opt out and instead buy private insurance. Percent Insured is 99.6% (There are about 300,00 uninsured individuals) Approximated 9% of Germans have supplemental insurance. The private, supplemental insurance covers items not paid for in the sickness fund benefit package. As mentioned above, only middle- and upper-class individuals can opt-out of the sickness funds. Of those eligible to opt out, only about 1/4 of individuals do decide to opt-out.

Germany has a population of 82.4 million with a life expectancy of 81.9 years in women and 78.7 years in men. In 2004, Germany spent US $ 3635 per person on health care. The US $ 300 billion total represents 10.6% of the GDP. Prior to 2007, the Social Health Insurance system covered approximately 88% of the population (72.5 million people), while 9.7% (8 million) purchased private health insurance in the marketplace. The remaining citizens were covered through other special state programs, such as care for military personnel. Germany has approximately 200,000 uninsured residents.

The German system, known as the Bismarck model, is the oldest in the world and was established in 1883.

2007 reform had four target goals:

(1) mandatory universal health insurance coverage;
(2) improvement of medical care;
(3) modernization of sickness funds; and
(4) reform of the health fund, the base of health care financing in Germany.

Emphasis on Equal Access

The current policy emphasizes solidarity, i.e. the idea that all citizens should have equal access to high quality health care, regardless of ability to pay. Health care financing in Germany currently follows an internal subsidy model. In this system, consumers pay both their solidarity tax and health insurance directly to the applicable sickness fund. The sickness fund then remits the solidarity fund contribution to the government health fund, while the solidarity fund distributes premium subsidies to the sickness funds. At present, the government subsidizes premiums for certain low-income or special classes of residents, in keeping with the solidarity principle. Basically, the total government subsidy to the sickness funds equals the difference between the aggregate solidarity contributions and premium subsidies. On average, though, employees contribute 7.6% of their salary for health insurance and employers contribute 6.6%.

Insurance plans that run at a deficit have the option of levying an additional premium on the insured, but it is capped at 1% of gross income. However, if the plan imposes the second premium, the insured is immediately free to change plans.

The 2007 financing reform has several goals. First, it attempts to increase transparency for consumers. It also standardizes the contribution rate for the mandatory insurance program. Flat-rate contributions already exist for long-term care, retirement, and unemployment insurance; now they will exist for the mandatory insurance program. The reform also tries to ensure equitable risk-sharing by risk-adjusting capitation payments. More importantly, the reform increases competition among insurers. For example, insurers have additional tools, such as discount negotiation rights and optional contribution rates, to increase their ability to economize.

Public and Private Sectors

Both public and private providers deliver in-patient hospital care. The majority of hospitals are enrolled in a hospital plan, which means that hospitals receive funding through the same mechanisms no matter the ownership. Sickness funds provide approximately 93% of the total funds, covering recurrent expenditures and maintenance costs. In addition, the sixteen state governments plan investments in hospitals, which are financed by both the state and local governments. These investments cover the remaining 7% of hospital financing. Hospital reimbursements are based on the German diagnosis-related groups. DRG over- or under-payments are adjusted marginally, at 65% withholding in the subsequent year and 60% reimbursement at years end, respectively.

German physicians number 133,000; of those, 118,000 are authorized providers in the Statutory Health Insurance system. Half of these providers are family practitioners, while the other 59,000 provide specialty care.

The 2007 Reforms

Currently, certain classes of citizens are insured by law. Workers who earn less than US$60,000 per year as well as pensioners, students, and persons who are unemployed, disabled, poor, or homeless are covered under the Social Health Insurance system. All insured in this system have equal access to benefits and services—in fact, statutory plans cannot refuse any applicant. Benefits include inpatient and outpatient care, all necessary medication, rehabilitation therapy, and even dental benefits. These plans include family insurance, so unemployed spouses and children of workers are coinsured for no additional charge. Access to private insurance is limited. Individuals who have made more than US $ 60,000 per year for three consecutive years or the self-employed may opt-out of social insurance and purchase private insurance instead. Civil servants are eligible for a 50% reimbursement on their health care costs if they purchase private insurance to cover the remainder. However, choosing private insurance coverage may be disadvantageous. In addition to risk-based premiums for all family members, opting for private coverage makes reenrolling in the social system difficult.

All eligible applicants must be accepted, and physicians have an obligation to treat. If patients are unable to pay their premiums, the welfare system will cover the payments. In addition, private insurance premiums will be capped at the average maximum contribution in the statutory system.

ISRAEL

The health care system in Israel has evolved into a highly technologically advanced system that provides universal coverage to all of its 6.4 million residents. Israelis enjoy high life expectancy at birth, reaching 82.6 and 78.5 years for females and males, respectively. The infant mortality rate is low, with 5.4 deaths per 1000. Israel spends approximately US $ 1890 per person on health care, which comprises about 9.1% of the GDP. The population growth in Israel has been due in large part to immigration. Today, 80% of the population is Jewish, with people of Arab descent comprising another 15%, and Christians and Druze making up the rest. Although the various populations have differences in health status, the health system itself does not differentiate between them.

Although the government provides universal coverage for its residents, it rations care to control costs, as do many nations. Government mandates do not offer totally comprehensive health care coverage. The national health insurance plans do not cover adult dental services, private physician fees, or privately ordered medications.

Employer contributions, tax revenues from residents and the national budget fund the Israeli health care system. Funding for health services primarily comes from two sources: (1) a monthly health insurance tax of up to 4.8% of income; and (2) employer contributions. The government also subsidizes health care costs through allocations in the national budget. Consumers make no premium payments by law. The National Insurance Institute serves as the central collection point and allocates the monies to the four sickness funds based on a capitation model. Premiums paid to each fund are risk-adjusted according to member age and disease status.

Sickness funds receive 3.5 times more money per person aged 75 years or older than for younger members. The plans also receive additional premiums payments for five specific diagnoses: (1) thalassemia; (2) Gaucher's disease; (3) end-stage renal disease; (4) multiple sclerosis; and (5) HIV/AIDS.

The sickness funds are precluded from denying any eligible applicant, as often as every twelve months. Enrollment periods begin on the first day of January and July of every year.

The sickness funds share risk with consumers through copayments, which are quite high compared to those in the European community.

A total of 354 general and specialty hospitals operate in Israel. The government network of hospitals provides approximately half of all beds in the country. The sickness funds also provide primary and secondary care through a number of outpatient clinics and other health-related centers.

Most of Israel's 26,000 physicians work as salaried employees of hospitals and sick funds. Israel has a physician-population ratio of 4.6 physicians per 1000 residents.

The Israeli government provides its citizens with universal coverage for a specific bundle of health care services, noted above. Patients unable to afford co-payments are not denied access; instead, government subsidies ensure that care is provided based on need, not ability to pay. Approximately 50% of the population chooses to purchase supplementary insurance to cover services not offered through sickness funds. The same insurance companies that administer the sickness funds are permitted to sell supplementary plans. Patients who purchase these plans tend to be wealthier and better-educated.

Like many developed nations, Israel's health system faces challenges due to rising health care costs and the aging population. Older adults in Israel make up 19.5% of the total population—a proportion higher than any country in the European Union or in the United States.

JAPAN

Japan has universal health insurance based around a mandatory, employment-based insurance. "The Employee Health Insurance Program requires all companies with 700 or more employees to provide workers with health insurance among some 1,800 'society-managed' plans. Nearly 85% of these plans cover a single company... Most of the rest of are industry-based. Small business workers join a government-run small business national insurance plan. The self-employed and retirees are covered by the Citizens Insurance Program administered by municipal governments. Japan has very generous health insurance benefits, significant provider choice, and high quality medical technology, but costs are not as high in the U.S. One reason for this is a significant level of cost sharing. The average Japanese household spends $2300 per year on out-of-pocket health care expenses (this figure excludes the payroll taxes used to finance health insurance premiums). Other reasons for lower health care costs is a healthy life-style, a lower incidence of disease and a general Japanese cultural aversion towards invasive procedures.

Another reason for lower costs is that the Japanese government sets a reimbursement fee schedule for all physician services. This has resulted in "assembly line medicine" where "two-thirds of patients spend less than 10 minutes with their doctor; 18 percent spend less than 3 minutes."

The health insurance plans are funded by an 8.5% (for large business) or an 8.2% (for small-businesses) payroll tax. The small business national health insurance program is also supplemented by government funds. Private supplemental insurance pays for less than 1% of health care costs. Hospital physicians are salaried employees but non-hospital physicians are paid on a fee-for-service basis. Hospitals and clinics are privately owned but the government sets the fee schedule, just as it does for private physicians. The fee-setting system, however, is very corrupt since there are over 3000 procedures whose price needs to be set. For instance, in 2004, a group of dentists was indicted for bribing the fee-setting board." Copayments are 10% to 30%, but generally closer to 30%. Copayments are capped at $677 per month for the average family.

Waiting times are a significant problem at the best hospitals. Many hospitals have been known to accept "under the table" payment to see patients quicker. Thus, the market may be working, whether or not policy-makers want it to do so.

Japan has a population of about 127.3 million, and the third largest economy in the world. The Health Insurance Law of 1922 first provided public health insurance to private sector employees. Now, Japan has broad health insurance coverage, featuring a private delivery system with a public financing scheme. The Ministry of Health, Labour and Welfare performs functions related to policy development, data collection, and health status and sector monitoring. The Ministry administers some of Japan's health insurance funds and undertakes quality and cost control initiatives. Among its most important functions is regulating the social insurance funding system. The Ministry facilitates negotiations about reimbursement levels. A national, fixed reimbursement schedule is one of the hallmark cost-containment measures in Japan. Nearly all health services are paid at the same fee-for-service rate, no matter who provides them or where they were provided. Certain hospitals, mostly long-term care or geriatric facilities, are reimbursed according to both the fee-for-service schedule and the Japanese diagnosis-procedure combination (DPC) group.

Consumers do not have a choice of plan. Premiums vary based on income even though the entitlements and their reimbursement rates are standard. All plans, however, contribute to the elderly care pool according to the proportion of elderly enrolled in a plan compared to the national average. For example, if the national average of elderly enrolment across plans is 9% and the elderly population of Plan A equals 3%, then Plan A would contribute 3 times more to the elderly care pool, in order to bring its costs in line with the national average.

Patient cost sharing varies based on age, income, and disease status. Premiums can vary from 6-9.5% of monthly income, while copayments typically range from 10-30%. All residents, with the exception of children, the elderly, and those with certain chronic diseases, have a 30% copayment. Most of those aged 70 and older contribute a 10% copayment. Children age 3 or younger pay 20%. The government insulates patients from excessive costs by capping copayments based on patients' ages and incomes.

A twenty-member council composed of payors, providers, and academics set the new reimbursement levels. More than 3000 service fees are revised individually to control utilization rates. Typically, fees for high-tech or over-utilized services are decreased—even below cost—to discourage their use, while rates for under-utilized, necessary services, typically found in ambulatory care, increase and even exceed cost.

94% 'Clinics' are Private

One-third of Japanese physicians work in office-based practices, called clinics. Ninety-four percent of the clinics are privately operated. Because these practitioners rarely have hospital admitting privileges, they tend to focus on primary care. The remaining two-thirds of physicians are hospital staff members and, with the exception of the physician owners, receive fixed salaries. Because hospital-based physicians are salaried and do not share hospital profits, they have little incentive to provide care based on profitability. Physicians also own a majority of the hospitals in Japan—in fact, the chief executive officer of any hospital must be a physician. Approximately 80% of hospitals are privately operated; however, the most prestigious are public sector or university-owned hospitals. In addition to their acute care function, many hospitals in Japan have long-term care units. Some have become *de facto* nursing homes. Reimbursement through the fixed fee schedule is the only method available. Balance billing is strictly prohibited. Moreover, should a physicians give unlisted care, the patient is responsible,

Patients have free access to any provider at any time. Lower-income patients pay a larger percent of their total income toward premiums and copayments, even with government assistance. The regressive nature of the system may make health care less affordable as costs continue to rise. More than one-third of all health expenditure is spent on health care for the elderly. At 30% copayments on top of employment-related taxes, Japanese patients bear a high burden of their health care costs.

NETHERLANDS

A country of approximately 16.6 million, the Netherlands recently enacted changes to its health insurance system. The Health Insurance Act 2006 is the most current of a string of market-oriented reforms that began in the early 1990s.

Dutch residents are required to purchase two kinds of health-related insurance: (1) insurance under the 2006 Health Insurance Act; and (2) insurance under the Exceptional Medical Expenses Act. Financing for the new system primarily comes from two sources. Employees contribute one-half of all revenues directly to the risk equalization fund through an income-based contribution calculated at 7.2% (or 4.4% for the self-employed and elderly) of the first €31,200 of annual income (2008). Employers are responsible for deducting the contribution directly from wages or allowances. Individual adults contribute 45% of the costs of the system in the form of community-rated premiums fixed according to province, which averaged €1100 per year in 2008. Under the 2006 Act, all adults also have a €150 per year deductible, excluding general practitioner services and maternity care. Those willing to assume more risk can lower premiums by paying a higher deductible, limited to €650 per year. For lower-income families, the state provides a "care allowance". About two-thirds of Dutch households receive the care allowance, which is triggered when the average community-rated premium exceeds a percentage of income (4% for single adults). The state also finances the premiums for children aged 18 years and younger. Private insurers may both receive funds from and pay into the risk equalization fund. The Health Care Insurance Board allocates funds to the insurers based on their case-mix severity, allocating additional funding for the high-risk insured. If, however, the insurers have low-risk insured profiles, they must pay an equalization amount back into the fund. No longer obligated to contract with every provider, insurers can negotiate for discounts with particular providers and use incentives to encourage patients to see preferred providers. Although each offers the same legally prescribed benefits package, they can adjust the coverage levels of the statutory benefits scheme. Insurers also may offer group discounts of up to 10% to members of any legal entity. However, they are not allowed to risk-adjust premium rates for consumers nor deny any applicant for basic coverage.

General Practitioners Provide Primary Care and Act as Gatekeepers

They are paid on both a capitation and consultation fee basis. Specialists receive a salary, a service fee, or both. Most work in hospitals and are self-employed. General practitioners also have expanded their traditional gatekeeper role. While each insured consumer must still register with a single general practitioner to authorize access to and coordinate care across specialties, these providers are also contracting directly with insurers, increasingly turning to integrated care. Integration with the insurance plans seeks to control costs, with forms of integration ranging from being on staff at an insurer-owned primary care center to participating in financial incentives, such as prescribing generics over brand-name drugs, and even risk-sharing. More than 90% of Dutch hospitals are privately owned; those that are publicly funded are typically university hospitals.

No one can be Denied Coverage

For those who cannot afford the premium, the government offers a subsidy to help cover the cost. To cover benefits excluded from the basic plan, such as adult dental care, eyeglasses, alternative medicine, or cosmetic surgery, 90% of consumers choose to purchase a supplementary policy. This supplementary policy does not have to be purchased from the same insurer that provides basic coverage, but patients often do purchase a combination package. Controlling costs is one of the main reasons the Dutch enacted health care reform. Health care costs are projected to increase to 5.5% annually during 2008-11. The government intends the reform to slow this growth and even reduce health spending.

The government hopes to combat premium defaults by allowing premiums to be deducted directly from wages or allowance, as are the income-related contributions. The penalty for triggering this mechanism will consist of paying a premium higher than any in that market. Also, even in light of the risk equalization payments, risk selection is a concern. Should the risk equalization formula prove inadequate, insurers will attempt to select only healthy, low-risk consumers into their risk pool. Finally, now that the Dutch have an institutional framework encompassing both universal coverage and managed competition, the Netherlands must develop quality, integrated delivery networks that meet consumer preferences.

SWEDEN

The goal of health care in Sweden is to provide equal access to good quality health care for all of its nine million citizens. Quite successful in meeting this goal, the Swedish system is the model of an effective and efficient universal health care system. Sweden delivers high-quality care at a modest cost. The country consistently ranks at or near the top for nearly all health outcomes when compared to other industrialized countries, with a particularly low infant mortality rate of 3 per 100,000 live births and a particularly high life expectancy (78 years for men and 82.8 years for women in 2005). while the United States spends US $ 5267 per capita on health care, Sweden spends less than half that amount (US $ 2517 per capita) yet achieves vastly better health outcomes.

The county councils' mandate includes purchasing health care delivery. Altogether, the county councils are responsible for nine regional hospitals, seventy county and provincial hospitals, and 1000 health centers across the country. While the councils have broad power to provide and manage the delivery of health care, health policy directives are made at the national level in Government and Parliament.

Health care costs consume approximately 9% of the total Swedish GDP (US $ 196.8 billion). Seventy-one percent of funds are raised through local income taxes levied by the county councils, taxed, on average, at 11% of income. The state subsidizes approximately 16% of overall health care costs through national taxation. Patient contributions account for a mere 3% of all health care funds, with the remaining 10% coming from other sources. Private providers deliver only about 10% of health care services, mainly in primary care.

Referrals may be Necessary

Within their own county council, patients are generally free to choose where to receive care. Referrals may be necessary if a patient wishes to receive care outside the home region, but referrals to specialists are not required within the council's jurisdiction. Prior to 2005, patients in Sweden experienced scheduling delays exceeding three months for pre-planned care such as cataract or hip replacement surgery. Patient dissatisfaction led the county councils and national government to establish a care guarantee. The 2005 guarantee promised that, if three months expired after the provider determined the necessary care, the patient could receive care elsewhere and the home county council would pay for both the care and any associated travel expenses. The county councils also provide other relatively comprehensive services. Basic services include comprehensive dental and mental health care. Other services include sex education, family planning counseling, and abortions.

Hospitals provide a disproportionate share of primary care, exacerbated by a shortage of primary care providers and short working hours for physicians. The decentralized system creates varying levels of efficiency, quality, and patient safety across the counties. Coordinating care between the municipal and county level is also difficult. Finally, the financing system is quickly becoming less sustainable. The income tax base may not grow quickly enough to support the aging population, and the flat cost-protection ceilings may need to be reassessed according to income or realigned with the real value of services.

SWITZERLAND

Switzerland's health care spending as a percentage of GDP is second only behind the U.S. Percent Insured is 99.5%. Insurance is purchased by individuals. Individuals generally must pay the full cost of premiums, but the government helps to finance insurance purchases for the poor. Thus, the Swiss government only pays for 24.9% of health care costs (compared with 44.7% in the U.S.). According to a WHO study, Switzerland ranks second only to the U.S. in terms of the ability of patients to choose their provider. This has lead to the Swiss paying for 31.5% throughout of pocket expenses.

The cantons generally fall within one of four regions, based on the predominant languages of French, German, Italian, or Romansh. Cultural differences among the regions are also evident in health care. Utilization varies significantly, with the French-speaking region often having the highest health services density and specialist utilization.

Although the federal tier of government set the standard basket of benefits required for each resident under the Federal Health Insurance Law, the organization and administration of the health care system falls within the purview of the cantons. Cantons are responsible for regulating and financing health care as well as accrediting hospitals. The cantons also engage in disease prevention and health regulation. The cantonal authorities delegate responsibility for nursing and home care services to the 3000+ local authorities under their collective jurisdiction.

Sickness funds collect most of the financing directly from the insured. All members of a fund contribute a flat premium based on broad age categories (0 to 18 years; 19 to 25 years; and 26+ years). Although the contribution is determined according to age group, it is not truly risk-adjusted, as it is community-rated and not modified directly based on disease status or health risk. In addition, premiums are regressive in that they are not based on ability to pay. In fact, only one-third of funds collected are based on ability to pay. However, those whose premiums exceed 8-10% of their income receive state assistance. Consumers are allowed to hedge risk and take a higher deductible for a decrease in premiums.

Most of the tax monies for health care are levied and collected at the cantonal and local levels of government. The Confederation contributes a mere 20% to the overall budget. The level of acceptable costs for which the government will provide subsidies is the funds' actual costs. The subsidies are given retrospectively. Although the sickness funds provide nearly half of the direct cost reimbursement, patient contributions, through premiums and copayments, make up 65% of total health care financing, according to WHO data from 1997.

Some funds offer plans through life insurance companies, which may inquire into health status. Others use managed care and physician gatekeepers to control cost. As in the United States, sickness funds are sometimes able to deny coverage for certain treatments. Some even go so far as to close offices in high-cost, unprofitable cantons. Competition among payors varies mostly on premium price and deductible levels, since the basic benefits package is set in law. All of the funds now offer HMO-style insurance for which the premiums are approximately 10-20% less expensive.

Two preferred provider models are relevant in Switzerland. In the first, physicians generally work on a salary basis for the insurance fund itself. While the fund-owned model is most common, physician-owned HMOs do exist. The second model is a network of independent providers who act as gatekeepers for the sickness fund to prevent unnecessary hospitalizations. The physicians are independent providers who contract with the funds under a risk-sharing agreement. The network physicians share in the yearly profit or loss. Losses are capped at SwF 10,000 per physician per year. Hospitals are excluded from managed care arrangements.

Coverage ranges from inpatient and ambulatory care to unlimited inpatient nursing home and hospital stays for the elderly and physically and mentally handicapped or disabled. Diagnostic and pharmaceutical treatments as well as complementary and alternative medicine are also guaranteed. Services that are not already included must be appropriate, clinically effective, and cost-effective to be offered as part of the standard benefits package.

Typically, between forty and seventy sickness funds operate in a given canton. Shopping around for the best rate is encouraged. Coverage for family members is not included in the standard benefits package, but sickness funds have low premiums for dependent children. Consumers are free to switch sickness funds twice yearly-open enrolment occurs as of the first of January and July. Funds must notify members of premium increases two months in advance. Should a fund increase member premiums, enrollees must give the plan one-month advance notice that they intend to switch.

Approximately 70% of the population in Switzerland purchases non-mandatory, supplemental health insurance for additional benefits not covered by the standard scheme.

GREAT BRITAIN

Great Britain represents all that is good and bad with centralized, single-payer health care systems. Health care spending is fairly low (7.5% of GDP) and very equitable. Long wait lists for treatment, however are endemic and rationing pervades the system. Patients have little choice of provider and little access to specialists. Percent Insured is 100%. 10% of Britons have private health insurance. Private health insurance replicates the coverage provided by the NHS, but gives patients access to higher quality care, and reduced waiting times. Most physicians and nurses are government employees. In 2004, the NHS negotiated lower salaries for doctors in exchange for reduced work hours. Few physicians are available at night or on weekends. Because of low compensation, there is a significant shortage of specialists. There are no deductibles and almost no copayments except for small copayments for prescription drugs, as well as for optical and dental care.

The National Health Service Act of 1946 set the framework for the health services finance and delivery system of the United Kingdom (UK). The National Health Service (NHS) began operating in 1948 under the principle that the state had the collective responsibility to provide equal access to a comprehensive health system free at the point of service. The central government sets health priorities for NHS as a whole and controls the overall pool of funds; NHS authorities, in turn, provide planning guidance to the health authorities in terms of service and financial networks. The ten strategic health authorities manage health care and disburse funds on a regional basis, linking the Department with the NHS.

Primary Care is Assured

The NHS is divided into primary and secondary care services. Primary care services are delivered by primary care trusts. The primary care trusts contract with local general practitioners, surgeons, dentists, and opticians to delivery primary care. These trusts receive about 75% of the overall NHS budget. Secondary care, or acute care, essentially refers to either emergent or elective care. Acute trusts manage the delivery of care in hospitals and ensure that hospitals deliver care efficiently. The 209 NHS hospital trusts oversee 1600 NHS hospitals and specialty care centers. With a budget of more than £90 billion, the NHS is the largest publicly funded health system in the world.

In 2006, 87% of health spending was financed by public funds—nearly 80% of the total budget is disbursed to primary care trusts. The Consolidated Fund of general tax revenues provided 81.5% of NHS financing in 1997. National Insurance contributions comprised another 12.2%. Patient charges accounted for 2.1%, and the remaining 4.2% came from repayments of NHS trust interest bearing debt (3.0%) and other sources (1.2%). That year, private funds accounted for 14.6% of total health expenditures.

The trusts are responsible for assessing the health care needs of its population and contracting for the appropriate level of services to meet those needs, all within a fixed budget. Private health insurance is mainly of two kinds: employment-based and individual insurance. More than half of those with private insurance have employer-based plans—around 59%. Individuals may purchase private insurance in the market, which is how 31% of those with private plans acquired them. The final 10% is comprised of umbrella organizations whose members voluntarily purchase coverage. Private coverage is drastically skewed toward those of higher socio-economic status. Only 10.8% of the population had private insurance in 1996.

General practitioners are the entry point to the NHS. More than 99% of the population has a registered general practitioner, and about 90% of all patient contact is with a general practitioner. These providers are generally self-employed—they work for the NHS as independent contractors rather than salaried employees. Contract negotiations occur between doctors' representatives and the government. Very little primary care in the UK is privately offered. District general hospitals are the foundation of hospital care in the United Kingdom. These hospitals are widely disbursed throughout NHS. Highly specialized tertiary facilities operate on more regional or supra-regional levels. Patients enter tertiary care facilities after being referred from the district hospitals. Community hospitals often provide long-term care, particularly for the elderly. More than 300 private hospitals operate in the United Kingdom. At times, NHS patients do have access to these private facilities.

Patients are free to choose their general practitioner within their region. Only through their general practitioner do patients have access to specialist care, unless in an emergency situation. The NHS does allow patients to upgrade their services without acquiring private insurance. Patients may receive an "amenity room," typically a private room, through the NHS for an additional fee. For privately insured patients who need care, NHS trusts also may offer these "pay beds" at NHS facilities.

Waiting Times: Waiting lists are a huge problem in Great Britain. Some examples: 750,000 are on waiting lists for hospital admission; 40% of cancer patients are never able to see an oncologist; there is explicit rationing for services such as kidney dialysis, open heart surgery and care for the terminally ill. Further, minimum waiting times have been instituted to reduce costs. "A top-flight hospital like Suffolk Est PCT was ordered to impose a minimum waiting time of at least 122 days before patients could be treated or the hospital would lose a portion of its funding."

SPAIN

The Spanish have one of the most centralized health care systems in the world. Patients have no choice of provider and there is almost no cost sharing. Like most centralized systems without cost-sharing, there are significant waiting times for procedures. This has resulted in a two-tiered system where 12% of the population receives higher quality care by purchasing private insurance. Spain ranks #7 on the WHO health care rankings and the Spanish are the second-most satisfied with the quality of their health care in Europe (behind France). Percent Insured is 98.7%. About 12% of the population has private health insurance (about 25% of people living in Madrid or Barcelona have private health insurance). Like in other countries, we see evidence of a two-tiered system. Private insurance payments account for 21% of total heat care expenditures. Further, a fair number of Spaniards pay out-of-pocket for care outside the national healthy system. Because of lower physician pay, Spain has fewer doctors and nurses per capital than most OECD countries. Spaniards can not choose their physician. They are assigned a primary care doctor who must refer the patient in the case that specialist services are needed. Patients are not allowed to change doctors unless they have private insurance. According to Tanner, "This has sparked an interesting phenomenon whereby sick Spaniards move in order to change physicians or find networks with shorter waiting lists." There are few copayments except for prescription drugs. Spain has about one-third as many MRI and CT units as the U.S.

Waiting lists are a significant barrier to care in Spain. The average wait to see a specialist in Spain is 65 days. Waiting times for procedures are also long, up to 62 days for a prostectomy and 123 days for a hip replacement. Rehabilitation and convalescence are not covered. Those with terminal illnesses are generally the responsibility of the patient's relatives.

NORWAY

All Norwegians are insured by the National Insurance Scheme. This is a universal, tax-funded, single-payer health system. Compared to France, Italy, Spain and Japan, Norway has the most centralized system. Percent Insured is 100%. All Norwegian citizens and residents are covered. The National Insurance Scheme is funded by general tax revenues. There is no earmarked tax for health care. The Norwegian tax burden is 45% of GDP. The government sets a global budget limiting overall health expenditures and capital investment. Norwegians can opt out of the government system and pay out-of-pocket. Many pay out-of-pocket and travel to a foreign country for medical care when waiting lists are long. Patients choose general practitioners (GPs) from a government list. These GPs then act as gatekeepers for specialist services. Patients can only switch GPs twice per year and only if there is no waiting list for the requested GP.

Hospital and non-hospital physicians generally are paid on a salaried basis. Some specialists can receive an annual grant and fee-for-service payments. Reimbursement rates, however, are set by the government and, unlike in France, the physician can not charge higher rates than the centrally-set reimbursement rate. There are no copayments for hospitals stays or drugs. There are small copayments for outpatient treatment.

There are significant waiting times for many procedures. Many Norwegians often go abroad for medical treatments. The average weight for a hip replacement is more than 4 months. "Approximately 23 percent of all patients referred for hospital admission have to wait longer than three months for admission." Also, care can be denied if it is not deemed to be cost-effective.

PORTUGAL

Portugal is similar to Norway in that it is a very centralized health care system. Despite the fact that Portugal ranks highly according to the WHO, there is widespread discontent with the Portuguese system. Most individuals in Portugal are insured by the state-run, single-payer National Health System. However, 25% of the population is insured through an occupation-based insurance scheme. These occupation-based schemes include most government, military and telecommunication workers. "These plans were originally intended to be incorporated into the NHS, but their powerful constituencies have prevented that from occurring."

Financing of the health care system is generated from general tax revenues. Health care spending accounts for 13% of government revenues. The National Health System (NHS) has an annual global budget, but it is often exceeded by a significant amount. Individuals in the occupation-based insurance schemes pay a premium of about 1% of their salary. About 10% of the population has private insurance. Private insurance pays for hospital stays and specialist care. Because there is no guaranteed renewability, premiums are often significantly raised or customers are dropped when they have very high claims amounts.

About half of primary care doctors are government employees and the other half work in private practice. Most specialists elect to go into private practice and are paid on a contractual basis by NHS. Patients must choose doctors from a list and can only change GPs with a written application. GPs act as gatekeepers. Referrals from the patient's GP is needed to access specialist care. For most services, there is no or little copayments. For diagnostic tests, hospital admissions, specialists visits and prescription drugs, however, copayments can run up to 40% or more. Waiting times are very long in Portugal. Further, there are often long waits for specialist visits.

GREECE

Greece has an employer-based health insurance system in which all Greek employers enroll their employees in one of the "social insurance funds." Due to strict regulation by the Greek Ministry of Social Health and Cohesion, Greece in essence has a single payer system. For instance, the Ministry controls employee contribution rates, insurance benefit packages, and the types of doctors a social insurance fund can employee. Also, employers can not choose among competing sickness funds as they can in Germany, they must choose an their industry-specific social insurance fund. The National Health Service (NHS) also operates its own health care services. For instance the NHS operates hospitals and employs some physicians. One can see the NHS as a backup for the social insurance funds, but in some rural areas, the NHS is the principal provider of care.

Similar to the U.S., only 83% of Greeks have health insurance covering primary care. Most Greeks (97%) do have health insurance for hospital care. About 8% of Greeks have private health insurance but this number has been growing rapidly in recent years. Greeks must have a referral from a GP in order to receive care at a public or NHS hospital. Wait times for medical care are very long in Greece. This is likely due to the provider shortages caused by low reimbursement rates. The wait for treatment at both public and NHS hospitals can be very long. There is a six month wait for some surgeries and the wait for appointments with specialists can be as long as 150 days. Simple blood tests often take a month.

Physician Compensation. About half of physicians are employed directly by the social insurance fund. The other half are in private practice, but are contracted on a fee-for-service basis by the insurance funds. Unlike in France, no balance billing is allowed. Despite this fact, many physicians demand under the table payments in exchange for treatment. Further, physicians often "actively attempt to persuade patients to move from a doctor's sickness fund contract to the doctor's private practice. Patients who switch pay out of pocket but receive faster and better care." In fact, one estimate claimed that informal out-of-pocket payments make up 42% of health care expenditures. Pay for doctors and nurses is fairly low and thus there are severe staffing shortages. In NHS hospitals, "it has been estimated that less than half of authorized medical positions are actually filled." The U.S. has twice as many MRI units per capita and 20% more CT units per capita.

Sources

Tanner, Michael D. (2008) "The Grass Is Not Always Greener: A Look at National Health Care Systems Around the World", Cato Policy Analysis No. 613.

Gerard, F. Anderson, Uwe, E. Reinhardt, Peter, S. Hussey, and Varduhi Petrosyan, "It's The Prices, Stupid: Why The United States Is So Different From Other Countries," *Health Affairs*, Volume 22, No. 3, 2003.

James, Banks, PhD, Michael Marmot, MD, Zoe Oldfield, MSc, and James P. Smith, PhD, "Disease and Disadvantage in the United States and in England," *JAMA*, May 3, 2006, Vol. 295, No. 17:2037-2045.

Paul, Belien, Health Care Reform in Europe, Centre for the New Europe, Brussels, November 1994.

Bianca, K. Frogner and Gerard, F. Anderson, Multinational Comparisons of Health Systems Data, 2005, The Commonwealth Fund (Publication No. 825), April 2006.

OECD Health Data 2006: Statistics and Indicators for 30 Countries.

James, L. Reed, Timothy, S. Barclay, and William, J. Fox, International Approaches to a Socialized Insurance System, Arizona Health Care Cost Containment System, August 27, 2001.

Cathy, Schoen, Karen, Davis, Sabrina, K.H. How and Stephen C. Schoenbaum. "U.S. Health System Performance: A National Scorecard," *Health Affairs*, 20 September 2006.

Health Reforms: Good Primary Health Care is the Way Forward

"The health care scenario is less than satisfactory all over the world, though the developed countries offer much better care than the third world countries. It is also a fact that need for primary health care (PHC) improvement is much more than secondary ot tertiary care in all these countries. There is no doubt every society requires most modern infrastructure and technology for its sick to be treated, in case they fall seriously ill. However, preventive care and primary care assumes greater significance in the context of large populations. Driven by the demographic, financial and social pressures of modernization, PHC increasingly share the aims of improved health equity, people-centered care, and a better protection of the health of their populations."

In recent years, powerful advances have been made in medicine and technology, impacting global health status worldwide. Nations across the globe are experiencing decreasing rates of child mortality, rising life expectancy and lowered incidence of chronic diseases. But the global health picture is not entirely positive. HIV/AIDS incidence still climbs, inadequate care for rural populations still prevails and access to essential medicines remains limited throughout the world. The PHC movement has seen a critical success in that it has contributed to the recognition of the social value of health systems, which has now taken hold in most countries in the world. This change of mindset has created a radically different health-policy landscape. Present-day health systems are a patchwork of components, many of which may be far removed from the goals set out 30 years ago.

Priority Areas for Future Action

The WHO has identified four priority areas for future action: ensuring value for money, poverty reduction, public health policy and strengthening national capabilities for emergency relief and humanitarian assistance. There is universal trend towards greater decentralization, pro-market economic policies, rapid expansion of the private health sector, introduction of user charges, and purchaser-provider splits. Developing countries like India are still struggling to expand their health infrastructure and provide basic health facilities to the entire population. If India is to progress towards equity, equality, comprehensiveness, universal accessibility and coverage, radical institutional reforms in the health sector are needed. The potential advantage from restructuring health care is that it can be extended to those who need it most.

The current era has been a time of clear change for health care delivery systems. Recent experiences of developed countries suggest that investment in decentralized population-based systems and health services research aimed at the developing evidence-based health care, rather than the emphasis on central, disease-based systems could yield substantial health gains for the populations. Despite some progress made in reduction of birth rate, and mortality rate, and increased life expectancy, India continues to have a poor performing health system as compared to Sri Lanka, China or Singapore.

Primary Care is Declining

Primary care is not yet available to every citizen because of poor planning and implementation. Even after 55 years of independence India does not have a National Health Service and is no-where close to achieving Health For All for its people. About 40% of population lives below poverty line and an equal number of people do not have access to even basic health care. We should learn from the tigers taking every opportunity to improve health care. Emphasis should be directed on developing an enabling policy and institutional environment in the health sector, and promoting an effective health dimension to social, economic, environmental and development policy. The objective should be to reduce child mortality; improve maternal health, combat HTV/AIDS, malaria, tuberculosis and other diseases, and provide access to affordable, essential drugs. More attention should be paid towards sustaining development and reducing poverty. A healthy population is a prerequisite for growth as much as a result of it. Investing in the health of poor people and promoting pro-poor health policies and practices should be a top priority. Precious investments in people's development lead to health equity and well-being.

Hospitals are not for just Disease Management

Today's challenging health care environment demands that hospitals and health systems continuously monitor, improve and refine how they deliver patient care efficiently. There are problems with the health care system. Many of these problems will require action by policy-makers. National health policy has been developed for many years on a fragmented, incremental basis. Our nation must choose wisely to ensure both high quality care and access for all of our citizens. Prevention and health is everybody's right and responsibility.

Syed Amin Tabish MD, says (in JK-Practitioner 2003; 10(2): 163-65) that "The universal goal of the health care system is to ensure adequate access to quality care at a reasonable price. The components of this goal include access, quality and price. Each of these factors cannot be dealt with in isolation. Each component would be maximized with the goal of improving health. The purpose of health services is to secure through the resources available the greatest possible improvement in the physical and mental health of the people. This warrants health services to bring health care closer to where people live, become more responsive to the needs and wishes of patients, get the most from the resources committed to it. We all need to take stock of what humankind has achieved during the past two millennia. We also need to assess the relative significance of the achievements of the past fifty years compared with the previous 2000 and our expectations for the next 20 years. The practice of medicine is becoming increasingly complex. It combines both science and art. Science-based technology is the foundation for the solution to many clinical problems. The combination of medical knowledge, intuition, and judgment defines the art of medicine."

Political Forces/Ideologies Play a Major Role

Health services comprise of medical care and public health services and are a function of the political system of a community. Political forces/ ideologies play a major role in determining the health policies of the country through decisions on resource allocation, human resource policy, choice of technology and the degree to which health services are to be made available and accessible to the population.. Health policies can also be used as a political lever to promote certain vested market invests.

The hospital is the predominant institutional provider. The hospital consumes the largest single share of personal health care resources and in some respects is the most visible and central organization in modern health care. Recently, the growth of the ambulatory care, especially within the context of technological advances and cost pressures, is causing the hospital to lose its historical pre-eminence. It has to evolve from the centre of excellence to community support. Humanity has undoubtedly achieved a great deal over the last 2000 years. Hospitals have benefited from the new technology, but have increasingly found themselves unable to keep up with the pace of the technology change. Today, hospitals are competing to acquire cutting-edge technology that, because of the relentless pursuit of technological perfection, will be obsolete within a few years. Perfection becomes a Utopian dream that is simultaneously too expensive to achieve and expensive not to pursue. The only means of achieving this dream is to ensure we have the latest technology at all times. Health care needs and medicine's capacity to respond are not static. If is necessary to determine the true current state of hospitals in order to increase their capability to respond to the population's needs. A key element is to develop and test a methodology for describing and comparing the state of hospital systems. It will begin to identify common issues and opportunities, with important policy implications.

Ambulatory Care includes a Wide Range of Services

Ambulatory care includes a wide range of services for the "walking" or non-institutionalized patient. Ambulatory care services play a key role as the initial and continuing point of contact with the system for more people. It also serves as a centre of the referral network for specialized hospital care. . . An increasing number of people have sought primary care from hospitals, sometimes because of lack of access to other care, taxing the ability of many facilities to respond. The result has been overcrowded facilities; the wrong mix of services, equipment, and personnel to respond to patient needs; and extremely dissatisfied consumers and providers. A hospital-based ambulatory care can provide comprehensive and accessible care and remove primary care patients from emergency rooms. Many hospitals have now successfully expanded outpatient services. Long-term or chronic care, along with mental health services, represents one of the greatest challenges for the future in health care. Mental health services involve a number of unique issues. Our society has yet to accept responsibility for solving the problems involving the mental health of our nation's citizens. The emphasis on both practice guidelines and evidence-based practice has yielded a further orientation towards outcome measures as indicators of community health. Accurate, comprehensive, and timely community health data are essential requisite of goal setting and programme performance monitoring. Health information is vital. The information revolution should allow better programme management and assessment. Information technology and consumerism will transform health care worldwide.

A system approach to health care is used to emphasize the interdependencies among the parts of the system and between the system's 'hard assets' and the organizational and financial arrangements that allow the system to function. A solid understanding of the system is essential for policy-maker, provider and consumer. The dynamic and interactive nature of the system should not be forgotten during planning and policy-making. Efforts to improve services should be based on modifying each element in the system. Today's health policy decision-makers must focus on health behaviour and health behavioural change to address contemporary health issues. The changing nature of the external environment, patterns of illness, and of the system's necessary responses should be outlined.

Why Health is Given a Back Seat in Governance?

Health is important among the objectives and values of most

individual human beings and that they expect their government and administrations to pursue policies that will afford them the opportunity to attain lives of optimum duration and quality. The health of its citizens is one of the most important resources needed by a nation for the pursuit of most other legitimate national objectives. National human behaviour requires some commensuration of the benefits and costs of all the options we seek to choose. India has experienced a faster growth in demand for health and medical care than in the resources it can easily make available for meeting that demand. Demographic and epidemiological changes, technological advances, the emergence of new threats to public health and the rising aspirations for a better life that are part of the evolving political development of our species, all sharpen the need to make choices and decisions about how the responsibilities and rewards of human activity are to be distributed. The public health is important enough to warrant planning for it. Improvement in health and reduction in death rates have occurred at most stages in life from birth through to old age. We live, on average, nearly as long as our counterparts in most other middle economies and developing nations. There is need to identify those public health priorities where there is sufficient evidence to conclude that action would have a significant benefit on health. Strategies for action must follow. Priorities must include those where both the evidence and the support for action is strong, those where the case for action is strong, but more evidence of the feasibility of implementation is still needed, and those where the case for action is strong, but where detailed recommendations are yet to be evolved.

Despite the progress made during the last five decades, grey areas still exist—inequality in health, social class and disease, quality of care, ever-increasing costs, etc. However, complacency cannot be justified. The aim of Health care delivery system and health policy should be to embrace the health of the public and protect and promote the health of all citizens in the interests both of those individuals and of the community, they comprise. It involves the promotion of health, the prevention of disease, the treatment of illness, the care of those who are disabled and the continuous development of the technical and social means for the pursuit of these objectives.

The health needs of the country are enormous and the financial resources and managerial capacity available to meet them fall somewhat short. National Health Policy had to make some hard choices between various priorities and operation options. The policy, while being holistic, undertakes the necessary risk of recommending differing emphasis on different policy components. The need to ensure that "equity" in the health sector stands as an independent goal has got desired attention. An expectation of significant improvement in the quality of services, and the consequential improved health status of the communities depends not only on increased financial and material outputs but also on a more empathetic and committed attitude in the service providers.

The health services would be expected to be responsive to the needs of all; cost-effective and affordable, and of high quality; humane, caring, and culturally acceptable; innovative in provision of services and exploitation of technology; sensitive to the wide spectrum of determinants of health (from nuclear biology to socio-economics) and the environment; based on sound ethical principles that define individual responsibility as much as the state's obligation, and able to measure the outcome of the investments.

Global Health Expenditure is Rising Fast

People expect their health authorities to secure their health and improve access to care, protect them against catastrophic expenditure and financial exploitation, and guarantee an equitable distribution of resources. The growth of the health sector provides financial leverage to do so, and globalization is offering some unprecedented opportunities to make use of that leverage. Opportunity for change is largely related to the flow of new resources into the health sector.

Across the world, expenditure on health is growing: between 1995 and 2005, it almost doubled from $ 2.6 to $ 5.1 trillion. The rate of growth is accelerating: between 2000 and 2005, the total amount spent on health in the world increased by $ 330 billion on average each year, against an average of $ 197 billion in each of the five previous years. Health expenditure is growing faster than GDP and faster than population growth. The net result is that, with some exceptions, health spending per capita grows at a rate of more than 5% per year throughout the world. Expenditure across countries in per capita expenditure, ranges from less than $ 20 per capita to well over $ 6000. These disparities stratify countries into three categories: high-expenditure health economies, rapid-growth health economies, and low-expenditure, low-growth health economies. The high-expenditure health economies, not surprisingly, are those of the nearly 1 billion people living in high-income countries. In 2005, these countries spent on average $ 3752 per capita on health, $ 1563 per capita more than in 1995: a growth rate of 5.5% per year.

Meager Outlay on Health Care: Rising out of the Pocket Cost

Low-income countries in Africa and South- and South-East Asia, i.e. total of 2.6 billion inhabitants, spent a mere $ 103 per capita on health in 2005, against $ 58 in 1995. In absolute terms, the growth has been disappointingly low. In the low-expenditure, low-growth health economies, out-of-pocket payments account for the largest share of the growth, while in rapid growth and high-expenditure health economies, increased government expenditure and prepayment mechanisms dominate. Where growth in health expenditure is through pre-payment mechanisms, there is greater opportunity to support PHC reforms: collectively pooled monies are more readily re-allocated towards interventions that provide a larger health return on investment than out-of-pocket payments. Conversely, countries where growth is primarily through out-of pocket expenditures have less leverage to support PHC reforms. Alarmingly, it is in countries where expenditure is the lowest and the burden of disease highest that there is a real lack of opportunities for harnessing the growth of their health sector for PHC reforms.

High-expenditure Health Economies

This group of countries funds almost 90% of its growth in health expenditure—an extra $ 200 per capita per year in recent years through increased government and private pre-payment funds. Expanding or changing the offer of services in these countries is less constrained by finances than by the relative lack of human resources to meet rising and changing demand. Their health systems are built around a strong and prestigious tertiary care sector that is important to the heavyweights of the pharmaceutical and medical supply industries. Out-of-pocket payments, though still significant at 15% of total expenditure, have been dwarfed by more progressive collective means of financing. The third-party payment institutions have, thus, become central actors while the longstanding autonomy of the health professionals is waning. Efforts to control costs, improve quality and access to disadvantaged groups have given rise to a widening public debate on which users and special interest groups have increasing influence. Nevertheless, the state carries more weight in the health sector of these countries than ever before, with increasingly sophisticated regulatory tools and institutions. Despite worries over their long-term sustainability, the solidarity mechanisms that finance these health systems enjoy considerable social consensus. The secular trend towards extension of coverage to all citizens, and, often reluctantly, to non-citizen residents as well, continues.

Rapid-growth Health Economies

In rapid-growth health economies, the challenge of engaging PHC reforms presents itself quite differently. The growing demand that comes with increased purchasing power is fuelling an expansion of services at unprecedented speed.

Assuming current growth rates continue through to 2015, per capita health expenditure will grow by 60% in the fast-growing health economies of the Americas compared to 2005 levels. In the same time period, that expenditure will double in Europe and the Middle-East and triple in East Asia.

Low-expenditure, Low-growth Health Economies

Inclusive coverage schemes need to be complemented by efforts: (i) to identify those who are excluded and set-up specifically tailored programmes to include them; and (ii) to tackle the social determinants of health inequalities through policy initiatives that cut across a large number of sectors, so as to translate the political commitment to health equity into concrete advances. In many of these countries, the shift in point of gravity from tertiary and specialized care to primary care is well under way. Better information and technological developments are creating new opportunities—and a market—for moving much of the traditionally hospital-based care into local services staffed by primary care teams or even into the hands of patients themselves. This is fuelling a change in perception of how health services should operate. It provides support for primary care, including self-care and home care.

Technological innovation is indeed a driver of improvement and current trends show that it is expanding the range of services offered by primary care teams. Technological innovation can, however, also be a driver of exclusion and inefficiency. The marked inter-country differences in the diffusion of medical technology are a reflection, not of rational evaluation, but of the incentives to providers to adopt these technologies, and the capacity to control that adoption.

The European Union's regulatory system, plays an increasing role in the harmonization of the technical requirements for registering new medicines or of product licensing, offering possibilities, among others, for more effective support to legal provisions encouraging generic substitution for pharmaceuticals in the private sector. Such mechanisms offer opportunities to increase safety and access, and thus create an environment in which national primary care reforms are encouraged.

Norway's strategy to reduce health inequalities illustrates that there is no single solution to this complex problem. Norway has identified a large number of determinants that influence the health of individuals: income, social support, education, employment, early childhood development, healthy environments and access to health services. These complex and interrelated determinants of health are not equally distributed in society, and it is, therefore, not surprising that this leads to inequities in health as well. The Norwegian strategy focuses on:

1. Reducing social inequities;
2. Reducing inequities in health behaviours and access to health services;
3. Targeted initiatives to improve social inclusion; and
4. Cross-sectoral tools to promote a whole-of-government approach to health.

Health Care is not a Standalone Sector

Working with other sectors, such as labour and finance, can create job opportunities and taxation systems that encourage more equitable distribution and redistribution of wealth, which can have a large impact on population health. In addition to universal approaches, social inclusion interventions targeted at providing better living conditions for the most disadvantaged are also critical in reducing the gaps between the most well-off and the least well-off members of society. In the long-run, however, a more pluralistic approach will be required with teams that include a variety of professionals with the instruments to provide coordination and continuity of care. That will require a different, more varied and more flexible cadre of health workers. The sustainability of primary care reforms in the category of high spending countries is questionable without: (i) a change in paradigm of the training of health personnel; and (ii) the necessary career, social and financial incentives to move health professionals to what in the past have been less prestigious and rewarding career options. Spurred by the growing awareness of global health threats and of the stratification of health outcomes along social fault lines, there is a major renaissance in public health. The connections between health and other sectors are better understood and are bringing health to the attention of all sectors. Research and information systems, demand for public health training and new discourses on public health are occupying the centre stage of public concerns.

In England and Wales, for example, a major primary care reform included an extensive public consultation through questionnaires addressed to more than 42,000 people, while over 1,000 individuals were invited to voice their interests and concerns in public hearings. This involvement facilitated consensus on a number of contentious parts of the reform, including shifts of resources to primary care and to underserved areas, while responsibilities were redistributed to improve cooperation and coordination.

Middle Income Countries

Biases towards highly sophisticated and specialized infrastructures that cater to the expectations of a wealthy minority are being further fuelled by a new growth market in medical tourism, whereby patients from high-expenditure health economies with high-fixed costs are out-sourced to these comparatively low-cost environments. This drains the supply of professionals for primary care, encouraging unprecedented rates of specialization within the workforce. In contrast with these developments, ministries of health in many of these countries are still organized around specific disease control efforts, and are ill-equipped to use the leverage of expanding resources to regulate health care delivery. The result is all too often a two-tiered system, with highly sophisticated and specialized health infrastructure that caters to expectations of a wealthy minority, in the presence of huge gaps in service availability for a large part of the population. Reforms that emphasize universal access to people-centered primary care can help to correct such distortions. These reforms can take advantage of technological innovations that facilitate rapid, simple, reliable and low-cost access to services that were previously inaccessible because they were too expensive or required complex supportive infrastructure. Such innovations include rapid diagnostic tests for HIV and gastric ulcers, better drugs that facilitate the shift from institution-based to primary care-based mental health, and advances in surgery that either eliminate or dramatically reduce the need for hospitalization. Combined with the multiplication of evidence-based guidelines, such innovations have considerably enlarged the problem-solving capacity of primary care teams, broadening the role of non-physician clinicians and the potential of self-care. Rapid expansion of people-centred care is thus possible in a context where the technological gap between close-to-client ambulatory care and tertiary institutions is less striking than it was 30 years ago. Chile, for example, has doubled the uptake of primary care services in a period of five years, along with a massive investment in personnel and equipment ranging from emergency dental care and laboratories to home-based management of chronic pain. The impact of this transformation can be amplified by targeting and empowering the large numbers of poor and excluded in these countries and by reforming public policies accordingly. In the rapid-growth health economies of the Americas and the European region less that one-third of the expected growth on current trends is through increased out-of-pocket expenditure on health. Two-third is through increased government expenditure, in combination, in the Americas, with expanded private pre-paid expenditure. The latter also plays a growing role in the Far East, whereas in the Middle East, around 40% of the growth, on current trends, will be in out-of-pocket expenditure. Leverage of PHC reforms will depend in part on the possibility to regulate and influence private pre-paid expenditure, and, particularly in Asia, to curb the reliance on out-of-pocket expenditure. In most of these countries, the level of expenditure compared to GDP or to total government expenditure remains low, offering financial room to further accelerate PHC reforms and underpin them through parallel, and equally important, moves towards universal coverage and reduced reliance on out-of-pocket payments. In many of these countries, public resources are allocated on a capitation basis as are, at least, part of pooled private pre-payment funds. This provides opportunities to include criteria, such as relative deprivation or unmet health needs in the capitation formulas. This effectively transforms resource allocation into an instrument for promoting health equity and for introducing incentives favouring conversion towards primary care and healthier public policies.

Expanding PHC and Reducing out of Pocket Expenditure is the Key

Some of the largest countries in the world—Brazil, for example—are now seizing these kinds of opportunities on a massive scale, expanding their primary care networks while diminishing their reliance on out-of-pocket payments. Such reforms, however, rarely come about without pressure from the user's side. Chile's health policy has defined a detailed benefit package, well publicized among the population as an enforceable right. People are being informed about the kind of services, including access to specialized care, which they can claim from their primary care teams. In combination with sustained investment, such unambiguous entitlements create a powerful dynamic for the development of primary care. Managed well, they have the potential to accelerate convergence while avoiding at least part of the distortions and inefficiencies that have plagued high-income countries in earlier years.

The persistence of high levels of maternal mortality in low health countries claim close to 90% of all maternal deaths. It is perhaps the clearest indication of the consequences of the under-funding of health on the performance of their health systems. Worryingly, growth in health expenditure in these countries is low and highly vulnerable to their political and economic contexts. In fragile states, particularly in those located in Africa, health expenditure is not only low but barely growing at all, and 28% of this little amount of growth in recent years is accounted for by external aid. Health expenditure in other countries of this group is growing at a stronger average rate of 6% to 7% per year. On current trends, by 2015, per capita health expenditure will have more than doubled in India compared to 2005, and increased by half elsewhere. In many countries, this represents significant leverage to engage PHC reforms, particularly where the growth is through increased government expenditure or, as in Southern Africa, through other forms of prepayment. In India, however, more than 80% of the growth will, on current trends, be in out-of-pocket expenditure, offering much less leverage. Countries in these regions accumulate a set of problems that in all their diversity share many characteristics.

Low Priority to Health Care in Low Income Countries

Efforts to establish sound public policies that promote health and deal with determinants of ill-health are limited at best. Unregulated commercialization of both—private and public—health care is quickly becoming the norm for urban and, increasingly, for rural populations, a much bigger and more underestimated challenge to PHC's values than the verticalism that so worries the international health community. In most of these countries, the state has had, in the past, the ambition to run the health sector on an authoritarian basis. In today's pluralistic context, with a multitude of different providers, formal and informal, public and private, only few have succeeded in switching to more appropriate steer-and-negotiate approaches. Instead, as public resources stagnated and bureaucratic mechanisms failed, *laissez-faire* has become the default approach to management of the health sector.

This has resulted in few or feeble attempts to regulate commercial health care provision—not only by the private, but also within the public sector, which has, in many instances, adopted the commercial practices of unregulated private care. Health authorities are, thus, left with an unfunded mandate for steering the health sector. Therefore, growing the resource-base is a priority: to refinance resource-starved health systems; to provide them with new life through PHC reforms; and to re-invest in public leadership. Prepayment systems must be nurtured now, discouraging direct levies on the sick and encouraging pooling of resources. This will make it possible to allocate limited resources more intelligently and explicitly than when health services are paid for out-of-pocket. While there is no single prescription for the type of pooling mechanism, there are greater efficiencies in larger pools: gradual merging or federation of pre-payment schemes can accelerate the build-up of regulatory capacity and accountability mechanisms. In a significant number of these low-expenditure, low-growth health economies, particularly in sub-Saharan Africa and fragile states, the steep increase in external funds directed towards health through bilateral channels or through the new generation of global financing instruments has boosted the vitality of the health sector. These external funds need to be progressively re-channeled in ways that help build institutional capacity towards a longer-term goal of self-sustaining, universal coverage. In the past, the bulk of donor assistance has targeted short-term projects and programmes resulting in unnecessary delays, or even detracting from the emergence of the financing institutions required to manage universal coverage schemes. The renewed interest among donors in supporting national planning processes as part of the harmonization and alignment agenda, and the consensus that calls for universal access, represent important opportunities for scaling up investments in the institutional apparatus necessary for universal coverage. While reduced catastrophic expenditure on health care and universal access are sufficiently strong rationales for such change in donor behaviour, the build-up of sustainable national financing capacities also offers an eventual exit strategy from donor dependence. Governments can do more to support the health sector in these settings.

Low Allocation on Health Care

Low growth health economies allocate only a small fraction of their government revenue to health. Even in sub-Saharan African countries, which have made progress and allocated an average of 8.8% of their government expenditure to health in 2005, the Abuja Declaration target of 15% is still a long way-off. Reaching that target would increase total health expenditure in the region by 34%. Experience of the last decade shows that it is possible to increase government revenues allocated to health rapidly. For example, following rising pressure from a broad range of civil society and political movements, India's general government expenditure on health—with a specific focus on primary health care—is expected to triple within the next five years. In a different context, the Ministry of Health in Burundi quadrupled its budget between 2005 and 2007 by successfully applying for funds that became available through debt reduction under the Enhanced Heavily Indebted Poor Countries (HIPC) initiative.

On average, in the 23 countries at completion point for the HIPC and Multilateral Debt Relief Initiative (MDRI), the annual savings from HIPC debt relief during the 10 years following qualification are equivalent to 70% of public spending on health at 2005 levels. While only part of that money is to be directed to health, even that can make a considerable difference to the financial clout of public-health authorities.

Millennium Development Goals (MDGs) are Crying for Attention

Opportunities arise not only from increased resources. The preponderance of pilot projects is gradually being replaced by more systematic efforts to achieve universal access, albeit often for a single intervention or disease programme.

These high visibility programmes, developed in relation to the MDGs, have revitalized a number of concepts that are key to people-centred care. Among them are the imperative of universal access to high quality and safe care without financial penalty, and the importance of continuity of care, and the need to understand the social, cultural and economic context in which all, in Mali, the primary care network is made up of community owned, community-operated primary care centres, backed up by government-run district teams and referral units. There is a coverage plan, negotiated with the communities, which, if they so wish, can take the initiative to create a primary care centre according to a set of criteria. The commitment is important, since the health centre will be owned and run by the community: for example, the staff of the health centre, a three to four person team led by a nurse or a family doctor, has to be employed (and financed) by the local community health association. The community can make an agreement with the Ministry of Health to obtain technical and financial support from the district-health teams, for the launch of the health centre and the supervision and back up of its subsequent operation.

The model has proved quite popular, despite the huge effort communities have had to put into the mobilization and organization of these facilities: by 2007, 826 such centres were in operation (up from 360, 10 years before), set-up at an average cost of US $ 17,000. The system has proved resilient and has significantly increased the production of health care: the number of curative care episodes managed by the health centres has been multiplied by 2.1. The number of women followed up in antenatal care has been multiplied by 2.7 and births attended by a health professional by 2.5, with coverage levels as measured through Demographic Health Surveys in 2006 standing at 70% and 49%, respectively; DTP3 vaccination coverage in 2006 was 68%. People obviously consider the investment worthwhile. Twice during the last 10 years, between 2000 and 2001 and 2004 and 2005, demand and local initiative for the creation of new centres was rising so fast that Mali's health authorities had to take measures to slow down the expansion of the network in order to be able to guarantee quality standards.

Integration is becoming a reality through approaches, such as the Integrated Management of Adolescent and Adult Illness (IMAI) and the community-based interventions emerging from the Onchocerciasis Control Programme (OCP).

Global initiatives are loosening their grip on disease-control mandates and are beginning to appreciate the importance of strengthening the system more generally, such as through GAVI Alliance's Health System Strengthening window, paving the way for better alignment of previously fragmented initiatives. Driven largely by demand, information technologies to support primary care, such as electronic medical records, are spreading much faster than anticipated.

Efforts to scale up HIV treatment have helped to expose the shortfalls in key systems inputs, such as the supply chain management of diagnostics and drugs, and build bridges to other sectors, such as agriculture, given the imperative of food security. Emerging awareness of the magnitude of the workforce crisis is leading to ambitious policies and programmes, including task shifting, distance learning and the innovative deployment of financial and non-financial incentives. In this context, the challenge is no longer to do more with less, but to harness the growth in the health sector to do more with more. The unmet need in these countries is vast and making services available is still a major issue. It requires a progressive roll-out of health districts—whether through government services or by contracting NGOs, or a combination of both. Yet the complexities of contemporary health systems, particularly, but not only in urban areas, call for flexible and innovative interpretations of these organizational strategies. In many of Africa's capitals, for example, public facilities of primary, and even secondary-level have almost or completely disappeared, and have been replaced by unregulated commercial providers. Creative solutions will have to build on alliances with local authorities, civil society and consumer organizations to use growing funds—pooled private pre-payment, social security contributions, funds from municipal authorities and tax-sourced funding—to create a primary care offer that acts as a public safety net, as an alternative to unregulated commercial care, and as a signal of what trustworthy, people centred health care can look like. What eventually matters is the experience of patients accessing services. Trust will grow if they are welcomed and not turned away; remembered and not forgotten; seen by someone who knows them well; respected in terms of their privacy and dignity; responded to with appropriate care; informed about tests; and provided with drugs and not charged a fee at the point of service.

What is Critical to Health?

Effective food security, education and rural-urban policies are critical for health and health equity: the health sector's influence on these policies depends to a large extent on its performance in providing quality primary care. Mobilizing the drivers of reform across all of the diverse national contexts in which PHC reforms must find their specific expression, globalization plays a major role. It is altering the balance between international organizations, national governments, non-state actors, local and regional authorities and individual citizens. The global health landscape is not immune to these wider changes. Over the last 30 years, the traditional nation state and multilateral architecture have been transformed. Civil society organizations have mushroomed, along with the emergence of public-private partnerships and global advocacy communities identified with specific health problems. Governmental agencies work with research consortia and consulting firms as well as with non-state transnational institutions, foundations and NGOs that operate on a global scale. National Diasporas have appeared that command substantial resources and influence with remittances—about US $ 150 billion in 2005—that dwarf overseas development aid. Illicit global networks make a business out of counterfeit drugs or toxic waste disposal, and now have the resources that allow them to capture and subvert the capacity of public agencies.

Power is gravitating from national governments to international organizations and, at the same time, to sub-national entities, including a range of local and regional governments and non-governmental institutions.

Mobilizing the Production of Knowledge

PHC reforms can be spurred and kept on track by institutionalizing PHC policy reviews that mobilize organizational imagination, intelligence and ingenuity. The know-how to conduct policy reviews exists, but requires more explicit articulations. They need to refocus on monitoring such progress with each of the four interlocking sets of PHC reforms; on identifying, as they unfold, the technical and political obstacles to their advancement; and on providing the elements for course corrections, where necessary. In a globalizing world, PHC policy reviews can take advantage of the emerging within and across-country collaborative networks to build up the critical mass that can lead and implement the necessary reforms. Indeed, for many countries, it is not realistic to find, within their own institutions, all the technical expertise, contextual knowledge and necessary capacity for dispassionate analysis that PHC policy reviews require. Open, inclusive and collaborative structures, such as the Latin American observatory models, can go a long way in harnessing the diversity of national resources. Such models also make it possible to derive further benefits from international collaboration and to overcome the scarcities within a single nation's capacities. Policy-makers today are more open to lessons from abroad than they may have been in the past, and are using them to feed national policy dialogue with innovative approaches and better evidence of what works and what does not. Embedding national institutions in regional networks that collaborate around PHC policy reviews makes it possible to pool technical competencies as well as information. Importantly, it can create regional mechanisms to get more effective representation in important but labour-intensive global bodies, with less strain on scarce national resources.

Building Network of Experts for PHC

More structured and intensive inter-country collaboration around PHC policy reviews would yield better international comparative data on variations in the development of health systems based on PHC, on models of good practice and on the determinants of successful PHC reforms. Such information is currently often either absent, hard to compare or outdated. By building on networks of experts and institutions from different regions, it is possible to produce consensus-based and validated benchmarks for assessing progress and easier access to international sources of information relevant to monitoring primary care. This could make a big difference in steering PHC reforms. Various initiatives in this direction, such as the Primary Health Care Activity Monitor for Europe (PHAMEU), a network of institutes and organizations from 10 European Union Member States, or the Regional Network on Equity in Health (EQUINET), a network of professionals, civil society members, policy-makers, and state officials in Southern Africa, are promising steps in that direction. There is a huge research agenda with enormous potential to accelerate PHC reforms that requires more concerted attention. Yet, currently, the share of health expenses devoted to determining what works best—to health services research—is less that 0.1% of health expenditure in the United States, the country that spends the highest proportion (5.6%).

Now, as the global health community moves away from vertical disease control, operational research is facilitating the shift. Recent studies involving 2.5 million people in 35 health districts in three countries have demonstrated that the community-directed treatment methods developed to combat river blindness can be utilized as a platform for integrated delivery of multiple primary health care interventions, including, bed-nets, malaria treatment and other basic health care interventions, with significant increases in coverage. For example, more than twice as many children with fever received appropriate anti-malarial treatment, exceeding 60% coverage on average. Critical to both the funding and execution of such research are the partnerships fostered with countries in the region, as well as other public, civil society and private institutions. The vision now is to make implementation and operations research an even more important element of global research agendas, so that new products may finally begin to yield their hoped-for health impact through sounder primary health care system implementation. Thus, the longstanding burden of deadly diseases, such as malaria, may be more effectively addressed—through global, regional and local knowledge-sharing and cooperation.

As another striking example, only US$ 2 million out of US $ 390 million in 32 GAVI Health System Strengthening grants were allocated to research, despite encouragement to countries to do so. No other $ 5 trillion economic sector would be happy with so little investment in research related to its core agenda: the reduction of health inequalities; the organization of people-centered care; and the development of better, more effective public policies. No other industry of that size would be satisfied with so little investment in a better understanding of what their clients expect and how they perceive performance. No other industry of that size would pay so little attention to intelligence on the political context in which it operates—the positions and strategies of key stakeholders and partners. It is time for health leaders to understand the value of investment in this area.

Mobilizing the Commitment of the Workforce

Each of the sets of PHC reforms emphasizes the premium placed on human resources in health. The expected skills and competencies constitute an ambitious workforce programme that requires a rethink and review of existing pedagogic approaches. The science of health equity and primary care has yet to find its central place in schools of public health. Pre-service education for the health professions is already beginning to build in shared curricular activities that emphasize problem-solving in multi-disciplinary teams, but they need to go further in preparing for the skills and attitudes that PHC requires. This includes creating opportunities for on-the-job learning across sectors through mentoring, coaching and continuing education. These and other changes to the wide array of curricula and on-the-job learning require a deliberate effort to mobilize the responsible institutional actors both within and across countries. However, as we have learned in recent years, the content of what is learned or taught, although extremely important, is but one part of a complex of systems that governs the performance of the health workforce. A set of systems issues related to the health workforce need to be guided to a greater degree by PHC reforms. For example, health equity targets for underserved population groups will remain elusive if they do not consider how health workers can be effectively recruited and retained to work among them. Likewise, grand visions of care coordinated around the person or patient are unlikely to be translated into practice if credible career options for working in primary care teams are not put in place. Similarly, incentives are critical complements in ensuring that individuals and institutions exercise their competencies when engaging health in all policies. The health workforce is critical to PHC reforms. Significant investment is needed to empower health staff—from nurses to policy-makers—with the wherewithal to learn, adapt, be team players, and to combine biomedical and social perspectives, equity sensitivity and patient centeredness. Without investing in their mobilization, they can be an enormous source of resistance to change, anchored to past models that are convenient, reassuring, profitable and intellectually comfortable. If, however, they can be made to see and experience that primary health care produces stimulating and gratifying work, which is socially and economically rewarding, health workers may not only come on board but also become a militant vanguard. Here again, taking advantage of the opportunities afforded by the exchange and sharing of experience offered by a globalizing world can speed up the necessary transformations.

Mobilizing the Participation of People

The history of the politics of PHC reforms in the countries that have made major strides is largely unwritten. It is clear, however, that where these reforms have been successful, the endorsement of PHC by the health sector and by the political world has invariably followed on rising demand and pressure expressed by civil society. There are many examples of such demand. In Thailand, the initial efforts to mobilize civil society and politicians around an agenda of universal coverage came from within the Ministry of Health. However, it was only when Thai reformers joined a surge in civil society pressure to improve access to care, did it become possible to take advantage of a political opportunity and launch the reform. In just a few years, coverage was extended and most of the population was covered with a publicly funded primary care system that benefit incidence analysis shows to be pro-poor. In Mali, the revitalization of PHC in the 1990s started with an alliance between part of the Ministry of Health and part of the donor community, which made it possible to overcome initial resistance and skepticism. However, sustained extension of coverage only came about when hundreds of local "community health associations" federated in a powerful pressure group to spur the Ministry of Health and sustain political commitment. In western Europe, consumer organizations have a prominent place in the discussions on health care and public policies relating to health, as have many other civil society organizations. Elsewhere, such as in Chile, the initiative has come from the political arena as part of an agenda of democratization.

In India, the National Rural Health Mission came about as a result of strong pressure from civil society and the political world, while, in Bangladesh, much of the pressure for PHC comes from quasi-public NGOs. There is an important lesson there: powerful allies for PHC reform are to be found within civil society. They can make the difference between a well-intentioned but short-lived attempt, and successful and sustained reform; and between a purely technical initiative, and one that is endorsed by the political world and enjoys social consensus. This is not to say that public policy should be purely demand-driven. Health authorities have to ensure that popular expectations and demand are balanced with need, technical priorities and anticipated future challenges. Health authorities committed to PHC will have to harness the dynamics of civil society pressure for change in a policy debate that is supported with evidence and information, and informed by exchange of experience with others, within and across national boundaries.

Stronger Case for Health Care Investment

Today, it is possible to make a stronger case for health than in previous times. This is not only because of intrinsic values, such as health equity, or for the sector's contribution to economic growth? however valid they may be, these arguments are not always the most effective—but on political grounds. Health constitutes an economic sector of growing importance in itself and a feature of development and social cohesion. Reliable protection against health threats and equitable access to quality health care when needed are among the most central demands people make on their governments in advancing societies. Health has become a tangible measure of how well societies are developing and, thus, how well governments are performing their role. This constitutes a reservoir of potential strength for the sector, and is a basis for obtaining a level of commitment from society and political leadership that is commensurate with the challenges. Economic development and the rise of a knowledge society make it likely, though not inevitable, that expectations regarding health and health systems will continue to rise—some realistic, some not, some self-serving, others balanced with concern for what is good for society at large.

The increasing weight of some of the key values underlying these expectations ? equity, solidarity, the centrality of people and their wish to have a say in what affects them and their health ? is a long-term trend. Health systems do not naturally gravitate towards these values, hence the need for each country to make a deliberate choice when deciding the future of their health systems. It is possible not to choose PHC. In the long-run, however, that option carries a huge penalty: in forfeited health benefits, impoverishing costs, in loss of trust in the health system as a whole and, ultimately, in loss of political legitimacy. Countries need to demonstrate their ability to transform their health systems in line with changing challenges as well as to rising popular expectations.

Health Care Sector Reforms in India

Sunil Nandraj says in his article, 'The Need for Health Sector Reform in India': India's health care system is characterized by a pattern of mixed ownership and with different systems of medicine—Allopathy, Ayurvedic, Unnani, Sidda and Homeopathy. Three major groups in health care in the country, the public health sector, the private health sector and the households who utilize health services. The public health sector consists of the central government, state government, municipal and local level bodies. Health is a state responsibility, however, the central government does contribute in a substantial manner through grants and centrally sponsored health programs/schemes. There are other ministries and departments of the government such as defense, railways, police, ports and mines who have their own health services institutions for their personnel. For the organized sector employees (public and private) provision for health services is through the Employee's State Insurance Scheme (ESIS).

The private health sector consists of the 'not-for-profit' and the 'for-profit' health sectors. The not-for-profit health sector includes various health services provided by Non-Government Organisations (NGO's), charitable institutions, missions, trusts, etc. Health care in the for-profit health sector consists of various types of practitioners and institutions. The licensed practitioners range from general practitioners (GPs) to the super specialists, various types of consultants, nurses and paramedics, licentiates, and rural medical practitioners (RMPs). The health care practitioners with no formal qualifications constitute the 'informal' sector which consists of faith healers, local medicine men/women, traditional birth attendants priests and a variety of unqualified persons (quacks). The private health subsector institutions are heterogeneous in the services they provide, their size and quality.

Indian Health Care System is Complex

D. Aggerwal says (*Indian Journal of Community Medicine,* Vol. 31, No. 4, October-December, 2006) that the importance of working on health sector reforms is paramount in Indian context. What do we mean by reforms in the health sector? Do we really need reforms in the health sector in India and how critical it is to build a consensus for a reforms agenda for the country? As far as the composition of the health system in the country is concerned, we know that the health system is highly heterogeneous and complex with multiple actors, the large number of treatment providers belonging to different pathies and in different settings. We have a wide range of providers: formal and non-formal, qualified and less than qualified, registered medical practitioners, etc. They are working in the outreach, home settings, stand alone dispensaries, nursing homes and corporate sector world-class hospitals. We have preventive and promotive care services in terms of immunizations, family planning, maternal health services, vertical disease control programme to name the few. We have a range of financing mechanisms to support health care. The Government spending on health is an attempt to subsidize health care. Large chunk of population has to make out-of-pocket expenditures to access health care. Health insurance is gradually growing and more players along with new products are going to be in the market given the conducive policy environment. Last decade has been witness to phenomenal growth in numbers of the medical colleges, nursing colleges and other similar training institutions. There are multiple institutional players in organizing health care. We have the panchayat system who are responsible for providing primary health care, the State Governments providing predominantly budgetary support, Central Government for setting broad policy frameworks and also budgetary support and several autonomous institutions, railways, army, ESI, etc. Also one can not ignore very impressive presence of private sector players especially as most states are promoting what they call as "medical tourism" to attract patients from neighbouring countries. We have 21 percent of global burden of disease. Twenty-five percent of all maternal deaths takes place in our country and same may be true for neonatal mortality.

Politics Influence Health System in Significant Manner

The goals, priorities, and the strategies, variations in the commitment are largely decided through the political contingencies. There are competing demands on the health systems. The evolution of the health systems is largely shaped by the culture, history, and norms. Any health system would have 3 important goals. Health sector or health system should work for improving the health status, but we know its difficult to measure. Indicators like life expectancy, DALYs, etc. are there. There are legitimate questions regarding use of these indicators and the inclusiveness. Averages mask the equity such as, the regional equity and the gender equity parameters and also the income quintiles.

Another goal of health system is customer satisfaction, which WHO refers to the health systems responsiveness. Health systems have to be responsive to the needs of the clients and the community. It is difficult to measure the customer satisfaction and gauze responsiveness of health systems.

Client satisfaction also depends on non-clinical aspects of care. One would expect that the customer satisfaction would largely depend on the clinical outcomes of care, but non-clinical outcomes of care do influence the customer satisfaction and that's what the health system have to worry about. Financial risk protection is another goal of health systems. We need to start thinking about how health systems are covering for the financial contingencies and financial risk. Are people protected against the high cost of medical care? So any health system should see to it that the financial protection is extended against the catastrophic illnesses and the poor people who are really worst affected with the high cost, are not constrained to seek care.

It is useful to pause and take stock of Indian health sector. We have improved life expectancy considerably from 49 years in 1970 to 63 years in 1998. Yet averages mask the equity dimensions. Clearly there are class and regional inequities. We also have high mortality and the burden of disease amongst the poor. An analysis of coverage with preventive and promotive interventions with special reference to income quintiles will highlight huge differentials. Several studies have indicated that poor don't seek care on account of poor purchasing power.

Client satisfaction is very high. As per NFHS-2 data, an overwhelming majority of clients are satisfied by the services delivered by the public systems. May be the expectations are low or may be our people are so courteous. But on the hand, we have the report from Transparent International, ranked the health system in India is the most corrupt system. It will be useful to see as how we are doing in terms of spending? Overall, Government spending is 0.9% of GDP, which is very low. WHO has pointed that we are really in the bottom quintile in the world in terms of public sector spending in the health care? Though the policy documents are explicit for increasing public spending to 2% and then 5% within next 10 years. It is also worrying that post-liberalization, one is seeing the greater decline of investment in social development sector including health sector since 1990 to 2000 or 2003 in the real terms. In terms of private expenditures 80 percent of all spending is on health from the private sides, it's kind of out-of-pocket expenditures because the health insurance is yet to catch imagination of masses.

There are wide interstate variations in terms of utilization of health care and out-of-pocket expenditures including risk of falling in debts after hospitalization.

This is important in context of taking forward the agenda of the reforms. Coming to delivery of public health services, it is important to know as who are the users?

Who uses the services? We thought the subsidy, which is given by the state would ultimately go to meet the needs of poor. What is happening? The richest quintile consumes three times more public health resources as compared to poor. It is poor who are subsidizing for rich in terms of uses of public health resources in the country, richest quintile consuming three times more services, more public health services as compared to poor. We have the data in terms of OPD care, as 80%-85% going in the private sector. Same is true for indoor care. So it is largely private sector which is dominating, in utilization of services and also largely unregulated. Health needs of urban poor, marginalized groups, tribal population, fringe populations, and other disadvantaged and vulnerable communities need to be addressed. What are the intermediate outcomes, those health systems should pursue in order to achieve ultimate outcomes. There are issues in terms of efficiency, quality, and access-related issues.

What do we mean by efficiency? What are the outputs, which we are producing? If we wish to provide 100% coverage for antenatal care, how we are going to produce such an output. Are we going to achieve it through the mobile services? Are we going to do it throughout reach services? Are we going to engage the private providers in deliveries of antenatal care? Are we going to talk of some paramedic model or some alternate service delivery or franchising model? Thus it is important to assess technical efficiency of our interventions. Allocative efficiency on the other hand will help us to know what do we produce, do we need to produce 100% antenatal care or do we need to produce 100% institutional delivery if our goal is to reduce maternal mortality. So those are the questions, which health systems and health sector need to answer, in case they are going to improve the health status and bring down the mortality and mobility burden. So what is being suggested here is look into technical efficiency of interventions and also look into allocative efficiency, i.e. where are you putting your money, Is your money in the right place? Technical efficiency, the essence of management and allocative efficiency is linked to political economy of health. So more decisions are taken in the context of political parameters in terms of political economy and not with reference to evidence base. So that's the kind of situation that we are still struggling whether we should train "Dais", or we should do 100% antenatal care, promote emergency obstetric care, do institutional deliveries, engage communities in safe motherhood, etc.

What is quality? Again quality is most abused term in health systems There are several definitions, lots of frameworks, different approaches and institutional mechanisms. There are multiple players in the quality. The management systems, the insurance companies, providers, third party administrators, health management organizations, clients, community are the different stakeholders. Quality influences both health status and satisfaction. If you provide good quality services, are you looking for the good clinical outcomes, improved health status or you are also looking for the client satisfaction? It is crucial to understand quality from the providers, management, and from the client and community prospective. The clinical and service quality dimensions of quality are important to focus and there are different budgets for different quality: If you have lower level allocation, lower level of budget, there is a quality curve, you are going to miss out either in the clinical quality or you are going to miss out in service quality. There is very limited information on QOC in health systems. Lately there are some efforts to incorporate quality monitoring in the programme designs. There have been some initiatives in the donor projects to work on the quality of care but apparently it has not gone much ahead. We are still monitoring coverage. We still monitor coverage for immunizations which is critical but we don't know, adverse events after immunizations. Service quality issues are important again but we really don't know how the privacy and confidentiality are addressed in the service delivery settings?

Access is another important element that needs to be considered. Access is dependent on availability of services such as physical availabilities of services, i.e. availability of providers. "Ghost PHCs" and sub-centres are common especially in remote districts. The women would come from all the way from a distant village to a sub-center or PHC, to only find out the sub centers are locked. So there is no effective availability of services. There are socio-cultural issues, gender of providers, the language, the jargon, which is used by providers, which makes it difficult for the poor women to access services. Economic barriers in access in terms of opportunity costs coming to a city seeking services with 2-3 relatives are also going to be quite significant. Utilization, which is a marker of demand, is also related to access and there are several factors, which influence utilization. Are outreach visits regular and predictable? So what is happening to the access for the primary reproductive health care services to the women? What is the package of services? Are we offering a complete package of say RCH services at one point? Can poor women negotiate the use of higher level health care services? Can she communicate to the providers in big hospitals?

Now after saying all that, what is the national context of health reforms which we should look forward? We all know that India is passing through demographic transition. There is very significant shift from high fertility and mortality to low mortality and fertility. We see there is a window of opportunity for India in terms of demographic bonus in case our adolescents are provided adequate skills and interventions are in place to promote their reproductive and sexual health. We also see the epidemiological transition taking place in country as we are still having communicable diseases, burden of malnutrition,, which have been controlled, eliminated from many other countries but we also have the lifestyle diseases the cardiovascular, the endocrinal diseases. So we have that kind of disease pattern, a double burden of disease. A responsive health system will incorporate this distinct shift. We also see the social transition-taking place. High literacy rates, the mobility is increasing, the expectations of the people of the health systems are going up. Technological transitions are also taking place. We are coming with the rapid diagnostic, auto disabled syringes, genetic engineering, IVF and emergence of non invasive technologies is also putting new demands on the health systems. Both National health policy documents, National population policy document, and several other Government documents talk of increasing allocation for health care in future. Clearly this is very much needed. What do we mean by reforms? Reforms encompass a range of those purposeful efforts to change the system for improving its performance. This is what the reforms would mean. You should make deliberate efforts, and conscious choices so that the changes in the system would lead to the improved performance in terms of those goals. Reforms have to be rational and logical, it can't be quick fix and knee jerk reaction. They have to rational, they have to be logical, they have to be specified. Do we have limited reforms with small changes here and there and just tinkering with the system, which is again possible and many countries had all these small reforms and have been successful. Or we go with a big bang theory with a big ticket reforms and change the way you financed the health care, organize services and delegation of technology, etc.

What should be the focus of reform in India. Decentralization is going to be the key element of the reform process. One size doesn't fit all is clearly the mantra. Alternate ways of financing health care should receive policy attention in a major way. Clearly there is scope of formulating demand side financing mechanisms so as to provide access to poor. Private sector should be seen as a national asset and alternate service delivery systems, e.g. social franchising should be considered. It is also critical to work with private sector in terms of certification and accreditation systems.

Sources

World Health Report, 2006, Working together for health. Geneva, World Health Organization, 2006.

Ezekiel, J.E. The perfect storm of overutilization. *JAMA*, 2008, 299:2789-91.

Halman, L *et al*. Changing values and beliefs in 85 countries. Trends from the values surveys from 1981 to 2004. Leiden and Boston MA, Brill, 2008 (European Values Studies, No. 11).

Lübker, M. Globalization and perceptions of social inequality. Geneva, International Labour Office, Policy Integration Department, 2004 (World Commission on the Social Dimension of Globalization, Working Paper No. 32).

National Health Accounts. Geneva, World Health Organization, 2008 (http//www.who.int/nha/country/en/index.html, accessed May 2008).

National strategy to reduce social inequalities in health. Paper presented to the Storting. Oslo, Norwegian Ministry of Health and Care Services, 2007 (Report No. 20 (2006-2007); http://www.regjeringen.no/en/dep/hod/Documents/regpubl/stmeld/2006-2007/Report-No-20-2006-2007-to-the-Storting.html?id=466505, accessed 19 July 2008).

Smith, G. *et al*. Genetic epidemiology and public health: hope, hype, and future prospects. *Lancet*, 2005, 366:1484-98.

Moran, M. Governing the health care state: a comparative study of the United

Kingdom, The United States and Germany. Manchester and New York, NY, Manchester University Press, 1999.

Heath, I. A general practitioner for every person in the world. BMJ, 2008, 336:861.

Busse, R., Schlette, S., eds. Focus on prevention, health and aging, and health professions. Gütersloh, Verlag Bertelsmann Stiftung, 2007 (Health Policy Developments 7/8).

Rothman, D.J. Beginnings count: the technological imperative in American Health Care. Oxford and New York NY, Oxford University Press, 1997.

PHC and mental health report. Geneva, World Health Organization, 2008 (in press).

Mullan, F., Frehywot, S. Non-physician clinicians in 47 sub-Saharan African countries.*Lancet*, 2007, 370:2158-63.

Achieving universal health coverage: developing the health financing system. Geneva, World Health Organization, 2005 (Technical briefs for Policy-Makers No. 1; WHO/ EIP/HSF/PB/05.01).

National Rural Health Mission. Meeting people's health needs in rural areas.

Framework for implementation 2005-2012. New Delhi, Government of India, Ministry of Health and Family Welfare (accessed 4 August 2008).

Heavily indebted poor countries (HIPC) initiative and multilateral debt relief initiative (MDRI)—status of implementation, 28 August 2007. Washington DC, International Monetary Fund, 2007 (http://www.imf.org/external/np/pp/2007/eng/082807.pdf, accessed 12 March 2008).

Integrated community-based interventions: 2007 progress report to STAC (30).

Geneva, United Nations Development Programme/World Bank/World Health Organization Special Programme for Research and Training in Tropical Diseases, 2008 (TDR Business Line 11).

Grodos, D. Le, District sanitaire urbain en Afrique subsaharienne. Enjeux, pratiques et politiques. Louvain-la-Neuve, Paris, Karthala-UCL, 2004.

Baser, H., Morgan, P. Capacity, change and performance. Maastricht, European Centre for Development Policy Management, 2008.

OECD reviews of health systems ? Switzerland. Paris, Organization for Economic Co-operation and Development/World Health Organization, 2006.

De Campos, F.E., Hauck, V. Networking collaboratively: the experience of the observatories of human resources in Brazil. Cahiers de sociologie et de démographie médicales, 2005, 45:173-208.

The PHAMEU project. Utrecht, Netherlands Institute for Health Services, 2008 (http://www.phameu.eu/). EQUINET Africa. Regional Network on Equity in Health in Southern Africa, Harare, 2008 (http://www.equinetafrica.org/).

Hamilton, M. III *et al*. Financial anatomy of biomedical research. JAMA, 2005, 294:1333-42.

Community-directed interventions for major health problems in Africa: a multi-country study: final report. Geneva, UNICEF/UNDP/World Bank/World Health Organization Special Programme for Research and Training in Tropical Diseases, 2008.
(http://www.who.int/tdr/publications/publications/pdf/cdi_report_08.pdf, accessed 26 August 2008).

UNESCO science report 2005. Paris, United Nations Educational, Scientific and Cultural Organization, 2005.

Tancharoensathien, V., Jongudomsuk, P., eds. From policy to implementation: historical events during 2001-2004 of UC in Thailand. Bangkok, National Health Security Office, 2005.

Biscaia, A., Conceição, C., Ferrinho, P. Primary health care reforms in Portugal: equityoriented and physician driven. Paper presented at: Organizing integrated PHC through family practice: an intercountry comparison of policy formation processes, Brussels, 8-9 October 2007.

Hughes, D., Leethongdee, S. Universal coverage in the land of smiles: lessons from Thailand's 30 Baht health reforms. *Health Affairs,* 2007, 26:999-1008.

Jongudomsuk, P. From universal coverage of health care in Thailand to SHI in China:what lessons can be drawn? In: International Labour Office, Deutsche Gesellschaft für Technische Zusammenarbeit (GTZ) Gmbh, World Health Organization. Extending social protection in health: developing countries' experiences, lessons learnt and recommendations. Paper presented at: International Conference on Social Health Insurance in Developing Countries, Berlin, 5-7 December 2005. Eschborn, Deutsche Gesellschaft für Technische Zusammenarbeit (GTZ), 2007:155-157 (http://www2. gtz.de/dokumente/bib/07-0378.pdf, accessed 19 July 2008).

Tangcharoensathien, V. *et al.* Universal coverage in Thailand: the respective roles of social health insurance and tax-based financing. In: International Labour Office, Deutsche Gesellschaft für Technische Zusammenarbeit (GTZ) Gmbh, World Health Organization. Extending social protection in health: developing countries' experiences, lessons learnt and recommendations. Paper presented at: International Conference on Social Health Insurance in Developing Countries, Berlin, 5-7 December 2005.

Maiga, Z., Traore Nafo, F., El Abassi, A. Health sector reform in Mali, 1989-1996. Antwerp, ITG Press, 2003.

Balique, H., Ouattara, O., Ag Iknane, A. Dix ans d'expérience des centres de santé communautaire au Mali, Santé publique, 2001, 13:35-48.

Chaudhury, R.H., Chowdhury, Z. Achieving the Millennium Development Goal on maternal mortality: Gonoshasthaya Kendra's experience in rural Bangladesh. Dhaka, Gonoprokashani, 2007.

FURTHER READINGS

Amin Tabish. Textbook of Hospital and Health Services Administration. Oxford University Press. New Delhi. 2002.

Amin Tabish. Looking after Health into the 21st Century. JK Practitioner. 1998; 5(2): 156-58.

Amin Tabish. Maternal and Child Health in developing countries: responding to the challenge. *J Applied Med.* 1998; 24(8): 579-84.

Amin Tabish. Health Services Organization and Public Health Delivery in India - Part I. *J Applied Med.* 1999; 25(4): 243-48.

Amin Tabish. Health Services Organization and Public Health Delivery in India - Part R *J Applied Med.* Sci. 1999 25(5): 323-26.

Amin Tabish. Towards Development of Professional Management. *J Management in Medicine,* England. 1995; 2(2): 178-87.

Amin Tabish. Holistic Approach to HFA By 2000. World Health Forum. Geneva. 1993; 14(2): 173-74.

Amin Tabish. Evidence-Based Medicine: linking research to practice. *J Med Sci.* 1999: 2(1): 2-3.

Amin Tabish. The Electronic Highway in Medicine. JK Practitioner. Editorial. 1999 6(4): 251.

Amin Tabish. Tackling Emerging Infectious Diseases. *J Med Sci.* 1999; 2(2): 12-16.

Maxcy-Rosenau-Last. Public Health and Preventive Medicine—14th ed. Prentice-Hall International Inc. USA 1998.

Richard Smith. Editorial. The Future of health care systems. *BMJ.* 314, 24 May 1997.

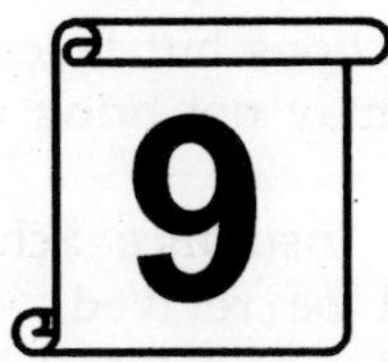

Political Commitment and Primary Health Care

"Health and education are basic in the nations' march to development, i.e. journey from a developing nation to a developed nation. USA is a living example of progress. Amartya sen advocated more attention to health and education. Political parties have also to make family planning, health care and education as election issues. In future the emphasis should shift from vote banks to welfare and development. Nothing is more important than the health and well-being of the citizens. In countries like USA where all political parties have health care as an important component of their election manifesto and political agenda the allocations to health care are massive. In developing countries like India, Pakistan, Bangladesh and others health care is a low priority and the allocations for public health are abysmally low. Primary health care has collapsed in these countries and most of the citizens depend on private health care, which is also of poor quality and unethical. Unless these countries have serious political commitment to health care the situation is unlikely to improve."

The population of India is in need of adequate health care and basic education for inclusive growth and realization of the potential. Unfortunately, health and education do not bring votes to the political parties, so these have never been the core issues in Indian elections, unlike US elections. But if you exclude health and education what is left in good governance? Economic growth bereft of adequate health care and good education cannot be called good governance. The nation is spending less than 1% of GDP on health though successive governments have promised to raise it to 3%. Similarly raising the expenditure from 3% to 6% of GDP has proved a tall talk despite repeated assurances. While the health care has collapsed in prosperous states like Punjab, education development has been limited to rise in number of the educational institutions, irrespective of the quality of education or the finished products. The cost of education has been steadily rising; with the result the burden on the parents has been unbearable. Education is a precursor to good health and health care.

Some political parties expressed their support to the following suggestions in the recent elections but failed in their emphasis since they fear that talk of health care may not bring votes:

1. Universal Health Insurance Scheme, launched by the NDA Government, will be revived, with the Central Government bearing the expense of medical insurance for all BPL families.
2. Total Sanitation Campaign, waste disposal and recycling, nutritional security to children, and eradication of communicable diseases will receive highest attention from the Government.
3. 50 essential medicines, which can take care of 90% of common diseases, will be distributed free to all needy citizens.
4. Each tehsil will have a well-equipped hospital with bed strength of at least 50.
5. Each district will have a modern multi-specialty hospital with an attached medical college. Public-Private Partnership model will be adopted for this purpose. This district will have a mobile extension service to cater to the needs of nearby rural areas.
6. Existing health care infrastructure, in which considerable public investment has already taken place, has enormous scope for improvement with minimal additional investment. Policy will be reformed to enable the private sector to partner in running this system.
7. Ayurveda will be given primacy in the overall health care plan. Over 7,00,000 practitioners of Ayurveda and other Indian systems of medicine have been making a major contribution to health care in rural and remote areas. They will be assisted to further expand and improve their services.
8. The entire health care system will be made more woman-centric and child-centric.
9. Considering the growing health care needs of senior citizens, the government will provide interest-free loans to young couples to build an extra room in their homes for their parents.
10. Every ministry in Government of India will incorporate health care as part of its plans and programmes.
11. Corruption in health care administration and medical education will be removed. Medical education will be made affordable.
12. In order to meet the enormous need for trained health care workforce in rural areas, the Government will start a new medical education course to create a large public health care cadre, who will work in rural areas.

13. Information Technology will be used innovatively and extensively to connect every hospital and every PHC in rural areas to the National Telemedicine Service Network.
14. Health tourism will be promoted in a big way.

Primary Health Care is the Key

As proposed at Alma Ata, the concept of PHC has socio-political implications. First, it explicitly stated the need for a comprehensive health strategy that not only provided health services, but also addressed the underlying social, economic, and political causes of poor health. Specifically, as conceived in the Alma Ata Declaration, such a strategy must promote a more equitable distribution of resources: Political commitment to Primary Health Care implies more than formal support from the government and community leaders.... For developing countries in particular, it implies the transfer of a greater share of health resources to the under-served majority of the population. At the same time, there is a need to increase the national health budget until the total population has access to essential health care.... Also, an explicit policy is required whereby the affluent countries commit themselves to a more equitable distribution of international health resources to enable the developing countries, and especially the least developed, to apply primary health care. PHC also emphasized the close link between health and development of the poorer sector of the community. Thus: Any distinction between economic and social development is no longer tenable.... Indeed, social factors are the real driving force behind development. The purpose of development is to permit people to lead economically productive and socially satisfying lives.... Community-based Health Programs which provided the inspiration for PHC were not just health initiatives. They were part of a larger struggle by marginalized people for their well-being and their rights. As such, they often ran into serious opposition. Even programs which may not have explicitly put social change on their agendas posed a threat to entrenched interests with their emphasis on addressing root causes of poor health and "putting the last first." The awareness raising and community organizing they conducted to this end was often seen as stirring up trouble by local authorities. Grassroots efforts to put health into the hands of the people posed a serious threat—not only to elites and governments—but also to the medical establishment, who for so long had maintained a powerful monopoly.

Root Cause is at Socio-economic Level

Although the challenges of addressing the socio-economic root causes of disease in developing countries may seem insurmountable, analyses of factors that contributed to health improvements in developed countries provide cause for optimism. The recommendations in a US report, embodied the essential elements of comprehensive primary health care—communicable disease control, promotion of child health, housing improvement, sanitation, training of community health workers, public health education, promotion of individual responsibility for one's own health, mobilization of community participation through sanitary associations, and creation of multi-disciplinary boards of health to assess needs and plan programs. Similarly, while reviewing factors that contributed to improvements in health in England, Thomas McKeown demonstrated that population health improved more because of investments in "environmental public health," political, economic, and social measures than from specific medical or therapeutic interventions. Decline in deaths from tuberculosis and from respiratory and water and foodborne diseases had already occurred before any effective immunizations or treatments were available.

Concrete Strategies and Processes

Of critical importance is the need to establish concrete strategies and processes, with clear targets, to reduce inequities in the allocation of resources for primary health care, and with a focus on both horizontal and vertical equity. The value of this proposal is illustrated by the striking success that has been achieved in social development and health by a few poor countries, notably Sri Lanka, Costa Rica, Cuba, China, and Kerala state in India. Mortality and malnutrition rates are much lower and life expectancy much higher in these countries than in other countries with similar economic characteristics and indeed some wealthier countries. In this regard, it is important to stress that the nature of the political system, its values, and its processes for participation define the frontiers of opportunity for health equity. Systems characterized by the absence of democracy and by pervasive corruption, violence, and sex discrimination are breeding grounds for inequities in health and in other social spheres.

Social Policies

International aid agencies and governments in developing countries should be aware that the pursuit of liberal macro-economic pro-growth policies has the tendency to provide better opportunities to those with resources and high levels of education while large segments of the population without these assets are unlikely to benefit and may in fact become casualties of economic transition. Thus, it is the duty of health policymakers to signal when other policies may undermine efforts to promote health equity.

Trained Health Personnel

Most importantly, to ensure the quality of primary health care, reform of the health sector under primary health care should include coherent human resource development plans at the village, district, state/regional, and national levels and strategies for retention of trained personnel in remote and rural areas. Primary health care systems in developing countries provide interventions that are already known to be effective. This means that achievement of quality in primary health care facilities requires the proper performance of these interventions according to prescribed standards to reduce mortality, morbidity, and disability. However, the most common challenge is that often these interventions are not properly executed. A recent study in southeast Nigeria, for example, revealed that inadequacy in the quality of services provided by community-based primary health care workers is a product of failures in a range of quality measures: structural, process failings, and lack of a protocol for systematic supervision of health workers. Thus, quality improvement in this context is not simply a matter of providing infrastructural resources but, rather, one of paying attention to improvement in process, especially through training and supervision.

Short-term measures are not sufficient to greatly alleviate the overall burden of disease in developing countries unless the socio-economic, political, and health system factors that underpin health and disease in these countries are challenged. The remedy lies in poverty alleviation, community participation, and the development of health systems and infrastructures to create and sustain health.

What the People Expect from their Governments

Primary health care, with universal access and social protection are the key expectations of the people all over the globe. People expect their governments to put into place an array of public policies that span local through to supra-national level arrangements, without which primary care and universal coverage lose much of meaning. These include the policies required to make health systems function properly; to organize public-health actions of major benefit to all; and, beyond the health sector, the policies that can contribute to health and a sense of security, while ensuring that issues, such as urbanization, climate change, gender discrimination or social stratification are properly addressed. What really determines the health status of poor people are wider social equity issues that can only be addressed by embracing the political dimensions of the problem. Solutions are not about health *per-se,* we are told, but about triggering organized popular demands for an overall fairer treatment in society. This is made clear through showing us examples of poor people's empowering initiatives from different continents. But they also show us how these initiatives systematically run into obstacles created by the existing national and international power structures.

Strongly reaffirming the values and principles of primary health care, including equity, solidarity, social justice, universal access to services, multi-sectoral action and community participation as the basis for strengthening health systems; World Health Organization urges Member States:

(1) To ensure political commitment at all levels to the values and principles of the Declaration of Alma-Ata, keep the issue of

strengthening health systems based on the primary health care approach high on the international political agenda, and take advantage, as appropriate, of health-related partnerships and initiatives relating to this issue, particularly to support achievement of the Millennium Development Goals;

(2) To accelerate action towards universal access to primary health care by developing comprehensive health services and by developing national equitable and sustainable financing mechanisms, mindful of the need to ensure social protection and protect health budgets in the context of the current international financial crisis;

(3) To put people at the centre of health care by adopting, as appropriate, delivery models focused on the local and district levels that provide comprehensive primary health care services, including health promotion, disease prevention, curative care and end-of-life services, that are integrated and coordinated according to need;

(4) To promote active participation by all people, in the processes of developing policy and improving health and health care, in order to support the renewal of primary health care;

(5) To train adequate numbers of health workers, able to work in a multidisciplinary context, in order to respond effectively to people's health needs;

(6) To ensure that vertical programmes, including disease-specific programmes, are developed and implemented in the context of integrated primary health care;

(7) To improve access to appropriate medicines, health products and technologies, all of which are required to support primary health care;

(8) To develop and strengthen health information and surveillance systems relating to primary health care in order to facilitate evidence-based policies and programmes and their evaluation;

(9) To strengthen health ministries, enabling them to provide inclusive, transparent and accountable leadership of the health sector and to facilitate multi-sectoral action as part of primary health care. (The World Health Report, 2008: Primary Health Care—now more than ever. Geneva, World Heath Organization)

PHC's Central Role in Health Care Systems Worldwide

Primary health care plays a central role in health care systems worldwide. It can offer families cost-effective services close to home, eliminating costly trips to specialists and hospitals. In developing countries, community health centers usually offer a broad range of services, including prenatal care, immunizations, treatment of childhood illnesses, treatment of malaria and other common infectious diseases, and other basic medical care. All too often, however, the coverage and effectiveness of primary care services are limited by insufficient resources and staff, erratic drug supplies, and faulty equipment. Governments increasingly recognize that adequate delivery of primary care services is fundamental to the effective functioning of health systems, to keeping families healthy, and to achieving national health goals.

Let us look at some public policies:

1. A first group of critical public policies are the health systems policies (related to essential drugs, technology, quality control, human resources, accreditation, etc.) on which primary care and universal coverage reforms depend. In Kenya, for example, children are now much better protected against malaria as a result of local services providing them with insecticide-treated bed nets. This has only been possible because the work of primary care was supported by a national initiative with strong political commitment, social marketing and national support for supply and logistics.
2. Some interventions, such as the fortification of salt with iodine, are only feasible at the regional, national or, increasingly at supra-national level. In the 23 developing countries that comprise 80% of the global chronic disease burden, 8.5 million lives could be saved in a decade by a 15% dietary salt reduction through manufacturers and a sustained mass-media campaign. Implementation of four measures from the Framework Convention on Tobacco Control (increased tobacco taxes; smoke-free workplaces; convention-compliant packaging, labeling and awareness campaigns about health risks; and a comprehensive advertising, promotion, and sponsorship ban) could save a further 5.5 million lives in a decade.
3. The third set of policies is "health in all policies". Population health can be improved through policies that are mainly controlled by sectors other than health. The health content of school curricula, industry's policy towards gender equality, or the safety of food and consumer goods are all issues that can profoundly influence or even determine the health of entire communities. In South Africa, a change in legislation increased women's access to a broad range of options for the prevention and treatment of unwanted pregnancy, resulting in a 91% drop in abortion-related deaths.

On a larger scale, transnational mechanisms, such as UNICEF's international procurement of vaccines, and the Global Drug Facility for tuberculosis treatment, afford considerable savings as well as quality assurances that countries on their own would be unlikely to negotiate. The realization that the health MDGs are contingent on bridging the massive health-worker shortfall in low-income countries has brought long overdue attention to a previously neglected area.

Human Resources for Health Care

Human resources for health are the indispensable inputs to effective implementation of primary care and universal coverage reforms, and they are also the personification of the values that define PHC. Yet, in the absence of a deliberate choice to guide the health workforce policy by the PHC goals, market forces within the health care system will drive health workers towards greater sub-specialization in tertiary care institutions, if not towards migration to large cities or other countries. When a country chooses to base its health systems on PHC—when it starts putting into place primary care and universal coverage reforms—its whole arsenal of system policies needs to be aligned behind these reforms: not just those pertaining to service delivery models or financing. It is possible to develop system policies that do not take account of the PHC agenda. It is also possible to choose to align them to PHC. If a country opts for PHC, effective implementation allows no half measures; no health systems building block will be left untouched.

Countrywide Public-health Initiatives

While it is essential that primary care teams seek to improve the health of populations at local level, this may be of limited value if national- and global-level policy-makers fail to take initiatives for broader, public policy measures, which are important in changing nutrition patterns and influencing the social determinants of health. Classical areas in which beyond-local-scale public-health interventions may be beneficial include: altering individual behaviours and lifestyles; controlling and preventing disease; tackling hygiene and the broader determinants of health; and secondary prevention, including screening for disease. This includes measures such as the fortification of bread with foliate, taxation of alcohol and tobacco, and ensuring the safety of food, consumer goods and toxic substances. Such national and transnational-scale public-health interventions have the potential to save millions of lives. The successful removal of the major risk factors of disease, which is technically possible, would reduce premature deaths by an estimated 47% and increase global healthy life expectancy by an estimated 9.3 years. Well-designed public-health policies can, however, reduce inequities when they provide health benefits to entire populations or when they explicitly prioritize groups with poor health.

Rapid Response Capacity

Humanitarian disasters or disease outbreaks demand a rapid response capacity that is crucial in dealing effectively with the problem at hand and is an absolute imperative in maintaining the trust of the population in their health system. Invoking quarantines or travel bans, rapidly sequencing the genome of a new pathogen to inform vaccine or therapeutic design, and mobilizing health workers and institutions without delay can be vital. While the advent of an "emergency" often provides the necessary good will and flexibility of these diverse actors to respond, an effective response is more likely if there have been significant investments in preparedness. The expectation of developing countries for equitable access to protection, including affordable access to anti-virals and vaccines in the event of a pandemic, is resulting in changes to national and global capacity strengthening: from surveillance and laboratories to capacity transfer for vaccine formulation and production, and capacity for stock-piling. Thus, the most equitable response is the most effective response, and the most effective rapid response capacity can only emerge from the engagement of multiple stakeholders in this global process of negotiation.

Commission on Social Determinants of Health (CSDH)

The final report of the CSDH contains a detailed series of recommendations for action, organized around the following three overarching recommendations.

1. Improve daily living conditions

Key improvements required in the well-being of girls and women; the circumstances, in which their children are born, early child development and education for girls and boys; living and working conditions; social protection policy; and conditions for a flourishing older life.

2. Tackle the inequitable distribution of power, money and resources

To address health inequities it is necessary to address inequities in the way society is organized. This requires a strong public sector that is committed, capable and adequately financed. This in turn requires strengthened governance including stronger civil society and an accountable private sector. Governance dedicated to pursuing equity is required at all levels.

3. Measure and understand the problem and assess the impact of action

It is essential to acknowledge the problem of health inequity and ensure that it is measured—both within countries and globally. National and global health equity surveillance systems for routine monitoring of health inequity and the social determinants of health are required that also evaluate the health equity impact of policy and action. Other requirements are the training of policy-makers and health practitioners, increased public understanding of social determinants of health, and a stronger social determinants focus in research. It starts by looking at the effects of agricultural, educational, environmental, fiscal, housing, transport and other policies on health. It then seeks to work with these other sectors to ensure that, while contributing to well-being and wealth, these policies also contribute to health. Other sector's public policies, as well as private sector policies, can be important to health. Some may lead to adverse consequences for health. Often such adverse consequences are identified retrospectively, as in the case of the negative health effects of air pollution or industrial contamination. Yet, it is also often possible to foresee them or detect them at an early stage. Decision-makers in other sectors may be unaware of the consequences.

Unsystematic Approach

The health sector's approach to improving public policies has been singularly unsystematic and guided by patchy evidence and muddled decision-making—not least because the health community has put so little effort into collating and communicating these facts. For all the progress that has been made in recent years, information on the effectiveness of interventions to redress, for example, health inequities is still hard to come by and, when it is available, it is confined to a privileged circle of concerned experts. A lack of information and evidence is, thus, one of the explanations for under-investment. Many public policy issues have a huge potential for unpopularity: whether it is reducing the number of hospital beds, imposing seatbelts, culling poultry or taxing alcohol, resistance is to be expected and controversy an everyday occurrence. Other decisions have so little visibility, e.g. measures that ensure a safe food production chain, that they offer little political mileage. Consensus on stern measures may be easy to obtain at a moment of crisis, but public opinion has a notoriously short attention span. Politicians often pay more attention to policies that produce benefits within electoral cycles of two to four years and, therefore, undervalue efforts where benefits, such as those of environmental protection or early child development, accrue over a time span of 20 to 40 years. If unpopularity is one intractable disincentive to political commitment, active opposition from well-resourced lobbies is another. An obvious example is the tobacco industry's efforts to limit tobacco control. Similar opposition is seen to the regulation of population growth, disposal of industrial waste and to the marketing of food to children. These obstacles to steering public policy are real and need to be dealt with in a systematic way.

Crisis management, short-term planning horizons, lack of understandable evidence, unclear inter-sectoral arrangements, vested interests and inadequate modes of governing the health sector reinforce the need for comprehensive policy reforms to realize the potential of public-health action. Fortunately, there are promising opportunities to build upon.

Better Information and Evidence

We know much about the relationship between certain behaviours—smoking, diet, exercise, etc.—and health outcomes, but much less about how to effect behavioural change in a systematic and sustainable way at population levels. Even in well-resourced contexts, the obstacles are many: the time-scale in achieving outcomes; the complexity of multi-factorial disease causation and intervention effects; the lack of data; the methodological problems, including the difficulties in applying the well-accepted criteria used in the evaluation of clinical methods; and the different perspectives of the multiple stakeholders involved. Even the elementary foundations for work on population health and the collection of statistics on births and deaths or diseases are deficient in many countries.

The growing global health "interdependence" is accompanied by a mushrooming of activities expressed at the global level. The challenge is, therefore, to ensure that emerging networks of governance are adequately inclusive of all actors and sectors, responsive to local needs and demands, accountable, and oriented towards social justice. The recent emergence of a global food crisis provides further legitimacy to an input from the health sector into the evolving global response. Gradually, a space is opening for the consideration of health in the trade agreements negotiated through the World Trade Organization (WTO).

In the European Union, the construction of health protection standards is shared between agencies and applied across Europe. Given the expense and complexity of drug safety monitoring, many countries adapt and use the standards of the United States Food and Drug Administration (FDA). WHO sets global standards for tolerable levels of many contaminants. In the meantime, countries must either undertake these processes themselves or ensure access to standards from other countries or international agencies, adapted to their own context.

Government as Broker for PHC Reform

The ultimate responsibility for shaping national health systems lies with governments. Shaping does not suggest that governments should—or even could—reform the entire health sector on their own. Many different groups have a role to play: national politicians and local governments, the health professions, the scientific community, the private sector and civil society organizations, as well as the global health community. Nevertheless, the responsibility for health that is entrusted to government agencies is unique and is rooted in principled politics as well as in widely held expectations. Politically, the legitimacy of governments and their popular support depends on their ability to protect their citizens and play a redistributive role. The governance of health is among the core public policy instruments for institutionalized protection and redistribution. In modern states, governments are expected to protect health, to guarantee access to health care and to safeguard people from the impoverishment that illness can bring. These responsibilities were progressively extended, incorporating the correction of market failures that characterize the health sector. Since the beginning of the 20th century, health protection and health care have progressively been incorporated as goods that are guaranteed by governments and are central to the social contract between the state and its citizens. The importance of health systems as a key element of the social contract in modernizing societies is most acutely evident during reconstruction after periods of war or disaster: rebuilding health services counts among the first tangible signs that society is returning to normal. The legitimacy of state intervention is not only based on social and political considerations.

There are also key economic actors—the medical equipment industry, the pharmaceutical industry and the professions—with an interest in governments taking responsibility for health to ensure a viable health market: a costly modern health economy cannot be sustained without risk sharing and pooling of resources. Indeed, those countries that spend the most on health are also those countries with the largest public financing of the health sector. Even in the United States, its exceptionalism stems not from lower public expenditure—but from its singularly high additional private expenditure. The persistent under-performance of the United States health sector across domains of health outcomes, quality, access, efficiency and equity, explains opinion polls that show increasing consensus of the notion of government intervention to secure more equitable access to essential health care.

Public Sector Stewardship Justified

A more effective public sector stewardship of the health sector is, justified on the grounds of greater efficiency and equity. This crucial stewardship role is often misinterpreted as a mandate for centralized planning and complete administrative control of the health sector. While some types of health challenges, e.g. public-health emergencies or disease eradication, may require authoritative command-and-control management, effective stewardship increasingly relies on "mediation" to address current and future complex health challenges. The interests of public authorities, the health sector and the public are closely intertwined. Over the years, this has made all the institutions of medical care, such as training, accreditation, payment, hospitals, entitlements, etc., the object of intensive bargaining on how broadly to define the welfare state and the collective goods that go with it. This means that public and quasi-public institutions have to mediate the social contract between institutions of medicine, health and society. In high-income countries today, the health care system and the state appear indissolubly bound together. In low- and middle-income countries, the state has often had a more visible role, but paradoxically, one that was less effective in steering the health sector, particularly when, during the 1980s and 1990s, some countries of them became severely tested by conflicts and economic recession. This resulted in their health systems being drawn in directions quite different from the goals and values pursued by the PHC movement.

Disengagement from Health Care

In many socialist and post-socialist countries undergoing economic restructuring, the state has withdrawn abruptly from its previously predominant role in health. China's deregulation of the health sector in the 1980s, and the subsequent steep increases in reliance on out-of-pocket spending, is a case in point and a warning to the rest of the world. A spectacular deterioration of health care provision and social protection, particularly in rural areas, led to a marked slowdown in the increase in life expectancy. This caused China to re-examine its policies and reassert the Government's leadership role—a re-examination that is far from over.

A similar scenario of disengagement has been noticed in India; where more than 80% care has been relegated to private out of pocket care. It has also been observed in many of the countries of central and eastern Europe and the Commonwealth of Independent States (CEE-CIS). In the early 1990s, public expenditure on health declined to levels that made administering a basic system virtually impossible. This contributed to a major decline in life expectancy. Catastrophic health spending became a major cause of poverty. More recently, funding levels have stabilized or even increased, but significant improvements in health outcomes have not followed and socio-economic inequalities in health and health care access are rising. Evidence and trends related to these rises, as well as increases in informal payment mechanisms for health care, indicate that re-engagement is still insufficient. Elsewhere, but most spectacularly in low income countries and fragile states, the absence or withdrawal of the state from its responsibilities for health reflects broader conditions of economic stagnation, political and social crisis and poor governance. In such conditions, public leadership has often become dysfunctional and de-institutionalized, a weakness that is compounded by a lack of financial leverage to steer the health sector. Global development policies have often added to the difficulties governments face in assuming their responsibilities.

Health Agency Focused around Diseases

For decades, the international community's health agenda—including that of WHO—has been structured around diseases and interventions rather than around the broader challenges being faced by health systems. While this agenda has certainly contributed to a better appreciation of the burden of disease affecting poor countries, it has also profoundly influenced the structure of governmental and quasi-governmental institutions in low- and middle-income countries. The resulting fragmentation of the governance of the health sector has diverted attention from important issues, such as the organization of primary care, the control of the commercialization of the health sector and human resources for health crises. The untoward consequences of this trend are most marked in aid-dependent countries because it has shaped the way funds are channeled. The disproportionate investment in a limited number of disease programmes considered as global priorities in countries that are dependent on external support has diverted the limited energies of ministries of health away from their primary role as mediator in the comprehensive planning of primary care and the public's health. As advocates have rightly argued in recent years, better inter-donor coordination is not going to solve this problem on its own: there is also an urgent need for reinvestment in governance capacity.

Participation and Negotiation

The necessary reinvestment in governmental or quasi-governmental institutions cannot mean a return to command-and-control health governance. Health systems are too complex: the domains of the modern state and civil society are inter-connected, with constantly shifting boundaries. Professions play a major role in how health is governed. Patients, protessions, commercial interests and other groups are organizing themselves in order to improve their negotiating position and to protect their interests. Ministries of health are, also, far from homogenous: individuals and programmes compete for influence and resources, adding to the complexity of promoting change. Effective mediation in health must replace overly simplistic management models of the past and embrace new mechanisms for multi-stakeholder policy dialogue to work out the strategic orientations for PHC reforms.

Social Accountability and Participation

As countries modernize, their citizens attribute more value to social accountability and participation. Throughout the world, increasing prosperity, intellectual skills and social connectivity are associated with people's rising aspiration to have more say in what happens at their workplaces and in their communities ? hence the importance of people-centeredness and community participation ? and in important government decisions that affect their lives ? hence the importance of involving civil society in the social debate on health policies. Another reason that policy dialogue is so important is that PHC reforms require a broad policy dialogue to put the expectations of various stakeholders in perspective, to weigh up need, demand and future challenges, and to resolve the inevitable confrontations such reforms imply.

Health authorities and ministries of health, which have a primary role, have to bring together the decision-making power of the political authorities, the rationality of the scientific community, the commitment of the professionals, and the values and resources of civil society. This is a process that requires time and effort. It would be an illusion to expect PHC policy formation to be wholly consensual, as there are too many conflicting interests. However, experience shows that the legitimacy of policy choices depends less on total consensus than on procedural fairness and transparency. Without a structured, participatory policy dialogue, policy choices are vulnerable to appropriation by interest groups, changes in political personnel or donor fickleness. Without a social consensus, it is also much more difficult to engage effectively with stakeholders whose interests diverge from the options taken by PHC reforms, including other sectors that compete for society's resources; for the "medico-industrial complex", for whom PHC reform may imply a realignment of their industrial strategy and for vested interests, such as those of the tobacco or alcohol industries, where effective PHC reform constitutes a direct threat.

Effective Policy Dialogue

The institutional capacities to enable a productive policy dialogue are not a must. They are typically weak in countries where, by choice or by default, *laissez-faire* dominates the approach to policy formation in health. Even in countries with mature and well-resourced health systems there is scope, and need, for more systematic and institutionalized approaches: negotiation between health authorities and professional institutions is often well established, but is much less so with other stakeholders and usually limited to discussions on resource allocation for service delivery. Policy dialogue must be built. How to do that depends very much on context and background. Experience from countries that have been able to accelerate PHC reforms suggests three common elements of effective policy dialogue:

1. making information systems instrumental to PHC reform;
2. systematically harnessing innovations; and
3. sharing lessons on what works.

Citizens need easier access to their own health records, which should inform them about the progress being made in their treatment plans and allow them to participate in decisions related to their own health and that of their families and communities. Communities and civil society organizations need better information to protect their members' health, reduce exclusion and promote equity. Health professionals need better information to improve the quality of their work, and to improve coordination and integration of services. Politicians need information on how well the health system is meeting society's goals and on how public money is being used. Information that can be used to steer change at the policy level is quite different from the data that most conventional health information systems currently produce. There is a need to monitor what the reforms are achieving across the range of social values and the associated outcomes that are central to PHC: equity, people-centeredness, protection of the health of communities and participation. That means asking questions is essential: is care comprehensive, integrated, continuous and effective? Is access guaranteed and are people aware of what they are entitled to? Are people protected against the economic consequences of ill-health? Are authorities effective in ensuring protection against exclusion from care? Are they effective in ensuring protection against exploitation by commercial providers?

The Need for Paradigm Shift

Better identification of priority health problems and trends is important (and vital to anticipate future challenges) but, from a policy point of view, the crucial information is that which allows identification of the operational and systemic constraints. In low-income countries in particular, where planning has long been structured along epidemiological considerations, this can provide a new and dynamic basis for orienting systems development. The report by the Bangladesh Health Watch on the state of the country's health workforce, for example, identified such systemic constraints and corresponding recommendations for the consideration of health authorities.

Thailand's "30 Baht" Universal Coverage

Leaders of Thailand's reform process organized a mutually reinforcing interplay between policy development at the central level and "field model development" in the country's provinces. Health workers on the periphery and civil society organizations were given the space to develop and test innovative approaches to care delivery, to see how well they met both professional standards and community expectations. Field model development activities, which were supported by the Ministry of Health, were organized and managed at provincial level; and extensively discussed and negotiated with provincial contracts. Each province developed its own strategies to deal with its specific problems. The large amount of flexibility given to the provinces in deciding their own work programmes had the advantage of promoting ownership, fostering creativity and allowing original ideas to come forward. It also built local capacities. The downside to the high level of autonomy of the provinces was a tendency to multiply initiatives, making it difficult to evaluate the results to be fed into the policy work in a systematic way. On balance, however, the difficulties due to the locally-driven approach were compensated for by the positive effects related to reform dynamics and capacity building. By 2001, nearly half of Thailand's 76 provinces were experimenting with organizational innovation, most of it around issues of equitable access, local health care systems and community health. Thailand's "30 Baht" universal coverage reform was a bold political initiative to improve health equity. Its transformation into a concrete reality was made possible through the accumulated experience from the field and through the alliances the fieldwork had built between health workers, civil society organizations and the public. This mutually reinforcing process of linking policy development with learning from the field is important for several reasons:

1. It taps the wealth of latent knowledge and innovation within the health sector;
2. Bold experiments in the field give front-line workers, system leaders and the public an inspiring glimpse of what the future might look like in a health system shaped by PHC values.
3. The linking of policy development with frontline action fosters alliances and support from within the sector, without which far-reaching reform is not sustainable; and
4. Such processes engage society both locally and at national level, generating the demand for change that is essential in building political commitment and maintaining the momentum for reform.

Critical Mass of Capacity

The stimulation of open, collaborative structures that supply reforms with strategic intelligence and harness innovation throughout the health system requires a critical mass of committed and experienced people and institutions. They must not only carry out technical and organizational tasks, but they must also be able to balance flexibility and coherence, adapt to new ways of working, and build credibility and legitimacy. However, that critical mass of people and institutions is often not available. Institutions in low-income countries that have suffered from decades of neglect and disinvestment are of particular concern. They are often short on credibility and starved of resources, while key staff may have found more rewarding working environments with partner agencies. Poor governance complicates matters, and is compounded by international pressure for state minimalism and the disproportionate influence of the donor community. The conventional responses to leadership capacity shortfalls in such settings, which are characterized by a heavy reliance on external technical assistance, toolkits and training, have been disappointing. They need to be replaced by more systematic and sustainable approaches in order to institutionalize competencies that learn from and share experience. Documented evidence of how individual and institutional policy dialogue and leadership capacities build up over time is hard to find, but a set of extensive interviews of health sector leaders in six countries shows that personal career trajectories are shaped by a combination of three decisive experiences.

1. At some point in their careers, all had been part of a major sectoral programme or project, particularly in the area of basic health services.
2. Many of them refer to this as a formative experience: it is where they learned about PHC, but also where they forged a commitment and started building critical alliances and partnerships.
3. Many became involved in national planning exercises, which strengthened their capacity to generate and use information and, again, their capacity to build alliances and partnerships. Few had participated personally in major studies or surveys, but those who had, found it an opportunity to hone their skills in generating and analyzing information.

These personal histories of individual capacity strengthening are corroborated by more in-depth analysis of the factors that contributed to the institutional capacities for steering the health sector in these same countries. Opportunities to learn from large-scale health-systems development programmes have contributed most, confirming the importance of hands-on engagement with the problems of the health sector in a collaborative environment. Especially noteworthy is the fact that the introduction of tools was rarely identified as a critical input, and respondents did not highlight inputs from experts and training. The implication is that the key investment for capacity building for PHC reforms should be to create opportunities for learning by linking individuals and institutions to ongoing reform processes. A further consideration is the importance of doing so in an environment where exchange, within and between countries, is facilitated. Unlike the conventional approaches to capacity building, exchange and exposure to the experience of others enhances self-reliance. This is not just a recipe for under-resourced and poorly performing countries. Portugal, for example, has organized a broad societal debate on its 2004-10 National Health Plan involving a pyramid of participation platforms from local and regional to national level, and substantial contributions to the plan from sources ranging from civil society and professional organizations to local governments and academia. At three critical moments in the process, international panels of experts were also invited from other countries to act as sounding boards for their policy debate: a collaboration that was a learning exercise for all parties.

The Political Process

PHC reforms change the balance of power within the health sector and the relationship between health and society. Success depends not only on a credible technical vision, but also on the ability to obtain the high-level political endorsement and the wider commitment that is necessary to mobilize governmental, financial and other institutional machineries. As a technical sector, health rarely has prominence in the hierarchy of the political arena. Ministries of health have often had enough to deal with simply trying to resolve the technical challenges internal to the sector. They are traditionally ill at ease, short of leverage and ill-equipped to make their case in the wider political arena, particularly in low- and low-middle-income countries. The general lack of political influence limits the ability of health authorities, and of other stakeholders in the PHC movement, to advance the PHC agenda, especially when it challenges the interests of other constituencies. It explains the frequently absent or overly cautious reactions against the health effects of working conditions and environmental damage, or the slow implementation of regulations that may interfere with the commercial interests of the food and tobacco industry. Similarly, ambitious reform efforts are often diluted or watered down under the influence of the donor community, the pharmaceutical and the health technology industries, or the professional lobbies.

Lack of political influence also has consequences within governmental spheres. Ministries of health are in a particularly weak position in low- and low-middle-income countries, as is evidenced by the fact that they can claim only 4.5% and 1.7%, respectively, of total government expenditure (against 10% and 17.7%, respectively, in upper-middle and high-income countries). The lack of prominence of health priorities in wider development strategies, such as the Poverty Reduction

Strategy Papers (PRSPs), is another illustration of that weakness. Equally, ministries of health are often absent in discussions about caps on social (and health) spending, which are dominated by debates on macro-economic stability, inflation targets or sustainable debt. It is telling that, in highly indebted countries, the health sector's efforts to obtain a share of the debt relief funds have been generally slow, less than forceful and unconvincing compared to education, foregoing possibilities for rapid expansion of their resource base. Despite these challenges, there is a growing indication that the political will for ambitious reforms based on PHC is taking place. India's health missions—"rural" and subsequently "urban"—are accompanied by a doubling of public expenditure on health. China is preparing an extremely ambitious rural PHC reform that also includes a major commitment of public resources. The size and comprehensiveness of PHC-oriented reforms in Brazil, Chile, Ethiopia, the Islamic Republic of Iran, New Zealand, Thailand and many other countries, reflect very clearly that it is not unrealistic to mobilize political will. Even in extremely unfavourable circumstances, it has proven possible to gain credibility and political clout through pragmatic engagement with political and economic forces. Experience across these countries shows that political endorsement of PHC reforms critically depends on a reform programme, that is formulated in terms that show its potential political dividends. To do that it has to respond explicitly to rising demand as well as to the health challenges and health system constraints the country faces, showing that it is not merely a technical programme, but one rooted in concerns relevant to society.

Resistance to Change is Universal

Creating the political alignment and commitment to reform, however, is only a first step. Insufficient preparation of its implementation is often the weak point. Of particular importance is an understanding of resistance to change, particularly from health workers. While the intuition of leadership has its merits, it is also possible to organize more systematic exercises to anticipate and respond to the potential reactions of stakeholders and the public: political mapping exercises, as in Lebanon; marketing studies and opinion polls, as in the United States; public hearings, as in Canada; or sector-wide meetings of stakeholders, as in the Etats Généraux de la Santé in French-speaking Africa. Delivering on PHC reforms requires a sustained management capacity across levels of the system, embedded in institutions that are fit for the purpose. In Chile, for example, administrative structures and competencies across the whole of the Ministry of Health are being redefined in line with the PHC reforms. Such structural changes are not sufficient. They need to be instigated in conjunction with changes in the organizational culture, from one of issuing decrees for change to a more inclusive collaboration with a variety of stakeholders across the levels of the health system. That in turn requires the institutionalization of policy-dialogue mechanisms drawing practice-based knowledge up from the ground level to inform overall systems governance, while reinforcing social linkages and collaborative action among constituencies at community level. This management capacity should not be assumed, it requires active investment.

Even with effective political dialogue to gain consensus on specific PHC reforms and the requisite management for implementation across levels of the system, many such reforms do not have their intended impact. The best-planned and executed policy reforms often run into unanticipated challenges or rapidly changing contexts. Broad experience in dealing with complex systems behaviour suggests that significant shortfalls or shifts away from articulated goals are to be expected. An important component to build into the reform processes is mechanisms that can pick up significant unintended consequences or deviations from expected performance benchmarks, which allow for course corrections during implementation. Widespread evidence on inequities in health and health care in virtually all countries is a humbling reminder of the difficulties confronting

Sources

Sen, A. Development as freedom. Oxford, Oxford University Press, 1999.

Fegan, G.W. *et al.* Effect of expanded insecticide-treated bednet coverage on child survival in rural Kenya: a longitudinal study. *Lancet*, 2007, 370:1035-1039.

Liu, Y. China's public health care system: facing the challenges. *Bulletin of the World Health Organization*, 2004, 82:532-538.

Kaufman, J.A. China's heath care system and avian influenza preparedness. Journal of Infectious Diseases, 2008, 197 (Suppl. 1):S7-S13.

Ståhl, T. *et al*, eds. Health in all policies: prospects and potentials. Helsinki, Ministry of Social Affairs and Health, 2006.

Berer, M. National laws and unsafe abortion: the parameters of change. *Reproductive Health Matters*, 2004, 12:1-8.

Grimes, D.A. *et al.* Unsafe abortion: the preventable pandemic. *Lancet*, 2006, 368:1908-1919.

Sommer, A., Mosley, W.H. East Bengal cyclone of November 1970: epidemiological approach to disaster assessment. *Lancet*, 1972, 1:1029-1036.

Bern, C. *et al.* Risk factors for mortality in the Bangladesh cyclone of 1991. *Bulletin of the World Health Organization*, 1993, 71:73-78.

Chowdhury, A.M. Personal communication, 2008.

Asaria, P. *et al.* Chronic disease prevention: health effects and financial costs of strategies to reduce salt intake and control tobacco use. *Lancet*, 2007, 370:2044-2053.

World abortion policies 2007. New York NY, United Nations, Department of Economic and Social Affairs, Population Division, 2007 (ST/ESA/SER.A/264, Wallchart).

Unsafe abortion. Global and regional estimates of the incidence of unsafe abortion and associated mortality in 2003, 5th ed. Geneva, World Health Organization, 2007.

Maternal health and early childhood development in Cuba. Ottawa, Committee on Social Affairs, Science and Technology, 2007 (Second Report of the Subcommittee on Population Health of the Standing Senate).

Evans, R.G., Thomas, McKeown, Meet Fidel Castro: physicians, population health and the Cuban paradox. *Health Care Policy*, 2008, 3:21-32.

Spiegel, J.M., Yassi, A. Lessons from the margins of globalization: appreciating the Cuban health paradox. *Journal of Public Health Policy*, 2004, 25:85-110.

The World Health Report—Health systems: improving performance. Geneva, World Health Organization, 2000.

Everybody's business—strengthening health systems to improve health outcomes. Geneva, World Health Organization, *Health Systems Services*, 2007.

Hogerzeil, H.V. The concept of essential medicines: lessons for rich countries. *BMJ*, 2004, 329:1169-1172.

Measuring medicine prices, availability, affordability and price components, 2nd ed. Geneva, Health Action International and World Health Organization, 2008 (http://www.haiweb.org/medicineprices/, accessed 20 August 2008).

Black, R.E., Morris, S.S., Bryce, J. Where and why are 10 million children dying every year? *Lancet*, 2003, 361:2226-2234.

Supply annual report 2007. Copenhagen, United Nations Children's Fund Supply Division, 2008.

Tambini, G. *et al*. Regional immunization programs as a model for strengthening cooperation among nations. Revista panamericana de salud pública, 2006, 20:54-59.

EPI Revolving Fund: quality vaccines at low cost. EPI Newsletter, 1997, 19:6-7.

Matiru, R., Ryan, T. The global drug facility: a unique, holistic and pioneering approach to drug procurement and management. Bulletin of the World Health Organization, 2007, 85:348-353.

Annual Report. Wellington, Pharmaceutical Management Agency, 2007.

The World Health Report 2006—Working together for health. Geneva, World Health Organization, 2006.

Victora, C.G. *et al*. Achieving universal coverage with health interventions. *Lancet*, 2004, 364:1555-1556.

Freitas do Amaral, JJ *et al*. Multi-country evaluation of IMCI, Brazil study. Ceará, Federal University of Ceará, ND.

Sontag, S. AIDS and its metaphors. New York, NY, Farrar, Straus and Giroux, 1988.

Mann, J.M. *et al*, eds. Health and human rights: a reader. New York NY, Routledge, 1999.

Friedman, S., Mottiar, S. A rewarding engagement? The treatment action campaign and the politics of HIV/AIDS. *Politics and Society*, 2005, 33:511-565.

Ottawa Charter for Health Promotion. In: First International Conference on Health Promotion, Ottawa, 21 November 1986. Geneva, World Health Organization, Department of Human Resources for Health, 1986 (WHO/HPR/HEP/95.1; http://www.who.int/hpr/NPH/docs/ottawa_charter_hp.pdf, accessed 2 July 2008).

Ezzati, M. *et al*. Comparative risk assessment collaborating group. Estimates of global and regional potential health gains from reducing multiple major risk factors. *Lancet*, 2003, 362:271-280..

Friel, S., Chopra, M., Satcher, D. Unequal weight: equity oriented policy responses to the global obesity epidemic. *BMJ*, 2007, 335:1241-1243.

Satcher, D., Higginbotham, E.J. The public health approach to eliminating disparities in health. *American Journal of Public Health*, 2008, 98:400-403.

The World Health Report 2008 Commission on Social Determinants 37. of Health. Closing the gap in a generation: health equity through action on the social determinants of health. Final report. Geneva, World Health Organization, 2008.

The World Health Report 2007—A safer future: global public health security in the 21st century. Geneva, World Health Organization, 2007.

Satterthwaite, D. In pursuit of a healthy urban environment. In: Marcotullkio PJ, McGranahan G, eds. Scaling urban environmental challenges: from local to global and back. London, Earthscan, 2007.

Taylor, C.E., Taylor, H.G. Scaling up community-based primary health care. In: Rohde J, Wyon J, eds. Community-based health care: lessons from Bangladesh to Boston. Boston, Management Sciences for Health, 2002.

WHO/Public Health Agency Canada Collaborative Project. Improving health equity through intersectoral action. Geneva, World Health Organization, 2008 (in press).

Puska, P. Health in all policies. *European Journal of Public Health*, 2007, 17:328.

Chami, Y., Hammou, J., Mahjour, J. Lessons from the Moroccan national trachoma control programme. Community Eye Health, 2004, 17:59.

Dye, C. *et al*. The decline of tuberculosis epidemics under chemotherapy: a case study in Morocco. *International Journal of Tuberculosis and Lung Disease*, 2007, 11:1225-1231.

Senegal: outbreak of lead intoxication in Thiaroye sur Mer 20 June 2008. Geneva, World Health Organization, 2008 (http://www.who.int/environmental_health_emergencies/events/Senegal2008/en/index.html, accessed 21 July 2008).

Muhlrad, N. Road safety management in France: political leadership as a path to sustainable progress. Paper presented at: Gambit 2004 Road Safety Conference, Gdansk, April 2004.

Our cities, our health, our future: acting on social determinants for health equity in urban settings. Geneva, World Health Organization, 2007.

Koivusalo, M. Moving health higher up the European agenda. In: Ståhl T *et al*, eds. Health in all policies: prospects and potentials. Helsinki, Ministry of Social Affairs and Health, 2006:21-40.

Gilson, L. *et al*. Challenging health inequity through health systems. Geneva, World Health Organization, 2007.

WHO report on the global tobacco epidemic, 2008: the MPOWER package. Geneva, World Health Organization, 2008.

Anaudova, A. Seventh Futures Forum on Unpopular Decisions in Public Health. Copenhagen, World Health Organization Regional Office for Europe, 2005.

Allin, S. *et al*. Making decisions on public health: a review of eight countries. Geneva, World Health Organization, European Observatory on Health Systems and Policies, 2004.

Setel, P.W. *et al*. on behalf of the Monitoring of Vital Events (MoVE) writing group. A scandal of invisibility: making everyone count by counting everyone. *Lancet*, 2007 (published online: DOI: 10.1016/S0140-6736(07)61307-5).

Mahapatra, P. *et al*. on behalf of the Monitoring of Vital Events (MoVE) writing group. Civil registration systems and vital statistics: successes and missed opportunities. *Lancet*, 2007 (published online: DOI: 10.1016/S0140-6736(07)61308-7).

AbouZahr, C. *et al*. on behalf of the Monitoring of Vital Events (MoVE) writing group. The way forward. *Lancet*, 2007 (published online: DOI: 10.1016/S0140-6736(07)61310-5).

Volmink, J. *et al*. A.M. Research synthesis and dissemination as a bridge to knowledge management: the Cochrane Collaboration. Bulletin of the World Health Organization, 2004, 82:778-783.

Halstead, S.B., Tugwell, P., Bennett, K. The International Clinical Epidemiology Network (INCLEN): a progress report. *Journal of Clinical Epidemiology*, 1991, 44:579-589.

Waters, E. *et al*. Cochrane Collaboration. Evaluating the effectiveness of public health interventions: the role and activities of the Cochrane Collaboration. *Journal of Epidemiology and Community Health*, 2006, 60:285-289.

Sweet, M., Moynihan, R. Improving population health: the uses of systematic reviews. New York NY, Milbank Memorial Fund, 2007.

Davies, P., Boruch, R. The Campbell Collaboration does for public policy what Cochrane does for health. *BMJ*, 2001, 323:294-295.

An idea whose time has come: New opportunities for HIA in New Zealand public policy and planning. Wellington, Public Health Advisory Committee, 2007.

Harris, P. *et al*. Health impact assessment: a practical guide. Sydney, University of New South Wales, 2007.

Wismar, M. *et al*. Implementing and institutionalizing health impact assessment in Europe. In: Ståhl T *et al*, eds. Health in all policies: prospects and potentials. Helsinki, Ministry of Social Affairs and Health, 2006.

Blau, J. *et al*. The use of health impact assessment across Europe. In: Ståhl T *et al*, eds. Health in all policies: prospects and potentials. Helsinki, Ministry of Social Affairs and Health, 2006.

Dannenberg, A.L. *et al*. Use of health impact assessment in the US: 27 case studies, 1999-2007. *American Journal of Preventive Medicine*, 2008, 34:241-256.

Wismar, M. *et al*, eds. The effectiveness of health impact assessment: scope and limitations of supporting decision-making in Europe. Geneva, World Health Organization, 2007.

Jewell, C.J., Bero, L.A. Developing good taste in evidence: facilitators of and hindrances to evidence-informed health policymaking in state government. *The Milbank Quarterly*, 2008, 86:177-208.

Communication from the Commission on Better Regulation for Growth and Jobs in the European Union. Brussels, European Commission, 2005 (COM (2005) 97 final).

Binder, S. *et al*. National public health institutes: contributing to the public good. *Journal of Public Health Policy*, 2008, 29:3-21.

Framework for the creation and development of national public health institutes. Helsinki, International Association of National Public Health Institutes, 2007.

Khaleghian, P., Das Gupta, M. Public management and the essential public health functions. Washington DC, The World Bank, 2004 (World Bank Policy Research Working Paper 3220).

Kickbusch, I. A new agenda for health. Perspectives in Health, 2004, 9:8-13.

World Trade Organization Declaration on the TRIPS Agreement and Public Health. Ministerial Conference, 4th Session, Doha, 9-14 November 2001. 2001 (WT/MIN(01)/DEC/2).

Wilk, E.A. van der *et al*. Learning from our neighbours - cross-national inspiration for Dutch public health polices: smoking, alcohol, overweight, depression, health inequalities, youth screening. Bilthoven, National Institute for Public Health and the Environment, 2008 (RIVM Rapport 270626001; http://www.rivm.nl/bibliotheek/rapporten/270626001.pdf, accessed 30 July 2008).

Porter, D. Health, civilization and the state. A history of public health from ancient to modern times. London and New York, Routledge, 1999.

The World Health Report 2000—Health systems: improving performance. Geneva, World Health Organization, 2000.

Waldman, R. Health programming for rebuilding states: a briefing paper. Arlington VA, Partnership for Child Health Care, Basic Support for Institutionalizing Child Survival (BASICS), 2007.

National health accounts. Geneva, World Health Organization (http//www.who.int/nha/country/en/index.html, accessed May 2008).

Schoen, C. *et al*. US health system performance: a national scorecard. *Health Affairs*, 2006, 25(Web Exclusive):w457-w475.

Jacobs, L.R., Shapiro, R.Y. Public opinion's tilt against private enterprise. *Health Affairs*, 1994, 13:285-289.

Blendon, R.J., Menson, J.M. Americans' views on health policy: a fifty year historical perspective. *Health Affairs*, 2001, 20:33-46.

Fox, D.M. The medical institutions and the state. In: Bynum WF, Porter R, eds. Companion encyclopedia of the history of medicine. London and New York, Routledge, 1993, 50:1204-1230.

Blank, R.H. The price of life: the future of American health care. New York NY, Colombia University Press, 1997.

Frenk, J., Donabedian, A. State intervention in health care: type, trends and determinants. Health Policy and Planning, 1987, 2:17-31.

Blumenthal, D., Hsiao, W. Privatization and its discontents—the evolving Chinese health care system. *New England Journal of Medicine*, 2005, 353:1165-1170.

Liu, Y., Hsiao, W.C., Eggleston, K. Equity in health and health care: the Chinese experience. *Social Science and Medicine*, 1999, 49:1349-1356.

Bloom, G., Xingyuan, G. Health sector reform: lessons from China. *Social Science and Medicine*, 1997, 45:351-360.

Tang, S., Cheng, X., Xu, L. Urban social health insurance in China. Eschborn, Gesellschaft für Technische Zusammenarbeit and International Labour Organization, 2007.

China: long-term issues and options in the health transition. Washington DC, The World Bank, 1992.

China statistics 2007. Beijing, Ministry of Health, 2007 (http://moh.gov.cn/open/statistics/year2007/p83.htm, accessed 31 May 2008).

WHO mortality database. Geneva, World Health Organization, 2007 (Tables; http://www.who.int/healthinfo/morttables/en/index.html, accessed 1 July 2008).

Suhrcke, M., Rocco, L., McKee, M. Health: a vital investment for economic development in eastern Europe and central Asia. Copenhagen, World Health Organization Regional Office for Europe, European Observatory on Health Systems and Policies (http://www.euro.who.int/observatory/Publications/20070618_1, accessed May 2008).

Collier, P. The bottom billion: why the poorest countries are failing and what can be done about it. Oxford and New York NY, Oxford University Press, 2007.

Grindle, M.S. The good government imperative: human resources, organizations, and institutions. In: Grindle MS, ed. Getting good government: capacity building in the public sectors of developing countries. Boston MA, Harvard University Press, 1997 (Harvard Studies in International Development:3-28).

Hilderbrand, M.E., Grindle, M.S. Building sustainable capacity in the public sector: what can be done? In: Grindle, M.S., ed. Getting good government: capacity building in the public sectors of developing countries. Boston MA, Harvard University Press, 1997 (Harvard Studies in International Development:31-61).

Goldsbrough, D. Does the IMF constrain health spending in poor countries? Evidence and an agenda for action. Washington DC, Center for Global Development, 2007.

Shiffman, J. Has donor prioritization of HIV/AIDS displaced aid for other health issues? *Health Policy and Planning*, 2008, 23:95-100.

Bill and Melinda Gates Foundation and McKinsey and Company. Global health partnerships: assessing country consequences. Paper presented at: Third High-Level Forum on the Health MDGs, Paris, 14-15 November 2005 (http://www.hlfhealthmdgs.org/documents/GatesGHPNov2005.pdf).

Stein, E. *et al.*, eds. The politics of policies: economic and social progress in Latin America. Inter-American Development Bank, David Rockefeller Center for Latin American Studies and Harvard University. Washington DC, Inter-American Development Bank, 2006.

Moran, M. Governing the health care state: a comparative study of the UnitedKingdom, the United States and Germany. Manchester, Manchester University Press,1999.

Saltman, R.B., Busse, R. Balancing regulation and entrepreneurialism in Europe's health sector: theory and practice. In: Saltman, R.B., Busse, R., Mossialos, E., eds. Regulating entrepreneurial behaviour in European health care systems. Milton Keynes, Open University Press for European Observatory on Health Systems and Policies, 2002:3-52.

McDaniel, A. Managing health care organizations: where professionalism meets complexity science. *Health Care Management Review*, 2000, 25:1.

World values surveys database. World Values Surveys, 2007 (V120, V121; http://www.worldvaluessurvey.com, accessed 15 October 2007).

Inglehart, R., Welzel, C. Modernization, cultural change and democracy: the human development sequence. Cambridge, Cambridge University Press, 2005.

Lopes, C., Theisohn, T. Ownership, leadership, and transformation: can we do better for capacity development? London, Earthscan, 2003.

Wasi, P. The triangle that moves the mountain. Bangkok, Health Systems Research Institute, 2000.

McKee, M., Figueras, J. Setting priorities: can Britain learn from Sweden? *British Medical Journal*, 1996, 312:691-694.The World Health Report.

Ammar, W. Health system and reform in Lebanon. World Health Organization Regional Office for the Eastern Mediterranean and Ministry of Health of Lebanon. Beirut, Entreprise universitaire d'Etudes et de Publications, 2003.

Stewart, J., Kringas, P. Change management—strategy and values. Six case studies from the Australian Public Sector. Canberra, University of Canberra, Centre for Research in Public Sector Management (http://www.dmt.canberra.edu.au/crpsm/research/pdf/stewartkringas.pdf).

Chalmers, I. From optimism to disillusion about commitment to transparency in the medico-industrial complex. *Journal of the Royal Society of Medicine*, 2006, 99:337-341.

Romanow, R.J. Building on values. The future of health care in Canada - final report. Saskatoon, Commission on the Future of Health Care in Canada, 2002.

Escorel, S., Arruda de Bloch, R. As conferências Nacionais de Saúde na Cobnstrução do SUS. In: Trinidade Lima, N. *et al*, eds. Saúde e democracia: história e perpsectivas do SUS. Rio de Janeiro, Editora Fiocruz, 2005:83-120.

Jongudomsuk, P. Achieving universal coverage of health care in Thailand through the 30 Baht scheme. Paper presented at: SEAMIC Conference 2001 FY, Chiang Mai, Thailand, 14-17 January 2002.

Galichet, B. *et al*. Country initiatives to lift health system constraints: lessons from 49 GAVI-HSS proposals. Geneva, World Health Organization, Department for Health System Governance and Service Delivery, 2008.

The state of health in Bangladesh 2007. Health workforce in Bangladesh: who constitutes the health care system? Bangladesh Health Watch (http://sph.bracu.ac.bd/bhw/, accessed June 2008).

Hemmings, J., Wilkinson, J. What is a public health observatory? *Journal of Epidemiology and Community Health*, 2003, 57:324-326.

Equity gauge profiles. Global Equity Gauge Alliance, 2008 (http:www.gega.org.za, accessed 24 April 2008).

De Campos, F.E., Hauck, V. Networking collaboratively: the experience of the observatories of human resources in Brazil. Cahiers de sociologie et de démographie médicales, 2005, 45:173-208.

Ashton, J. Public health observatories: the key to timely public health intelligence in the new century. *Journal of Epidemiology and Community Health*, 2000, 54:724-725.

Intelligent health partnerships. York, *Association of Public Health Observatories*, 2008 (http://www.apho.org.uk/resource/item.aspx?RID=39353 accessed 10 June 2008).

Robinson, M., Baxter, H., Wilkinson, J. Working together on coronary heart disease in Northern and Yorkshire. *Stockton-on-Tees, Northern and Yorkshire Public Health Observatory*, 2001.

Bell, R. *et al*. Perinatal and infant health: a scoping study. Stockton-on-Tees, *Northern and Yorkshire Public Health Observatory*, 2001.

Grant, S., Wilkinson, J., Learmonth, A. An overview of health impact assessment. Stockton-on-Tees, *Northern and Yorkshire Public Health Observatory*, 2001 (Occasional Paper No. 1).

Bailey, K. *et al*. Towards a healthier north-east. *Stockton-on-Tees, Northern and Yorkshire Public Health Observatory*, 2001.

Beal, J., Pepper, L. The dental health of five-year-olds in the Northern and Yorkshire Region. *Stockton-on-Tees, Northern and Yorkshire Public Health Observatory*, 2002.

Thailand's health care reform project, 1996-2001: final report. Bangkok, Ministry of Health, Thailand Office of Health Care Reform, 2001.

Tancharoensathien, V., Jongudomsuk, P., eds. From policy to implementation: historical events during 2001-2004 of UC in Thailand. Bangkok, National Health Security Office, 2005.

Baser, H., Morgan, P. Capacity, change and performance. Maastricht, European Centre for Development Policy Management, 2008.

Macq, J. *et al*. Quality attributes and organisational options for technical support to health services system strengthening. Background paper commissioned for the GAVI-HSS Task Team, Nairobi, August 2007.

Boffin, N., De Brouwere, V. Capacity building strategies for strengthening the stewardship function in health systems of developing countries. Results of an international comparative study carried out in six countries. Antwerp, Institute of Tropical Medicine, Department of Public Health, 2003 (DGOS-AIDS Impulse Programme 97203 BVO "Human resources in developing health systems").

Carrolo, M., Ferrinho, P, Perreira Miguel, J. (rapporteurs). Consultation on Strategic Health Planning in Portugal. World Health Organization/Portugal Round Table, Lisbon, July 2003. Lisbon, Direcção Geral da Saùde, 2004.

Forss, K. *et al*. Evaluation of the effectiveness of technical assistance personnel. Report to DANIDA, FINNIDA, NORAD and SIDA, 1988.

Fukuda-Parr, S. Capacity for development: new solutions to old problems. New York NY, United Nations Development Programme, 2002. Messian L. Renforcement des capacités et processus de changement. Réflexions à partir de la réforme de l'administration publique en République Démocratique du Congo. BTC Seminar on Implementing the Paris Declaration on Aid Effectiveness, Brussels, 2006.

OECD. StatExtracts [online database]. Paris, Organisation for Economic Co-operation and Development, 2008 (http://stats.oecd.org/WBOS/Index.aspx accessed June 2008).

Irwin, A. Beyond the toolkits: bringing engagement into practice. In: Engaging science: thoughts, deeds, analysis and action. London, Wellcome Trust, 2007:50-55.

Rowe, A.K. *et al*. How can we achieve and maintain high-quality performance of health workers in low-resource settings? *Lancet*, 2005, 366:1026-1035.

Blaise, P., Kegels, G. A realistic approach to the evaluation of the quality management movement in health care systems: a comparison between European and African contexts based on Mintzberg's organizational models. *International Journal of Health Planning and Management*, 2004, 19:337-364.

Lippingcott, D.F. Saturation training: bolstering capacity in the Indonesian Ministry of Finance. In: Grindle, M.S., ed. Getting good government: capacity building in the public sectors of developing countries. Boston MA, Harvard University Press, 1997 (Harvard Studies in International Development:98-123).

Krause, E. Death of the guilds. professions, states and the advance of capitalism, 1930 to the present. New Haven and London, Yale University Press, 1996.

World health statistics 2008. Geneva, World Health Organization, 2008.

Poverty Reduction Strategy Papers, their significance for health: second synthesis report. Geneva, World Health Organization, 2004 (WHO/HDP/PRSP/04.1 2004).

World Bank Independent Evaluation Group. Debt relief for the poorest: an evaluation update of the HIPC Initiative. Washington DC, The World Bank, 2006 (http://www.worldbank.org/ieg/hipc/report.html, accessed June 2008).

Pangu, K.A. Health workers' motivation in decentralised settings: waiting for better times? In: Ferrinho, P., Van Lerberghe, W., eds. Providing health care under adverse conditions. Health personnel performance and individual coping strategies. Antwerp, ITG Press, 2000:19-30.

Mutizwa-Mangiza, D. The impact of health sector reform on public sector health worker motivation in Zimbabwe. Bethesda MD, Abt Associates, 1998 (Partnerships for Health Reform, Major Applied Research 5, Working Paper No. 4).

Wiscow, C. The effects of reforms on the health workforce. Geneva, World Health Organization, 2005 (background paper for The World Health Report 2006).

Rigoli, F., Dussault, G. The interface between health sector reform and human resources in health. Human Resources for Health, 2003, 1:9.

Road map for a health justice majority. Oakland, CA, American Environics, 2006 (http://www.americanenvironics.com/PDF/Road_Map_for_Health_Justice_Majority_AE.pdf, accessed 1 July 2008).

10

Outsourcing as a Health Care System: Health Tourism

"Health tourism has assumed the role of a health care system to fulfil the unmet medical needs from developed as well as developing countries. Health tourism can be broadly defined as provision of 'cost effective' private medical care in another country, in collaboration with the tourism industry for patients needing surgical and other forms of elective specialized health care. This process is being facilitated by the corporate sector involved in medical care as well as the tourism industry—both private and public. It entails patients going to a different country for either urgent or elective medical procedures, and is fast becoming a worldwide, multibillion-dollar industry. The reasons patients travel for treatment vary. Many medical tourists from the United States are seeking treatment at a 10th of the cost at home. From Canada and UK, it is often people who are frustrated by long waiting times. For others, becoming a medical tourist is a chance to combine a tropical vacation with elective or plastic surgery."

Health Tourism is not New

Health tourism is actually thousands of years old. In ancient Greece, pilgrims and patients came from all over the Mediterranean to the sanctuary of the healing god, Asklepios, at Epidaurus. In Roman Britain, patients took the waters at a shrine to bathe, a practice that continued for 2000 years. From the 18th century wealthy Europeans traveled to spas from Germany to the Nile. In the 21st century, relatively low-cost jet travel has taken the industry beyond the wealthy and desperate. The most recent trend in privatisation of health services is medical tourism, which is gaining prominence in developing countries. Globalisation has promoted a consumerist culture, thereby promoting goods and services that can feed the aspirations arising from this culture. This has had its effect in the health sector too, with the emergence of a private sector that thrives by servicing a small percentage of the population that has the ability to "buy" medical care at the rates at which the "high end" of the private medical sector provides such care. This has changed the character of the medical care sector, with the entry of the corporate sector. Corporate run institutions are seized with the necessity to maximise profits and expand their coverage. These objectives face a constraint in the form of the relatively small size of the population in developing countries that can afford services offered by such institutions. In this background, corporate interests in the Medical Care sector are looking for opportunities that go beyond the limited domestic "market" for high cost medical care. This is the genesis of the "medical tourism" industry. With global revenues estimated at $2.8 trillion, the health care industry is the world's largest industry. The Indian health care industry has the potential to show the same exponential growth that the software and pharmaceutical industries have shown in the past decade. Countries that actively promote medical tourism include Cuba, Costa Rica, Hungary, India, Israel, Jordan, Lithuania, Malaysia and Thailand. Belgium, Poland and Singapore are now entering the field. South Africa specializes in medical safaris-visit the country for a safari, with a stopover for plastic surgery, a nose job and a chance to see lions and elephants.

Need for Health Tourism as a System of Health Care

Medical tourism covers a broad spectrum of medical services. It mixes leisure, fun and relaxation together with wellness and health care. The idea of the health holiday is to offer you an opportunity to get away from your daily routine and come into a different relaxing surrounding. Here you can enjoy being close to the beach and the mountains. At the same time you are able to receive an orientation that will help you improve your life in terms of your health and general well-being. It is like rejuvenation and cleanup process on all levels—physical, mental and emotional. Many people from the developed world come to India for the rejuvenation promised by yoga and Ayurvedic massage, but only a few consider it a destination for hip replacement or brain surgery. However, a nice blend of top-class medical expertise at attractive prices is helping a growing number of Indian corporate hospitals lure foreign patients, including a few from developed nations such as the UK and the US.

As more and more patients from affluent nations with high Medicare costs look for effective options, India is pitted against Thailand, Singapore, Malaysia and some other Asian countries, which have good hospitals, salubrious climate and tourist destinations. While Thailand and Singapore with their advanced medical facilities and built-in medical tourism options have been drawing foreign patients of the order of several lakhs per annum, the rapidly expanding Indian corporate hospital sector has been able to get a few thousands for treatment. But, things are going to change drastically in favour of India, especially in view of the high quality expertise of medical professionals, backed by the fast improving equipment and nursing facilities, and above all, the cost-effectiveness of the package. As Indian corporate hospitals are on par, if not better than the best hospitals in Thailand, Singapore, etc there is scope for improvement.

Scope of Health Tourism

With internationally recognized health care professionals, holistic medicinal services and low cost of treatment, India has the potential to attract over one million health tourists every year, according to confederation of Indian industry (CII). The country offers a unique mix of systems such as yoga, ayurveda and meditation and modern medical system. This, along with world-class experts and the cost advantage, can help earn $5 billion every year, a CII release said. While a heart surgery costs $30,000 in the US, it costs $6,000 in India. Similarly, a bone marrow transplant costs $26,000 here compared to $250,000 in the US. If a liver transplant costs in the range of Rs. 60 lakhs-70 lakhs in Europe and double that in the US, a few Indian hospitals, such as Global in Hyderabad, have the wherewithal to do it in around Rs. 15 lakh-20 lakhs. Similarly, if a heart surgery in the US costs about Rs. 20 lakhs, the Chennai-headquartered Apollo Hospitals Group does it in roughly Rs. 2 lakhs. Knee surgery (on both knees) costs 350,000 rupees ($7,700) in India; in Britain this costs £10,000 ($16,950), more than twice as much. Dental, eye and cosmetic surgeries in Western countries cost three to four times as much as in India. Take the rising popularity of "preventive health screening". At one private clinic in London a thorough men's health check-up that includes blood tests, electro-cardiogram tests, chest x-rays, lung tests and abdominal ultrasound costs £345 ($574, €500). By comparison, a comparable check-up at a clinic operated by Delhi-based health care company Max Health Care costs $84. The Indian government predicts that India's $17-billion-a-year health care industry could grow 13 per cent in each of the next six years, boosted by medical tourism, which industry watcheRs. say is growing at 30 per cent annually. Price advantage is, of course, a major selling point. The cost differential across the board is huge: only a tenth and sometimes even a sixteenth of the cost in the West.

Citing the example of Thailand, CII said India should aggressively publicize its traditional medicinal system and surgical services in association with the tourism authorities. Indians, NRIs and tourists from around the world are beginning to realize the potential of modern and traditional Indian medicine. Indian hospitals and medical establishments have also realized the potential of this niche market and have begun to tailor their services for foreign visitors. At a regional level, this nascent industry came to limelight with the arrival of 'Naby Noor' from Pakistan, who came by the Indo-Pak bus service and got a red-carpet treatment at a hospital in Bangalore. Several Indian state governments have realized the potential of this 'industry' and have been actively promoting it. Visitors, especially from the west and the middle-east find Indian hospitals affordable and viable option to grappling with insurance and National medical systems in their native lands. Many prefer to combine their treatments with a visit to the 'exotic east' with their families, however, the country would have to improve its health care infrastructure, connectivity between major cities and streamline immigration procedure for medical visitors. Accreditation of Indian hospitals is also essential for attracting such tourists, it added.

Government as well as Corporate Sector Need to Promote Health Tourism

Close on the heels of introducing a medical visa, the Government has started overseas marketing of India as a medical tourism destination. According to senior Government officials, they hope to complete the process of price-banding of hospitals in various cities. By marketing India as a global medical tourism destination, the Government hopes to capitalize on the low-cost, high-quality medical care available in the country. Medical tourism focuses on treatment of acute illness, elective surgeries such as cardiology and cancer, among others. Statistics suggest that the medical tourism industry in India is worth $333 million (Rs. 1,450 crore) while a study by CII-McKinsey estimates that the country could earn Rs. 5,000-10,000 crore by 2012. Probably realizing the potential, major corporates such as the Apollo, the Tatas, Fortis, Max, Wockhardt, Piramal, and the Escorts group have made significant investments in setting up modern hospitals in major cities. Many have also designed special packages for patients, including airport pickups, visa assistance and board and lodging, health care industry officials said. While the trickle of foreigners coming to India for treatment has started, officials are hopeful that this will become a flood once the various initiatives being taken by the Government take off. Apart from receiving patients from those parts of the globe that have poor medical facilities, India has also been getting some medical visitors from the West for a variety of reasons including the long waiting period there for treatment in Government hospitals there. Indian Government has introduced the following policy measures to encourage medical tourism.

National Health Policy recognizes the treatment of international patients as an export, which allows private hospitals treating such patients to enjoy benefits such as lower import duties, increase in the rate of depreciation (from 25 per cent to 40 per cent) for life-saving medical equipment, and several other tax sops.

- India's relatively developing medical tourism segment has been anointed by health care and tourism industry pundits as the next 'best' thing for the country.
- There are plenty of challenges that need to be addressed for India to become the world's preferred health care destination.
- Prominent among them being the need for proper accreditation and requisite standardization systems in place, a tripartite synergy between hospitals, tour operators and respective state governments.

- They spoke about the various challenges impeding the growth of the medical tourism industry and emphasized the need for a synergy between hospitals, state government and international tour operators.
- India will have to project itself as being a holistic medical destination to get an edge over other countries.
- We need to club together a couple of 'pathies' because we have a very strong base of alternative healing therapies like yoga, naturopathy, ayurveda, etc.
- Creating awareness about India's facilities is a must to establish credibility in foreign markets.
- Standardization of a price band for graded hospitals and a quality assurance model should be taken up immediately to take medical tourism ahead.
- The private health care industry is quietly facilitating a revolution to enable India to emerge as a health destination.
- STARK contrasts are no surprise in urban India, and in the health care sector, the difference between what is available (world-class techniques and service, at a price) and what the common denominator urgently needs is no less so.
- Private sector health care centers are gleaming "islands of excellence", as the industry calls them, all too often surrounded by seas of medical neglect.
- When the mix is just right (support from the government in the form of incentives and tax breaks, international health care accreditation standards in place, breakthroughs in insurance coverage for overseas patients, and savvy promotion of India as a tourism-plus-medical tech destination) the sector is certain the numbers will fall into place.
- What's more, the beneficiary of such growth will be the country's desperately overburdened public health system, say industry associations such as the Confederation of Indian Industry (CII) and the Federation of Indian Chambers of Commerce and Industry (FICCI), which see medical tourism a mirror of the early years of India's info-tech growth.
- Look at the possibility of the public hospitals being technologically upgraded to world-class standards with this source of income.
- Such optimism apart, India's three-tier public health system—primary health centers (PHC) in villages, district hospitals, and tertiary care hospitals—is increasingly unable to attend to the medical needs of the population.
- There is no doubt that a technology-centric approach to health care, such as that promoted by the major private hospitals, will inevitably affect the cost of care to the common man.

India Moving Ahead to Develop Health Tourism as a System

India is considered one of the leading countries promoting medical tourism—and now it is moving into a new area of "medical outsourcing," where sub-contractors provide services to the overburdened medical care systems in western countries. India's top-rated education system is not only churning out computer programmers and engineers, but an estimated 20,000 to 30,000 doctors and nurses each year. The largest of the estimated half-dozen medical corporations in India serving medical tourists is Apollo Hospital. Dr. Prathap C. Reddy, the chairman of the company, began negotiations in the spring of 2004 with Britain's National Health Service to work as a sub-contractor, to do operations and medical tests for patients at a fraction of the cost in Britain. Apollo now has 37 hospitals, with about 7,000 beds. The company is in partnership in hospitals in Kuwait, Sri Lanka and Nigeria. Apollo has also reacted to criticism by Indian politicians by expanding its services to India's millions of poor.

India will be happy to provide fixed-price treatment packages, integrating all transport, medical and living costs into one price. Plus a vacation at any of India's fabulous destinations. India is hoping to expand its tourist industry—to include visitors with heart conditions and cataracts. The sight of the country's overcrowded public hospitals, open sewers and garbage-littered streets would unsettle most visitors' confidence about public sanitation standards in India. Though the quality of health care for the poor in countries like India is undeniably low, private facilities offer advanced technology and procedures on par with hospitals in developed nations.

Vishal Bali, of Wockhardt Hospitals, points out as proof of quality that the US private health insurers Blue Cross and Blue Shield insure patients treated at his group's hospitals. The British health insurer Bupa also insures the costs of treatment at Wockhardt hospitals. Mr Bali adds that Wockhardt is in talks with Britain's National Health Service about outsourcing the treatment of British patients to India. Early this year Rosemarie—who is into tourism business—encountered a leg ailment which curtailed her active life. She made extensive enquiries with the Turkish hospitals. She wanted to know what exactly was wrong with her leg, what are the corrective procedures available, what are the latest advances in the field, what is the success rate and how long will it take her to bounce back to her active life. Around this time, she happened to read "Stern," a popular German magazine, which had a special feature on India. It featured India's advancement in medical field. She will have to undergo special hip resurfacing surgery, she landed in Mumbai. Rosemarie speaking from Workhardt Hospital, Mumbai where she is undergoing post-surgery physiotherapy told that her entire medical experience in India was wonderful.

Indo-US Health

If you or a loved one have a health problem that is causing concern about the cost and quality of available care, IndUShealth suggests you consider the excellent, high-quality treatment options available to you in India at a fraction of the cost in a U.S. hospital. IndUShealth's case managers and alliance of physicians in North America are ready to work with you to evaluate your needs and provide the necessary guidance that will help you take advantage of the exceptional care options available to you at one of our partner super-specialty hospitals in India.

At IndUShealth, we strive to make each patient's experience nothing short of an outstanding success. Any patient seeking affordable, high quality medical care can benefit from the IndUShealth system. However, those who may benefit the most are uninsured individuals who may face staggering medical bills for serious procedures. It's notable that half of U.S. bankruptcies are a direct result of catastrophic medical events and their associated costs.

- Patients seeking treatments that are routinely performed in India, but not approved in the U.S. (robot assisted joint replacement as an example).
- Patients that want to take personal accountability for their health care decisions, and make the best choice from global, rather than local options.
- Wait-listed patients with chronic pain or disability, e.g. Canada.

Advent Medical Services

Advent Medical Services group is a leading medical service provider based in India with accomplished and distinguished physicians and surgeons with a vast experience in variety of disciplines including cardiothoracic surgery cosmetic and plastic surgery, laparoscopic surgery, endoscopic surgery, microsurgery, joint replacements and highly advanced form of ophthalmic and ear surgery. Advent is closely affiliated with world-class medical laboratory and research facilities. The group offers the best of class and personalized medical care in a cost-effective manner. It provides a risk free concept of medical evaluation. After completing the registration, he/she can complete the medical history form which is securely transmitted to expert team of Board Certified physicians and surgeons in India. Team evaluates the patient's medical history and provides a professional opinion and an estimated cost for the treatment.

Every year 1 billion dollars are spent by Nigerians, on Medical Care in US and Europe. This expenditure can be reduced as much as 50% or more, through quality service available in India. The package offers free Preventive Health Care Program (PHP) for one person accompanying the patient. This package includes Echocardiography; CT scan; Ultrasonography; Treadmill testing; X-ray Hormonal levels, Liver, Kidney and Pulmonary function tests, Blood Urine and Stool investigations or any other relevant investigation.

India's Health Care Tourism

The health care sector in India has witnessed an enormous growth in infrastructure in the private and voluntary sector. The private sector which was very modest in the early stages has now become a flourishing industry equipped with the most modern state-of-the-art technology at its disposal. It is estimated that 75-80% of health care services and investments in India are now provided by the private sector. An added plus had been that India has one of the largest pharmaceutical industries in the world. It is self sufficient in drug production and exports drugs to more than 180 countries.

- Bone Marrow Transplant
- Brain Surgery
- Cancer Procedures (Oncology)
- Cardiac Care
- Cosmetic Surgery
- Dialysis and Kidney Transplant
- Drug Rehabilitation
- Gynaecology and Obstetrics
- Health Checkups
- Internal/Digestive Procedures
- Joint Replacement Surgery
- Nuclear Medicine
- Neurosurgery and Trauma Surgery
- Preventive Health Care
- Refractive Surgery
- Osteoporosis
- Spine Related
- Urology
- Vascular Surgery
- Dental jobs

A typical package will consist of:

- Assessment of medical history
- Patient received at the airport/Package inclusive of accompanying person.
- Transfer to a hotel.
- Escorted to the specialty hospital as per appointments for admission.
- Treatment administered.
- Rejuvenation holiday begins.
- Post-treatment check-up.
- Transfer to airport and departure.

Dental Care Packages

Following are some of the procedures offered under Dental care packages:

- Veneers
- Filling and Asthetic reconstruction
- Dental Implants
- Bleaching
- Crowns and Bridges
- Cast partial dentures
- Periodontal Surgery
- Oral Surgery
- Pedodontics

Eye Care

India's ophthalmologists offer you custom made solutions for all your eye care problems. From corrective eye disorders to Diabetic retinopathy, Glaucoma, Cornea and Refractive Surgery to Low-stress cataract surgery. The eye surgery techniques have now become so advanced that the cataract surgery can be done in a day. LASIK (Laser Assisted Stromal *In-situ* Keratomileusis), a method of re-shaping the external surface of the eye to correct low, moderate and high degrees of nearsightedness, astigmatism and far-sightedness is also offered. The cost of such treatment in the UK is Pound 4000 and in the USA $ 5000 as against $ 1200 or less in India for the same treatment with highly experienced Indian doctors. A cataract surgery in the UK costs about Pounds 3000 and in the USA about $11000. In India in one of the best eye hospitals the cost is about Pound 400 or $ 700. This includes all investigations including the A scan on the IOL Master, the best intraocular lenses (Alcon Acrysof and the Allergan Sensar from USA, Pharmacia Tecnis Wavefront IOL from Sweden and also the Acritec from France) hospital stay, surgeon's fee, pre- and post-operative treatment as well as follow ups. Chandigarh has a centre of excellence in eye care at Advanced eye centre, PGI. Several private clinics also offer world class services.

A Worldwide Market

While, India has attracted patients from Europe, the Middle East and Canada, Thailand has been the goal for Americans. India mainly attracted people who had left the country for the West; Thailand treated western expatriates across Southeast Asia. Many of them worked for western companies and had the advantage of flexible, worldwide medical insurance plans geared specifically at the expatriate and overseas corporate markets. With the growth of medical-related travel and aggressive marketing, Bangkok became a centre for medical tourism. Bangkok's International Medical Centre offers services in 26 languages, recognizes cultural and religious dietary restrictions and has a special wing for Japanese patients.

The medical tour companies that serve Thailand often put emphasis on the vacation aspects, offering post-recovery resort stays.

Cuba, for example, first aimed its services at well-off patients from Central and South America and now attracts patients from Canada, Germany and Italy. Malaysia attracts patients from surrounding Southeast Asian countries; Jordan serves patients from the Middle East. Israel caters to both Jewish patients and people from some nearby countries. One Israeli hospital advertises worldwide services, specializing in both male and female infertility, *in-vitro* fertilization and high-risk pregnancies. South Africa offers package medical holiday deals with stays at either luxury hotels or safaris.

The newest and fastest-growing area of medical tourism is a visit to the dentist, where costs are often not covered by basic insurance and by only some extended insurance policies. India, Thailand and Hungary attract patients who want to combine a filling, extraction or root canal with a vacation.

Procedure Charges in India and US (US $)

Procedure	*Cost (US$)*	
	United States	*India*
Bone Marrow Transplant	2,50,000	69,000
Liver Transplant	3,00,000	69,000
Heart Surgery	30,000	8,000
Orthopedic Surgery	20,000	6,000
Cataract Surgery	2,000	1,250

Here's a brief comparison of the cost of few of the Dental treatment procedures between USA and India

Dental procedure	*Cost in US ($)*		*Cost in India ($)*
	General Dentist	*Top End Dentist*	*Top End Dentist*
Smile designing	-	8,000	1,000
Metal Free Bridge	-	5,500	500
Dental Implants	-	3,500	800
Porcelain Metal Bridge	1,800	3,000	300
Porcelain Metal Crown	600	1,000	80
Tooth impactions	500	2,000	100
Root canal Treatment	600	1,000	100
Tooth whitening	350	800	110
Tooth coloured composite fillings	200	500	25
Tooth cleaning	100	300	75

Facilities Available in India

Indian corporate hospitals excel in cardiology and cardiothoracic surgery, joint replacement, orthopedic surgery, gastroenterology, ophthalmology, transplants and urology to name a few. The various specialties covered are Neurology, Neurosurgery, Oncology, Ophthalmology, Rheumatology, Endocrinology, ENT, Pediatrics, Pediatric Surgery, Pediatric Neurology, Urology, Nephrology, Dermatology, Dentistry, Plastic Surgery, Gynecology, Pulmonology, Psychiatry, General Medicine and General Surgery

The various facilities in India include full body pathology, comprehensive physical and gynecological examinations, dental checkup, eye checkup, diet consultation, audiometry, spirometry, stress and lifestyle management, pap smear, digital Chest X-ray, 12 lead ECG, 2D echo colour doppler, gold standard DXA bone densitometry, body fat analysis, coronary risk markers, cancer risk markers, carotid colour doppler, spiral CT scan and high strength MRI. Each test is carried out by professional M.D. physicians, and is comprehensive yet pain-free.

There is also a gamut of services ranging from General Radiography, Ultra Sonography, Mammography to high end services like Magnetic Resonance Imaging, Digital Subtraction Angiography along with intervention procedures, Nuclear Imaging. The diagnostic facilities offered in India are comprehensive to include Laboratory services, Imaging, Cardiology, Neurology and Pulmonology. The Laboratory services include biochemistry, hematology, microbiology, serology, histopathology, transfusion medicine and RIA.

Questions and Answers on Health Tourism

Que.: Is India really a better place to get medical treatment?

Ans.: Yes, Currently India receives patients from over 50 countries across the world. Here are some reasons behind its emergence as the preferred health care destination: India has a vast reservoir of skilled doctors. Many of them have proved their mettle in the US and UK and returned to India to work in hospitals here. The caliber of other doctors practicing in India is also of a very high order.

Que: Why should patients come from USA for treatment to India?

A recent film 'Sicko' has indicted the American health care system; the insurance and pharma companies are exploiting the American citizens. Those who are not insured cannot afford treatment at home and hence come to India for world class health care at a fraction of cost.

Que.: I always thought India was a poor nation of snake charmers and rope tricks. How then can it offer world-class health care, that too at minimal costs ?

Ans.: India has all along been a knowledge-oriented nation. However, it never had a chance to showcause its expertise. The revolution in

Information Technology changed the rules of the game. And India made complete use of the knowledge base built by its English-speaking engineers to come out and display its immense capabilities.

And now for the costs. India is a diverse economy where a family of four can live comfortably, without debt, on a monthly income of just $300. As a result, the costs of services and products too have stayed at extremely low levels.

Now, thanks to the world becoming inter-connected and people being more willing to explore other nations, India has emerged as a preferred source of low cost health care. An extremely welcome alternative to the prohibitive costs prevalent in the western countries.

Que.: I don't know anyone in India. I'm already ill. Then how am I to cope with travel, stay and surgery in India ?

Ans.: It's ok if you don't know anybody in India. After all, Mediescapes India brings you comprehensive, custom-built schemes for health care. This includes:

++Getting second opinions from well-known board certified doctors in India

Offering all support information on

++Your ailment

++Recommended mode of surgery

++The hospital that will perform the surgery

++Costs involved

++Mediescapes India has entered into exclusive affiliate arrangements with a leading hospital in India. This means that you can count on special and personalized attention when you come to India for medical treatment through Mediescapes India.

Que: I just need a second opinion. I don't intend to come to India. Is it possible to get an opinion alone from one of your affiliated hospitals?

Ans.: Yes, of course. Just pay $ 50 and get a second opinion from one of our affiliate hospitals. You are not obligated to have your surgery in India through Mediescapes India just because you have asked for a second opinion.

Que.: Do I have to pay any fees or commissions for your services ?

Ans.: We do not charge any fees or commissions from people who want to use the services of our health care partners.

Que.: How do I pay the costs of surgery ?

Ans.: You pay the costs of surgery directly to the hospital. The benefits of such a payment are:

Your money is paid directly to the service provider, i.e. the hospital and not to any intermediary

Our health care partner have been rich expertise in treating patients from almost all parts of the world. Hence, the Payment systems are well in place in the partner hospital to accept payments from almost any part of the world.

Que.: What are the surgeries offered by your partner hospital and what are the rates?

Ans.: Click here to find the spectrum of hospitals as well as surgeries/treatments our partner hospitals/clinics offer.

*- Costs exclude travel, visa and any other incidental costs. Cost only include cost of surgery, boarding and lodging for the package period for the patient and the boarding and lodging expenses of ONE accompanying person.

Que.: I want to get my surgery/medical treatment done in India. How should I go about it?

Ans.: Here's suggested step-by-step process:

Ist Step—With your initial medical enquiry sent to us, submit your name, e-mail address, postal address and contact phone numbers.

IInd Step—Complete the second opinion questionnaire (Medical Quote Request Form) that we send to you by email. Basically this Medical Quote Request Form covers current nature of your ailment/your need for second medical opinion/various types of Diagnostic reports available with you and other medical records such as CT Scan/MRI Scans/back home hospital or clinic or your personal doctor's conducted test reports/X-Rays, etc. All these past or current medical history of a patients' information's helps our board certified medical specialists in answering your medical query with full details.

IIIrd Step—If further asked by our attending medical specialists/doctors for better understanding your medical conditions then send scanned copies of all your diagnostic reports/pathological reports/MRI/CT-Scans/OPG Images/Dental Moulds/X-Rays/Angiograms, etc. to facilitate out specialists second opinion. You can also use our postal address to send CD's or Xerox copies of all reports or use our Telefax or can also use postal mail or courier to send these.

IVth Step—Based on all above receive full information from our board certified attending specialist doctor's/medical consultants advice on your medical treatment approximate cost for rough planning purposes and total duration of your stay required at the hospital with pre-operative and post-operative extra stay requirement, etc. based on your posted surgery/medical treatment in India medical enquiry.

Vth Step—Also receive full details about cost of your stay at respective treatment city using a hotel or service apartment or guest house from us. Also receive full details about your treating institution/hospital in India with profile of attending doctor's/specialist and respective department at the Hospital where your medical treatment is suggested for your approval/consent and for planning purposes.

VIth Step—Acquire consent of your local physician to fly down to India. Inform us about consent/medical trip making condition.

VIth Step—Enter into the required agreements (Pre -Registration/ Indemnity or Consent Bond or Agreement) with the hospital in India for your firm medical treatment with them.

VIIIth Step—Enter into similar agreements (Indemnity Bond) with chosen hotel/service apartment/guest house in India for pre-operative and post-operative stay duration.

IXth Step—Pay the surgery/medical treatment full cost/full fees to the hospital directly via us to book OT/doctors' appointment/ward or room category chosen by you booking, etc.

Xth Step—Receive details of your date of surgery/medical treatment via email support form us.

XIth Step—Proceed for India Medical Visa (given for special medical emergencies). Here you have to carry confirm appointment with your Indian medical specialist/India hospital booking, etc. papers given by us for speedy India Visa clearance (we can issue you medial visa recommendation letter)

XIIth Step—Book tickets to fly to India. Inform us about your international arrival/departure flight timings and flight number, etc.

XIIIth Step—Fly down to India. receive by our representative. Orientation of your treatment city/hotel or service apartment or guest house stay, etc. are undertaken by us for your familiarization.

XIVth Step—Meet the attending specialist/treating doctor at the hospital/treating Institution where you will undergo surgery/your medical treatment and proceed on your specific treatment/medical surgery there.

XVth Step—On completion of treatment/medical procedure/ discharge from the hospital with final medical bill clearance and as per post-operative stay requirement suggested by your attending Indian medical specialist/doctor stay at the pre-booked hotel or service apartment or guest house and ones full clearance received from attending medical specialist/ doctor is received either fly back home or enjoy a recuperative holidays in India for few weeks or as per opted choice.

XVIth Step—Carry medications or prescriptions for generic medicines/drugs recommended by your attending medical specialist/doctor to carry home. Afterwards continue your post treatment follow-up if any, through email with attending medical specialist/doctor.

India's Health Tourism System has Some Unique Strengths

The scope and concept of Medical Tourism (MT) has today transgressed and evolved from healing by mineral and hot spring in the Neolithic and Bronze Age to today's health farms. India should provide the best of Eastern and Western health care systems. Ayurveda, Yoga and Siddha can be India's gift to the world. "Ayurveda is recognised as an official health care system in Hungary. Doctors in the West are increasingly prescribing Indian Systems of Medicine. More than 70 per cent of the

American population prefer a natural approach to health," Dr Bhaskar Shah, said. Americans are said to spend around USD 25 bn on non-traditional medical therapies and products. Addressing the same conference organized by INDIAN EXPRESS, Anil Maini, said, "MT has gained prominence with the advent of cutting edge technologies in India in specialties like cardiology, oncology, neurology, molecular and receptor imaging, which have improved sensitivity and specificity, early diagnosis, accurate and precise staging in oncology, significant input in decision making, evaluation of treatment outcome and improved morbidity and mortality." The main deterrents to MT are poor airports and infrastructure, non-medical people getting into the business, unnecessary investigation and treatment, no replies to follow-ups and Indian doctors not providing sufficient information to patients. The threats to India are the practice of Indian hospitals raising their prices every now and then, while treatment in Eastern European countries like Poland and Hungary are good and cheap, with France being just around 25 per cent costlier.

The Key "Selling Points" of the Medical Tourism

"Cost effectiveness, world class treatment" and its combination with the attractions of tourism are the key selling points. The latter also uses the ploy of selling the "exotica" of packaging of health care with traditional therapies and treatment methods. For example open-heart surgery could cost up to $70,000 in Britain and up to $150,000 in the US; in India's best hospitals it could cost between $3,000 and $10,000. The outcome of such a surgery in Indian hospitals matches with the best in the world. India is now moving into a new area of "medical outsourcing," where sub-contractors provide services to the overburdened medical care systems in western countries. India's Policy declares that treatment of foreign patients is legally an "export" and deemed "eligible" for all fiscal incentives extended to export earnings. Anil Kamath, pointed out that good news about India is that medical tourism is growing at a rate of 7.5 per cent to 8.0 per cent with health care growing at a rate of 20 per cent. MT has also received a boost with corporatisation of the hospitals sector and interest of international players with reference to investment and foreign direct investment. The medical tourism market is estimated to grow by USD 2.2 bn with a corresponding increase in the health care market by USD 60 bn by 2012. The growing international competition is another attribute with India facing a stiff competition with the East Europe having approximately half of US tariffs, Thailand having approximately 1/8th of US tariffs and India having 1/10th US tariffs.

National Health Policy

National Health Policy recognizes the treatment of international patients as an export, which allows private hospitals treating such patients to enjoy benefits such as lower import duties, increase in the rate of depreciation (from 25 per cent to 40 per cent) for life-saving medical equipment, and several other tax sops. Medical corporations in India serving medical tourists led by Apollo Hospital Enterprises are aggressively moving into medical outsourcing.

The following points merit attention:

- We need to club together 'pathies' because we have a very strong base of alternative healing therapies like yoga, naturopathy, ayurveda, etc.
- Creating awareness about India's facilities abroad is a must to establish credibility in foreign markets.
- Standardization of a price band for graded hospitals and a quality assurance model should be taken up immediately to take medical tourism ahead.
- India's relatively developing medical tourism segment has been anointed by health care and tourism industry pundits as the next 'best' thing for the country.
- There are plenty of challenges that need to be addressed for India to become the world's preferred health care destination.
- There is a need for a synergy between hospitals, state government and international tour operators. India will have to project itself as being a holistic medical destination to get an edge over other countries
- The private health care industry is quietly facilitating a revolution to enable India to emerge as a health destination.
- STARK contrasts are no surprise in urban India, and in the health care sector, the difference between what is available (world-class techniques and service, at a price) and what the common denominator urgently needs is no less so.
- Private sector health care centres are gleaming "islands of excellence", as the industry calls them, all too often surrounded by seas of medical neglect.
- When the mix is just right (support from the government in the form of incentives and tax breaks, international health care accreditation standards in place, breakthroughs in insurance coverage for overseas patients, and savvy promotion of India as a tourism-plus-medical tech destination) the sector is certain the numbers will fall into place.
- The beneficiary of such growth will be the country's desperately overburdened public health system, say industry associations such as the Confederation of Indian Industry (CII) and the Federation of Indian Chambers of Commerce and Industry (FICCI).
- Look at the possibility of the public hospitals being technologically upgraded to world-class standards with this source of income.
- India's three-tier public health system—primary health centres

(PHC) in villages, district hospitals, and tertiary care hospitals—is increasingly unable to attend to the medical needs of the population.

- Technology-centric approach to health care, such as that promoted by the private hospitals, will affect the cost of care to the common man.
- "If we can build our brand, there will be no stopping us," says Dr Prathap Reddy, chairman of the Apollo Group.
- Price-banding exercise by a cii-affiliated industry body, the Indian Health Care Federation, completed late last year, indicates fair prices for standard treatments in a good hospital. This was preceded by complaints of wide variation in prices and indiscriminate fee-hikes.
- Imminent launch of campaign using brochures and advertorials by the tourism ministry to project Indian health care, will disseminate case-studies and the new pricing information. Targeting GP practices in western countries, especially those run by Indian doctors.
- Growing interest by foreign governments and public health care bodies in checking out Indian health care. Side-trip to hospitals being included in official itineraries, like the now-mandatory visit to Infosys.
- Satisfied customers and free publicity in the western media for top Indian hospitals for delivering on price and quality.
- A newly-created autonomous Indian accreditation board to set standards in safety and patient care. Expects to accredit 50 hospitals this year. Simultaneously, a drive for American accreditation by leading hospitals.

What's not Happening?

- Industry and government not working in a coordinated manner. Progress so far driven mainly by individual players and ministries. Inter-ministerial taskforce on medical tourism, with representatives from six ministries and the private sector, set-up two years ago, has little to show.
- The much-touted new 'medical visa' is a disaster, say facilitators, more expensive and cumbersome than a regular visa, and requiring an array of documents.
- Medical tourists still negotiate snake-like immigration queues at airports, despite promises of a fast-track for the last two years. Recently, a Pakistani child needing a liver transplant took an hour and a half to clear at Delhi airport.
- Government failing to deliver on quality of airports, roads and infrastructure which don't make India look like a destination for "world class" medical treatment.

- Much more needs to be done to enforce norms, standards and ethical practices in a notoriously unregulated health care sector.
- Big breakthroughs depend on insurance companies, corporations and public health care bodies like Britain's has picking up the tab for medical treatment in India. Such deals have so far proved elusive, but the industry maintains they will happen.
- Handful of top doctors' names crop up in testimonials by medical tourists. Hospitals will have to maintain quality as numbers increase. It takes thousands of testimonials to build a brand, but just a few brickbats can destroy one.

Noises from a Global Health Care Bazaar

"We have no health insurance. My wife suffers constantly with her back pain. We cannot even begin to think about treatment here in the US because of the extremely high cost. After seeing your operations on 60 Minutes, we both have new hope. Please contact us." Shortly after it was featured in the American TV programme 60 Minutes, e-mails began hitting the inbox of Delhi's Indraprastha Apollo Hospital, seconds apart from each other. From Illinois, Florida, Washington, Texas, New Mexico, California, Oregon, Oklahoma, Tennessee, Virginia, from British Columbia and Alberta, Canada. Curious, hopeful or frankly desperate, they were all looking for deals, asking prices, checking out packages: what will a new hip cost, by itself, and with bigger breasts thrown in? What about a package for two-a facelift for me, Lasik eye surgery for my companion? How much for a bridge, a root canal, IVF, angioplasty, gastric bypass surgery.... This is my budget, what can I get for it?

It might sound discordant, this price-tagging of body parts, but for Indian private hospitals, nothing is more musical than these noises from a global health care bazaar. They demonstrate that an idea that seemed absurd at the start of this decade has entered the realm of reality: that people from the West will travel thousands of miles, to so-called cholera country, for medical treatment—if the price is right, and the quality is right. It's an idea with big money attached to it: medical tourism is forecast to become a $2.3 billion business for India by 2012. Some analysts predict it could be the next major driver of the Indian economy after information technology—if the industry and the government play their cards right.

Western TV crews accompanied often elderly people to India, filmed them hobbling out of Third World airports, with bhangra on the soundtrack, and driving into First World tertiary hospitals with the best technology money could buy. They showed them being "swamped by staff" and "feeling like kings", as one delighted patient described it, and seen by western-qualified senior consultants within an hour of arrival—which could be 2 a.m.

The crews tracked the pilgrims' progress, finding their way into an operating theatre where a surgeon obligingly delivered a tribute to the

British system that trained him. But the main message came through loud and clear: white people getting knees replaced, hips resurfaced, and dental work done at bargain-basement prices by experienced doctors who knew their job. British tabloids went to town on teenager Elliot Knott who successfully underwent spine surgery here last August after being told to wait a year for an operation by the National Health Service U.K. Most private hospitals saw a marked upward trend in western arrivals last years, most of them from the UK, US and Canada.

The Apollo Group saw an overall five per cent increase in the number of western medical tourists, according to executive director (finance) Sunita Reddy, despite no special effort to market to them. But at Apollo's flagship Delhi hospital, which gets more medical tourists than its other hospitals, the arrivals from some countries seem to have doubled. For example, it got around 80 American patients from April to November 05, more than the entire number in the previous financial year. Any international marketing executive—and every upmarket private hospital now has one—can recite the numbers in her sleep: 8,50,000 waiting for a hospital bed in the UK, 47-million plus uninsured in the US. Medical value-travellers, as hospitals like to call them, are also people looking for body shapes that insurance companies won't pay for and dreams that even efficient public health care systems won't deliver, like those of the 5 feet 4 tall Frenchman who recently came to India for a leg-lengthening operation. Many are also in quest of treatments not available at home, like hip resurfacing, less radical than hip replacement, but yet to be approved by the US Food and Drug Administration.

Foreign Medical Tourists

Agonizing pain kept his wife in bed for 16 to 20 hours a day, and the wait for an appointment with the right kind of doctorwas no less painful. Google took Smith to India. "Much of Marlene's pre-operative pain has gone. We're 100 per cent satisfied. We paid $19,000, including airfare. In the US, the metal alone would have cost $40,000."

Marlene and Paul Smith; Canadians:

Treatment: Spinal fusion surgery

Contrary to the popular stereotype, not every medical tourist is dying to see the Taj. He could be someone for whom a hospital room is the only piece of India he can handle. In a month's stay at Apollo Hospital for complicated surgery to correct his wife Marlene's curved spine, Paul Smith, from Barrie, a small picture-postcard town in Ontario, left the hospital only once, on a trip to the airport to sort out ticketing. "With Marlene in bed, why would I want to sightsee?" he said. In December, however, thanks to Elliot, and other high-profile visits arranged by their start-up, Taj Medical Group, they were able to send 27. They are going home in a few hours and they won't be returning. One giant leap into the unknown was probably enough. And yet, they couldn't be more grateful, raving about their doctor, dreaming about a better life for Marlene, determined to spread the word about India. Fortunately for the tourism ministry not all medical tourists confine themselves to hospital rooms.

Dr. Trehan says American citizens not covered by insurance—or those in countries such as the United Kingdom where there are long waiting lists for many National Health services—prefer to receive treatment in a country like India where top-tier institutions can provide high-quality health care at a fraction of the cost. Trehan recently operated on an 83-year old Canadian cardiac patient who needed a valve replacement with a bypass, but had been turned down by doctors back home. "No doctor was willing to do it for him. It's my specialization, patients with 10 or 20 per cent heart function. I told him the risk was less than five per cent," said Trehan.

Language is another big advantage in India, says Howard Staab, who spent more than three weeks in Escorts Hospital and at a resort, recuperating after surgery: "Doctors and nurses were all Indians, and many of the doctors were trained in the United States and Britain and most of them spoke very good English. I did not have any trouble understanding them." Howard Staab's partner Maggie Grace, who accompanied him on his medical trip to India, is writing a book about their experience. "We want to help people in the United States know they have choices," says Mr. Staab. "There will be our book coming out very soon. My partner Maggie Grace is writing it. The book title is "Patient Pilgrimage: A True Story of the First Americans Travel to India for Heart Surgery" and the website is www.howardsheart.com." Howard Staaab says one key to his trip's success was that it combined a high degree of medical excellence with a human touch.

Amitabh Kant, the bureaucrat who led 'Incredible India' and helped successfully reinvent Kerala as God's own Ayurvedic paradise, is leading the ministry's initiative to promote India as a "global health care destination". So, after incredible temples, incredible tigers and incredible yoga, it's now going to be incredible doctors backed by incredible technology. Glossy brochures, prepared with the help of ad agency Ogilvy and Mather, feature men and women in spotless white coats bending over patients against backdrops of sleek medical hardware. The patients in the brochure seem mostly white and middle-aged, for a reason: Kant is aiming way beyond the harried middle classes from SAARC countries, Afghanistan and poorer African countries who have been flocking to India for specialized medical care which their countries lack. They, too, are coming in rising numbers, especially from Afghanistan and Africa, and sure, hospitals want their custom. But for reasons of both prestige and money, what really excites both government and industry is the fatter wallets in western countries with ageing populations and rising health care costs and the Gulf, where seekers are finding it harder to access medical treatment in the West, post 9/11.

It's definitely not the titled rich that are showing up here. Cosmetic surgeon Mohan Thomas's upcoming patients include a pair of London cabbies, husband and wife, coming for facelifts. But even a school teacher from Bognor Regis can book a nice room when a hip replacement costs less than half of what it does back home. If they like the main course, western patients will also splurge on side dishes. Like Briton Barry Peters, who came to get a hip replaced, and got his teeth done as well, paying less for the whole treatment, including airfares, than just the dental would have cost him in London. Or Serena Taylor from California, who came to look after her friend seeking plastic surgery, and decided to buy an eyelift. It must be like eyeing a pricey handbag for several weeks and suddenly finding it at 80 per cent off. What else can you say but, "I'll have that"?

"A hospital cannot replace a hotel. We should not keep these patients in hospital a minute more than required, we must send them to a place where they can recuperate," says Apollo group chairman Dr Prathap Reddy. In Bangalore, patients can check out of leading private hospitals, and convalesce in places like Soukya, a sprawling health farm on the outskirts of the city. With an in-house team of ayurvedic physicians and allopathic doctors on call, when needed, its medical director, homeopath Dr Isaac Mathai, claims to have the "lowest doctor-patient ratio in the world". It's the detox destination for Indian software and media tycoons, and its international guests.

Scot Johnson: American

Treatment: Cervical disc replacement

"I heard about medical treatment in India from the TV show 60 Minutes. Big American hospitals are full of Indian doctors, that's how I knew they'd be good."

Howard looked into state-of-the-art cardiac facilities in India, Argentina and Texas, where top U.S.-trained doctors do the same procedures for a fraction of the cost. Of course, Howard would prefer to stay in the Triangle to be near his son and wide circle of friends. But who could resist these other options? After much deliberation Howard and his partner, Maggi, will fly to India for the surgery as soon as they can obtain the appropriate visas. Indian Hospitals Lure Foreigners with $6,700 Heart Surgery.

Dhanyavaad

Staab was rolled into Escorts' operating room on Sept. 28. Grace, who'd picked up a smattering of Hindi, wrote "dhanyavaad," for "thank you," on his bare chest with purple marker. The surgeons first decided to repair Staab's mitral valve. A day later, the valve walls thickened and obstructed blood flow. Staab went in for a second operation on Sept. 30, and doctors replaced the valve. He was ready to leave on Oct. 8 when blurry vision from suspected blood clots kept him for another two days to thin his blood. Staab and Grace returned to the U.S. on Oct. 24. Grace says finding out about India was the tough part. If not for Srivastava, she and Staab never would have figured out where to look, let alone gather the courage to make the trip. Back in North Carolina, Staab had an opportunity to compare health care in the U.S. with his treatment in India. An early November checkup found that his blood was still too thick, and he entered Durham Regional Hospital.

Grace says she had to ask for sheets to make Staab's bed and get him water herself. The bathroom wasn't cleaned, and they had to ask twice for the intravenous bag containing blood-thinning heparin to be changed when it became empty, she says. Carol Clayton, senior public relations specialist at Durham Regional, says the hospital addresses patient concerns as soon as they are brought to the staff's attention.

In April, Ian Stuart Crombie, 64, couldn't finish his round of golf at the Bonny Island course in Rivers State, Nigeria, because of pain in his right hip. Doctors gave him two choices: live on painkillers or undergo surgery. Crombie opted for a route that more Europeans and Americans are taking. He looked beyond a decrepit airport and teeming streets and chose India for medical care. In September, the British citizen flew 5,159 miles (8,303 kilometers) from his home in Winchester to Apollo Hospital in Chennai. Doctors performed a hip resurfacing, which involved shaving his thighbone and fitting it with a metal head that was then anchored in his hip socket. With the operation, Crombie joined the international clientele flocking to India for cut-rate services that include telephone call centers, software design and financial analysis. Indian hospitals are a very cheap option where patients get the same quality they're used to back home," says Sanjay Dongre, who manages the equivalent of $237 million of shares at UTI Asset Management Co. in Mumbai, which owns Apollo stock.

For Crombie, who was working as a human resources manager in Africa, Apollo presented a low-cost option. He says his medical plan didn't cover the hip operation. He didn't bother with the U.K. National Health Service because of its waiting list and decided not to pursue treatment in Nigeria. A private hospital back home would charge 15,000 pounds ($27,965), he says. Instead, Crombie paid a total of 5,000 pounds for his India trip, including the operation, airfare and a stay at the $130-a-night Park Hotel in Chennai. Crombie was familiar with India, where his job had taken him to recruit workers in Cochin, Mumbai and New Delhi. He found Bose on the Internet and checked his credentials with doctors Bose had worked with in the U.K. He decided on India after e-mail exchanges persuaded him that hip resurfacing rather than hip replacement would give him a better shot at playing golf again. "I can imagine someone who's not been to India before may find it intimidating," Crombie says.

On vacation in India in September, Brown experienced chest pain again and was rushed to Wockhardt Hospital in Bangalore. Wockhardt performed an angioplasty the next day, inserting a wire mesh tube called a stent to prop open an artery. "The hospital could have been in London," Brown recalls. "It was immaculately clean and had good standards." Back in England, Brown says, he got a letter from the National Health Service in November asking him to come in for his initial test—two months after he'd had the surgery in India.

Some Middle Eastern patients began choosing India after the Sept. 11, 2001, attacks on New York and Washington, says Suneeta Reddy, 45, director of finance at Apollo Hospitals and daughter of founder and Executive Chairman Prathap Reddy, 71. In November, Waleed Khalid Al-Zadjali, 40, a doctor in Oman, picked Apollo for his father's angioplasty and his mother's knee replacement. Oman hospitals often refer patients to India for complicated procedures because the country is familiar, closer than the U.S. or Europe and cheap, he says. "After 9/11, people were scared to go to the U.S.," he says.

Healthy Competition in Health Care

Top private hospitals are also vying with each other in other ways to attract an international clientele. As in an accelerated race for the latest hardware-you can't miss the giant boards advertising the latest scanner—and for that prized certificate by the Joint Commission International (JCI) in the United States, a non-governmental body that accredits international hospitals meeting exacting American standards. The early birds who have it, such as Apollo in Delhi and Wockhardt in Mumbai, display it big, and other hospitals are in the queue. "The fact that we are JCI-accredited is a symbol of quality assurance for patients in the western world. The hospital room is changing too, with globalization clearly the spur, though all CEOs maintain that demanding Indian patients are driving the changes, too. John Connell, a primary school teacher from Southampton in the UK, who came to Wockhardt in Mumbai earlier this month for a new minimally invasive procedure to treat a hole in his heart, had the following in his hospital room: a computer, internet, a DVD player with regional compatibility that could play British DVDs, a mini-bar, a coffee-maker, a cell-phone. The hospital also offered him and wife Amanda "virtual family visits"—that is, a video of them shot in the room and uploaded for their families back home. A hospital car was made available for them to move around in the neighbourhood. John's room still managed to look like a hospital room, but at new hospitals like the Max Devki Devi Heart and Vascular Institute in Delhi, it's all blonde wood, expensive blinds, and leather sofas, the work of a British designer hired by the company to get the look right. And prices? Ashmeena Ghei, international marketing head, who is already facilitating visits by a stream of international patients, quotes them in dollars: $150 for a room, $300 for a suite.

But the 2.3 billion dollar question is: Will the Stream turn into a Flood?

Judging by the talk on the hospital circuit, it won't be long before every upmarket private hospital offers ayurvedic massages, aromatherapy, mudbaths, pranic healing, yoga, the works. And full-fledged departments of alternative medicine, with homeopaths, naturopaths, and unani medicine specialists on board to deliver that authentic dose of India. The BPO sector, in comparison, earned $5.2 billion last year. (*Source*: CII-McKinsey report) The government hopes to encourage a budding trade in medical tourism, selling foreigners the idea of travelling to India for low-cost but world-class medical treatment. Naresh Trehan, executive director of Escorts Heart Institute and Research Centre, a leading private health care provider, says India has established world-class expertise in practices such as cardiac care, cosmetic surgery, joint replacements and dentistry. Merging medical expertise and tourism became government policy when finance minister Jaswant Singh, in this year's budget, called for India to become a "global health destination". If foreigners respond, a new medical tourism industry could be generating revenues of Rs. 100 bn ($2.1 bn, €1.9 bn, £1.3 bn) by 2012, according to a report by McKinsey Consultants and the Confederation of Indian Industry, a business group.

Take the rising popularity of "preventive health screening". At one private clinic in London a thorough men's health check-up that includes blood tests, electro-cardiogram tests, chest x-rays, lung tests and abdominal ultrasound costs £345 ($574, €500). By comparison, a comparable check-up at a clinic operated by Delhi-based health care company Max Health Care costs $84.

According to Hari Prasad, vice-president of Apollo Hospitals in Hyderabad, foreigners should have confidence in India's medical system because many Britons and Americans are accustomed to being treated by expatriate Indian doctors. In any case, most private health care providers hold modest ambitions about which foreign patients would come to India seeking treatment. For instance, of the 5,200 hospital beds run by the Apollo hospital group, about 100 beds are usually occupied by foreign patients, mostly from the Middle East, Africa and countries of south Asia. Indeed, demand for medical tourism is most likely to come from among the 25m-strong Indian Diaspora, says Deep Kalra, chief executive officer of travel agency makemytrip.com. Mr Kalra says wealthy first- and second-generation expatriate Indians are aware of the rise of India's high quality, low-cost hospitals. He estimates there is a potential market of some 12m expatriate Indians who would combine regular visits to India and save time and money by undergoing non-emergency procedures such as eye operations, dental work, cosmetic surgery and knee surgery. Mr Kalra's agency plans to launch a medical tourism package later this year. Still, some remain skeptical about medical tourism's potential. Sumanjit Chaudhry, an executive at India's Max Health Care group, says: "I imagine if someone is sick and ill they won't want to have a holiday. You'll hardly see a guy who comes here for heart surgery leaping off and going to the beach."

Maharashtra Medical Tourism Council (MTC)

Initially the MTC plans to woo foreign patients who pay for private health care in their own countries. But it also plans to work with state-run systems. For instance, Anapum Verma, the council's honorary secretary, believes Britain has a "huge potential" for medical tourism owing to its long waiting lists for surgery. He has already had exploratory conversations with some British National Health Service managers about the possibility of sending patients to India. For the MTC, its plans are the next chapter in globalization and the outsourcing of work to India. As Sanjay Agarwala, the Hinduja's chief neurosurgeon, says: "Wherever you can offer better services at a more competitive price, that is the place that is going to win in the end." Contrary to the claims of the council, Dr Baru believes there will be no trickle down of money to the impoverished public health system, which currently receives just 0.9% of India's gross domestic product. The MTC's plans may well benefit the doctors and patients involved, but it is currently unclear how a country that still suffers from malaria and TB will reap the rewards of a new wave of medical tourists coming to India.

In recent years Indian Medical Tourism Sector has exhibited tremendous potential. Studies reveal that the Sector is growing at an exaggerated rate of 15% for last five years. It is expected that with the current growth rate the Industry will reach Rs. 270,000 crores by 2012. Statistics show that the medical tourism industry in India is worth $333 million at present (Rs. 1,450 crore), while a study by CII-McKinsey estimates that the country could earn Rs. 5,000-10,000 crore by 2012. Probably realizing the potential, major corporates such as the Tatas, Fortis, Max, Wockhardt, Piramal, and the Escorts group have made significant investments in setting up modern hospitals in major cities. Many have also designed special packages for patients, including airport pickups, visa assistance and board and lodging, health care industry officials said. Foreigners have already started trickling into India for medical treatment thus officials are hopeful that this will become a flood once the various initiatives being taken by the Government take off. With world-class medical care, equipment and facilities now available in India, patients from the United States and other developed countries are going there for treatment. A number of private hospitals in India offer packages designed to attract foreign patients, with airport-to-hospital bed transfer service, Internet access, and other facilities. Some packages include add-ons, such as a yoga holiday or a trip to the world-famous Taj Mahal.

Religious Tourism: As an Engine of Growth of Health Tourism in India

Synergy of religious tourism and medical tourism can work. It can improve health care for the countrymen and earn dollars from foreign medical tourists. It will not put any burden on the state exchequer or burden the country with debts. It will be self financing as well as fulfilling to the community. This is in consonance with Indian tradition to help the people in pain and disability. If the donations from all over the country are channelised to health care, it will not only lead to health care for all in India, but also make it attractive for the medical tourists from abroad.

Various religious sects and their heads have to come forward to further a common cause that is good for the humanity. See appendix on the list of religious places in India.

Agra Moving Forward

While the states of Karnataka, Maharashtra, Gujarat, Tamil Nadu, and Andhra Pradesh are quite ahead in tourism promotion, other states are also making efforts to march ahead. Agra is definitely moving in the direction of a well developed medical tourism centre. With the new international airport coming up soon, and competent city doctors working abroad, this process will start soon enough. "Medical facilities in Agra have expanded immensely. Earlier we referred our patients to hospitals in Delhi, now with the latest gadgetry and facilities available locally, patients take advantage and save both money and time."

Apollo Hospitals has also entered into partnership with Pankaj Mahendru's medical outfit. The new venture is called Apollo Pankaj. Said Apollo Pankaj director Pankaj Mahendru: "Earlier during the British and Mughal empires also, Agra was the main centre of health services. Now embassies and corporate houses are referring patients to hospitals here which have a fairly competent base of manpower and facilities." An American company Mefcom Agro Ind has acquired stakes in Kamayani Patients Care India, a multi-specialty hospital, providing specialty cancer treatment. Metro, Heritage, Pushpanjali, Shanti Ved, Pareek's, Nawal Kishore's, GG Nursing Home and Sarkar's, the oldest nursing home in Agra, are some of the other hospitals that have broken new ground in Agra by modernizing their infrastructure and facilities. To support the fast growing medical tourism industry, at least a dozen training institutes for paramedic staff as well as research centres have come up. The Agra Mental Hospital is conducting several programmes to train personnel for this specialised sector. Even the 150-year-old S.N. Medical College now presents a new profile in a bid to attract patients from the rest of India and even abroad.

Rajasthan Enterprise

For this, land would be provided at special prices to all new private medical institutions, including medical and dental colleges, diagnosis centres, blood banks, and nursing and paramedical training institutes. The policy will also boost other medical streams like ayurveda, homoeopathy and naturopathy. A "land bank" will be created to give land to medical institutions that are promoting and practicing alternative medical therapies.

To benefit from the policy, nursing and paramedical institutions will have to make an investment of at least Rs. 50 million. Similarly, nursing homes and 15-bed hospitals planning a facility within 50 km from regional headquarters or 20 km from district headquarters or in a village or town with a population of less than 50,000 will have to invest at least Rs.5 million. Investors will also have to abide by environment protection rules for hospital waste disposal and follow the rules and regulations set by the committee of standards.

Obesity Treatment looks Attractive: Gujarat Story

In a development that could bring patients from US and Europe to the country, a private hospital today launched a world class bariatric surgery clinic in Gujarat to treat people suffering from severe obesity, a disease that is fast attaining epidemic proportions in India. The star-studded launch of the clinic at Apollo Gleneagles Hospitals here saw at least 25 people queuing up for surgery to get rid of excessive body weight and in turn associated diseases like high blood pressure, diabetes and cardiac ailments. 'The new facility, first of its kind in India after sporadic attempts elsewhere in the country, is also eyeing patients from the west, where the cost of treatment is more and the waiting time enormous. "The facility, being backed by a support group for obese people, is a comprehensive unit, which will benefit not only domestic patients but also thousands of patients in the Americas and Europe, who are showing interest in flying down to get operated," says laparoscopic and bariatric surgeon, who heads the clinic. Quoting the WHO, he says 17 per cent of men and 15 per cent women in India were confirmed to be obese and the numbers were growing by leaps with changing lifestyles and eating habits. "Globally, over 1.7 billion people are affected by the disease. In the US, over 300,000 people die of obesity while in Europe around 250,000 people are killed by the scourge," he warned.

India's Global Fame: Singing Paeans?

India's tertiary health care sector is on the road to global fame. A growing number of spotlessly clean private hospitals are on the threshold of a boom in medical tourism, positioning themselves as the best destinations for procedures ranging from coronary bypasses to orthopedic surgery at the most affordable costs. These hospitals offer high-quality care for international patients, whose numbers are reportedly rising 15 per cent annually; the prices that they charge are a fraction of what prevails in the developed world. India's corporate hospitals are fully equipped, up market and efficient. With their toll-free helplines, interactive websites, online quotes and time-bound treatment access, they appear to be a world apart from the overburdened, often badly managed and poorly funded public health system.

Just three major corporate hospital groups, Fortis Health Care, Wockhardt and Apollo Hospitals run 26 hospitals in the subcontinent and that number is growing. They are forming partnerships with international insurance and tourism companies that will send both insured and uninsured patients for low cost treatment. With some friendly policies from the Government, some analysts think, the private health care sector can transform the potential of medical tourism into a very profitable reality. One oft-cited report that endorses this optimistic outlook is "Health Care in

India: The Road Ahead", produced by the Confederation of Indian Industry and McKinsey and Company. It puts a number to the promise: tertiary hospitals, with a 25 per cent growth rate in revenues from foreign patients (comparable to institutions such as Bumrungrad in Thailand), could generate additional earnings of Rs. 5,000 crore to Rs. 10,000 crore by 2012. That potential is based, in part, on the low cost of care in international price terms, competent medical personnel and absence of long waiting times for procedures, says the report.

Stories of foreign nationals undergoing complicated surgery in the country are frequently featured in the media. Those who come now are not just from other developing countries (the first lady of Guyana brought a group of 15 patients for cardiac treatment to Frontier Lifeline hospital in Chennai), but also from the United Kingdom, Europe and North America. Tanzania and Iraq have a Memorandum of Understanding with the Madras Medical Mission.

Many opt to undergo surgery in India for reasons that range from long waiting times in the U.K., high costs or lack of insurance cover in the U.S., to plain lack of expertise in many Asian, African and West Asian countries.

The CII-McKinsey report says that the allopathic system can offer treatment in specialities such as cardiac, liver, renal and orthopaedic procedures, while Indian systems of medicine could attract patients from even the developed world to treat "lifestyle diseases" such as stress and rheumatism. Many visitors who come for such de-stressing and health-building treatment may also choose to visit tourist spots. Such tourism potential holds the key to Kerala's plans. The Ayurveda State has declared 2006 the year of medical tourism and is actively supporting its well-known traditional medicine and tourism sectors, as they reach out to more potential visitors.

Elsewhere, development plans, both State-led and in the private sector are being pursued actively: Karnataka, which gets about 8,000 patients a year and forecasts an annual growth rate of 25 per cent, will promote a massive health park near a new international airport in Bangalore; non-resident Indians have formed a medical tourism company in Vadodara and international property developers are venturing into the health care sector to participate in the construction boom. In Maharashtra, the State Government is part of the Medical Tourism Council that has members from Association of Hospitals and FICCI.

The Spin-off

Explaining the view, Anupam Verma, honorary secretary of the Medical Tourism Council of Maharashtra and a director of Mumbai's Hinduja Hospital, says, "Look at the possibility of the public hospitals being technologically upgraded to world-class standards with this source of income. Also, with exposure to the paid medical service market, the spirit of competition will germinate in public hospitals ...(to) enhance their efficiency and service delivery levels."

Such optimism apart, India's three-tier public health system—primary health centres (PHC) in villages, district hospitals, and tertiary care hospitals—is increasingly unable to attend to the medical needs of the population.

Government expenditure on public health infrastructure is shrinking. At present, India spends about a per cent of its gross domestic product (GDP) on health care, lower than the average of 2.8 per cent of GDP spent by some less developed countries. Yet, as the National Human Development Report (2001) points out: "There has been a misplaced emphasis on maintenance and strengthening of private health care services ... at the expense of broadening and deepening of a public health care system targeted at controlling the incidence of disease, particularly of communicable diseases, in rural areas." Private health care is indeed expanding rapidly to fill the need for services. According to a World Bank study released in January 2004, nearly 82 per cent of all health spending in India is private.

Now, private health care groups are lobbying for the adoption of measures they say will encourage growth—some of these are tax allowances for rural doctors, relaxations in the norms for setting up medical colleges, and relaxation in indirect taxes on purchase of equipment, medicines, medical consumables and devices. "The challenge," says Dr. Trehan, "is to try and match the cost of creation with ability to pay. Thus to incentivise hospitals to come up in rural areas, the government needs to go much beyond this." S.K. Venkataraman emphasises that the industry urgently needs infrastructure status "with attendant benefits like a tax holiday, concessional utilities and preferential land allotments, in order to create an enabling environment for the healthy growth of this sector".

These demands are questioned by health policy analysts. Ravi Duggal, health researcher with Mumbai's Centre for Enquiry into Health and Allied Themes, points out that private hospitals have obligations for their not-for-profit status under the Public Trust Act to provide health care free to the extent of 20 per cent of their resources. "Where is the accountability of this provision?" he asks.

Certainly, the view from ground zero of a public hospital's out-patient's department is uniformly grim. Under-funded, undermanned and under-equipped, Mumbai's severely overburdened public hospitals have borne the brunt of public rage.

What the critiques say about health tourism as a system of health care.

Here is a complex case for a debate involving health care tourism. The entrepreneurs, medical community, and government agencies have to make choices that touch the national conscience. To what extent should Indian entrepreneurs and the medical community promote medical tourism? Should the government play any role in encouraging medical tourism?

Governments should have no role in promoting health care tourism since it negatively impacts the people they are supposed to represent. And the private sector needs self-regulation.

The buzz in the Western news media is health care tourism and the role of India's medical establishment in providing affordable health care. According to the National Coalition on Health Care, there are 46.6 million uninsured Americans. The number of Americans travelling overseas for health care is increasing each year. Health Care costs in the United States are skyrocketing. Insurance premiums and health care costs are growing at more than three times the overall inflation, averaging at least a nine per cent increase in each of the last five years. Even in socialistic medical systems such as in Europe and Canada, the wait for critical surgery is supposedly long and painful. The private health care system is so expensive that many have little option but to seek medical services from low-cost countries such as India. the cost for critical heart bypass in India is just 7.7 per cent of the cost in the U.S. The costs for other surgeries including hip replacement are less than 20 per cent of that in the U.S. Even after adding first class airfare and five star facilities, Westerners are better off seeking medical services in India (there may be some long term risks, which we will ignore for the time being).

The Indian medical tourism industry is in its infancy and the potential for growth is substantial. Obviously, capitalists are ready to exploit such opportunities and the massive cost differentials. And why not? Numerous state-of-the-art hospitals are popping up in major Indian cities to service foreign clientele.

But, here is the conundrum. In its latest report, World Health Organisation (WHO) identifies India along with other poorest nations in Africa and South Asia as having the greatest shortage of health care professionals. India has around 650,000 physicians with a density of 0.60 physicians per 1000 people. In comparison, the U.S. has 2.56 per 1000 and most Western nations have at least four times higher density of doctors than India. China has 1.05 physicians per 1000. More troubling is that India has a large numbers of patients with tuberculosis, malaria, AIDS/HIV, leprosy, and other contagious diseases. India lags far behind the Western world in average life expectancy and has much higher infant mortality rates. So, we can safely assume the demand for health care professionals in India far exceeds the supply.

India has low public health care spending. Based on WHO data, government spending as a percentage of total health care costs of most Western nations—including the U.S.—is higher than India's. In India, more than 75 per cent of the health care spending is in the private sector (for the U.S. it is 44.6 per cent). The percentage of out-of-pocket spending on private health care is a whopping 97 per cent. In the U.S., it is just 24.5 per cent and in most European countries it is even lower.

Thus, the massive gap between the demand and the supply and significantly higher private spending on health care raises numerous questions as medical tourism takes firmer roots. Private cost of health care services may rise since health care tourism amplifies the gap between the demand and the supply. The need for five-star hospital services and advanced medical devices will increase investment levels, which will force providers to seek higher revenue generating foreign clients. Since some of the major hospital groups are publicly traded, there will be greater pressure for increasing shareholder value. Since doctors' reputations attract patients, there will be a bidding war for well-known doctors. All this can be expected to increase the cost of health care services for the local population.

While various States and industry associations are aggressively promoting medical tourism, one needs to step back and ask ethical questions and consider social implications. Is it in the best interests of the nation? While the private sector has the right to pursue what is best for its shareholders and investors, what role should government play in promoting or encouraging medical tourism? How will medical tourism impact the large middle and upper income population that generally avoids government facilities?

There are stories of families spending their life savings to keep their loved ones alive. That is, health care is something that cannot be negotiated. That is why most Western nations have a socialistic system. In the U.S., there is a government-supported health care safety net for the poor and retirees. But, a socialistic payment system collides with a capitalistic provider system. Health care costs have become a national debate. As the percentage of senior citizens in the West continues to increase, there will be a greater demand for health care services that can impact the cost in India.

Some will quickly argue that controlling medical tourism is regressive. But, consider the following hypothetical situation to evaluate the ethical dilemma. Let's assume a massively spreading disease creates global shortage of food-grains such as wheat, rice, and lentils. the global shortage makes it appealing for Indian traders to export to rich countries. Should India allow export of essential food-grains for enormous profits? If you agree with the export ban, then you need to accept a ban on medical tourism given the abysmal health care access. If you think otherwise, how do you justify the skyrocketing costs that the common man has no way of paying? If you assume that this is the way things are, then you must also be prepared for social unrest, political upheaval, and violence! Thus, decisions under these complex situations cannot be purely for short-term economic gain. They have social and political ramifications. Entrepreneurs and hospitals argue that a high-paying Western clientele can subsidize the cost of providing services for the local population. This is a sound argument if we ignore the severe shortage of medical professionals. Further, foreign clientele will expect more than the required resources since the long-term risks involved are higher. Thus, hospitals and doctors will spend disproportionately more resources for foreign (or wealthy) patients. It is hard to conceive how resources can be allocated for poor patients under severe deficit.

Health care is an essential service and, therefore, the government can interfere to impose constraints on health care tourism since it takes away capacity from the local population and imposes costs on the entire population. But, it then raises counter arguments. Where should the government impose constraints? Should the government prevent doctors and nurses from leaving the country? Since there is a severe shortage of teachers and professors, should the government prevent teachers from leaving the country? The same applies to engineers, scientists, and managers. Obviously, it is hard to draw a line.

Private investors and shareholders have the right to demand higher returns for their investments. However, is it prudent for the government to support health care tourism? Should government allow unlimited medical tourism? Should the government impose taxes on medical tourism dollars?

Medicine is called a noble profession since it directly impacts people's lives. However, health care tourism is about providing access to those who can afford it. These actions can lead to severe negative outcomes. The entrepreneurs, the medical profession, and all the enablers such as industry associations and State governments need to tread carefully. This is a great case that tests the national conscience.

They feel strongly that governments should have no role in promoting health care tourism since it negatively impacts the people they are supposed to represent. Health care is an essential service and the government has the right to interfere in the event of scarcity. Democracy will force governments to avoid unaffordable costs or access. However, my views for the private sector are mixed. It is undesirable to impose constraints that may not be in the best interests of the shareholders. However, the medical community cannot turn a blind eye to the realities and the implications for overall costs. They need to balance their resources and openly commit access to the common man at subsidized rates. The private sector needs to self-govern with transparency and controls. If not, the government may reconsider non-profit status or impose taxes on revenues from medical tourism. Obviously, this is a case for socially responsible governance. The question we should pose to the entrepreneurs and the medical community is whether they will create transparency and standards for socially responsible medical tourism, or work only towards profits?

Appendix I

WORLD HEALTH REPORT 2008: ADVANCING AND SUSTAINING UNIVERSAL COVERAGE

People expect their health systems to be equitable. The roots of health inequities lie in social conditions outside the health system's direct control. These root causes have to be tackled through inter-sectoral and cross-government action.

At the same time, the health sector can take significant actions to advance health equity internally. The basis for this is the set of reforms that aim at moving towards universal coverage, i.e. towards universal access to health services with social health protection.

The central place of health equity in PHC

"If you get sick, you have to choose: you either go without treatment or you lose the farm."[1] Nearly a century ago, the unforgiving reality of life in rural Canada prompted Matthew Anderson (1882-1974) to launch a tax-based health insurance scheme that eventually led to countrywide adoption of universal health care across Canada in 1965. Unfortunately, equally shocking lose-lose situations abound today across the world. More than 30 years after the clarion call of Alma-Ata for greater equity in health, most of the world's health care systems continue to rely on the most inequitable method for financing health care services: out-of-pocket payments by the sick or their families at the point of service. For 5.6 billion people in low- and middle-income countries, over half of all health care expenditure is through out-of-pocket payments. This deprives many families of needed care because they cannot afford it. Also, more than 100 million people around the world are pushed into poverty each year because of catastrophic health care expenditures.[2] There is a wealth of evidence demonstrating that financial protection is better, and catastrophic expenditure less frequent, in those countries in which there is more pre-payment for health care and less out-of-pocket payment. Conversely, catastrophic expenditure is more frequent when health care has to be paid for out-of-pocket at the point of service. While equity marks one of PHC's boldest features, it is one of the areas where results have been most uneven and where the premium for more effective reforms is perhaps the greatest. Out-of-pocket payments for health care are but one of the sources of health inequity. Deeply unequal opportunities for health combined with endemic inequalities in health care provision lead to pervasive inequities in health outcomes.[3]

Growing awareness of these regressive patterns is causing increasing intolerance of the whole spectrum of unnecessary, avoidable and unfair differences in health.[4] The extent of health inequities is documented in much more detail today. They stem from social stratification and political inequalities that lie outside the boundaries of the health system. Income and social status matter, as do the neighbourhoods where people live, their employment conditions and factors, such as personal behaviour, race and stress.[5] Health inequities also find their roots in the way health systems exclude people, such as inequities in availability, access, quality and burden of payment, and even in the way clinical practice is conducted6. Left to their own devices, health systems do not move towards greater equity. Most health services—hospitals in particular, but also first-level care—are consistently inequitable providing more and higher quality services to the well-off than to the poor, who are in greater need.[7,8,9,10]. Differences in vulnerability and exposure combine with inequalities in health care to lead to unequal health outcomes; the latter further contribute to the social stratification that led to the inequalities in the first place. People are rarely indifferent to this cycle of inequalities, making their concerns as relevant to politicians as they are to health system managers.

It takes a wide range of interventions to tackle the social determinants of health and make health systems contribute to more health equity.[11] These interventions reach well beyond the traditional realm of health-service policies, relying on the mobilization of stakeholders and constituencies outside the health sector.[12] They include[13]: reduction of social stratification, e.g. by reducing income inequality through taxes and subsidized public services, providing jobs with adequate pay, using labour intensive growth strategies, promoting equal opportunities for women and making free education available, etc.; reduction of vulnerabilities, e.g. by providing social security for the unemployed or disabled, developing social networks at community level, introducing social inclusion policies and policies that protect mothers while working or studying, offering cash benefits or transfers, providing free healthy lunches at school, etc.; protection, particularly of the disadvantaged, against exposure to health hazards, e.g. by introducing safety regulations for the physical and social environment, providing safe water and sanitation, promoting healthy lifestyles, establishing healthy housing policies, etc.); mitigation of the consequences of unequal health outcomes that contribute to further social stratification, e.g. by protecting the sick from unfair dismissal from their jobs. The need for such multiple strategies could discourage some health leaders who might feel that health inequality is a societal problem over which they have little influence. Yet, they do have a responsibility to address health inequality. The policy choices they make for the health sector define the extent to which health systems exacerbate or mitigate health inequalities and their capacity to mobilize around the equity agenda within government and civil society. These choices also play a key part in society's response to citizens' aspirations for more equity and solidarity. The question, therefore, is not if, but how health leaders can more effectively pursue strategies that will build greater equity in the provision of health services.

Moving towards universal coverage

The fundamental step a country can take to promote health equity is to move towards universal coverage: universal access to the full range of personal and non-personal health services they need, with social health protection. Whether the arrangements for universal coverage are tax based or are organized through social health insurance, or a mix of both, the principles are the same: pooling pre-paid contributions collected on the basis of ability to pay, and using these funds to ensure that services are available, accessible and produce quality care for those who need them, without exposing them to the risk of catastrophic expenditures.[14,15,16] Universal coverage is not, by itself, sufficient to ensure health for all and health equity—inequalities persist in countries with universal or near-universal coverage—but it provides the necessary foundation9. While universal coverage is fundamental to building health equity, it has rarely been the object of an easy social consensus. Indeed, in countries where universal coverage has been achieved or embraced as a political goal, the idea has often met with strong initial resistance, for example, from associations of medical professionals concerned about the impact of government-managed health insurance schemes on their incomes and working conditions, or from financial experts determined to rein in public spending. As with other entitlements that are now taken for granted in almost all high-income countries, universal health coverage has generally been struggled for and won by social movements, not spontaneously bestowed by political leaders. There is now widespread consensus that providing such coverage is simply part of the package of core obligations that any legitimate government must fulfil *vis-à-vis* its citizens. In itself, this is a political achievement that shapes the modernization of society.

Industrialized countries, particularly in Europe, began to put social health protection schemes in place in the late 19th century, moving towards universalism in the second half of the 20th century. The opportunity now exists for low- and middle-income countries to implement comparable approaches.

Costa Rica, Mexico, the Rebublic of Korea, Thailand and Turkey are among the countries that have already introduced ambitious universal coverage schemes, moving significantly faster than industrialized countries did in the past. Other countries are weighing similar options.[14] The technical challenge of moving towards universal coverage is to expand coverage in three ways. The breadth of coverage—the proportion of the population that enjoys social health protection—must expand progressively to encompass the uninsured, i.e. the population groups that lack access to services and/or social protection against the financial consequences of taking up health care. Expanding the breadth of coverage is a complex process of progressive expansion and merging of coverage models. During this process, care must be taken to ensure safety nets for the poorest and most vulnerable until they also are covered. It may take years to cover the entire population but, as recent experience from a number of middle-income countries shows, it is possible to move much faster than was the case for industrialized countries during the 20th century.

Meanwhile, the depth of coverage must also grow, expanding the range of essential services that are necessary to address people's health needs effectively, taking into account demand and expectations, and the resources society is willing and able to allocate to health. The determination of the corresponding "essential package" of benefits can play a key role here, provided the process is conducted appropriately. (Box 2.2)

The third dimension, the height of coverage, i.e. the portion of health care costs covered through pooling and pre-payment mechanisms must also rise, diminishing reliance on out-of pocket co-payments at the point of service delivery. In the 1980s and 1990s, many countries introduced user fees in an effort to infuse new resources into struggling services, often in a context of disengagement of the state and dwindling public resources for health. Most undertook these measures without anticipating the extent of the damage they would do. In many settings, dramatic declines in service use ensued, particularly among vulnerable groups,[20] while the frequency of catastrophic expenditure increased. Some countries have since reconsidered their position and have started phasing out user fees and replacing the lost income from pooled funds.

Box 2.1: Best practices in moving towards universal coverage Emphasize pre-payment from the start. It may take many years before access to health services and financial protection against the costs involved in their use are available for all: it took Japan and the United Kingdom 36 years.[14]

The road may seem discouragingly long, particularly for the poorest countries, where health care networks are sparsely developed, financial protection schemes embryonic and the health sector highly dependent on external funds. Particularly in these countries, however, it is crucial to move towards pre-payment systems from a very early stage and to resist the temptation to rely on user fees. Setting up and maintaining appropriate mechanisms for pre-payment builds the institutional capacity to manage the financing of the system along with the extension of service supply that is usually lacking in such contexts. Coordinate funding sources. In order to organize universal coverage, it is necessary to consider all sources of funding in a country: public, private, external and domestic. In low-income countries, it is particularly important that international funding be channeled through nascent pre-payment and pooling schemes and institutions rather than through project or programme funding. Routing funds in this way has two purposes. It makes external funding more stable and predictable and helps build the institutional capacity to develop and extend supply, access and financial protection in a balanced way.

Combine schemes to build towards full coverage. Many countries with limited resources and administrative capacity have experimented with a multitude of voluntary insurance schemes: community, cooperative, employer-based and other private schemes, as a way to foster pre-payment and pooling in preparation for the move towards more comprehensive national systems.[18] Such schemes are no substitute for universal coverage although they can become building blocks of the universal system.[18] Realizing universal coverage means coordinating or combining these schemes progressively into a coherent whole that ensures coverage to all population groups[15] and builds bridges with broader social protection programmes.[19]

This has resulted in substantial increases in the use of services, especially by the poor.[20] In Uganda, for example, service use increased suddenly and dramatically and the increase was sustained after the elimination of user fees.[22,23] Pre-payment and pooling institutionalizes solidarity between the rich and the less well-off, and between the healthy and the sick. It lifts barriers to the uptake of services and reduces the risk that people will incur catastrophic expenses when they are sick. Finally, it provides the means to re-invest in the availability, range and quality of services.

Challenges in moving towards universal coverage

All universal coverage reforms have to find compromises between the speed with which they increase coverage and the breadth, depth and height of coverage. However, the way countries devise their strategies and focus their reforms very much depends on their specific national contexts. In some countries, a very large part of the population lives in extremely deprived areas, with an absent or dysfunctional health care infrastructure. These are countries of mass exclusion typically brought to mind when one talks about "scaling up": the poor and remote rural areas where health care networks have not been deployed yet or where, after years of neglect, the health infrastructure continues to exist in name only. Such patterns occur in low-income countries.

Box 2.2: Defining "essential packages": what needs to be done to go beyond a paper exercise?

In recent years, many low- and middle-income countries (55 out of a sample of 69 reviewed in 2007) have gone through exercises to define the package of benefits they feel should be available to all their citizens. This has been one of the key strategies in improving the effectiveness of health systems and the equitable distribution of resources. It is supposed to make priority setting, rationing of care, and trade-offs between breadth and depth of coverage explicit. On the whole, attempts to rationalize service delivery by defining packages have not been particularly successful.[24] In most cases, their scope has been limited to maternal and child health care, and to health problems considered as global health priorities. The lack of attention, for example, to chronic and non-communicable diseases confirms the under-valuation of the demographic and epidemiological transitions and the lack of consideration for perceived needs and demand. The packages rarely give guidance on the division of tasks and responsibilities, or on the defining features of primary care, such as comprehensiveness, continuity or person-centeredness.

A more sophisticated approach is required to make the definition of benefit packages more relevant. The way Chile has provided a detailed specification of the health rights of its citizens[25] suggests a number of principles of good practice. The exercise should not be limited to a set of predefined priorities: it should look at demand as well as at the full range of health needs.

- It should specify what should be provided at primary and secondary levels.
- The implementation of the package should be costed so that political decision-makers are aware of what will not be included if health care remains under-funded.
- There have to be institutionalized mechanisms for evidence-based review of the package of benefits.
- People need to be informed about the benefits they can claim, with mechanisms of mediation when claims are being denied. Chile went to great lengths to ensure that the package of benefits corresponds to people's expectations, with studies, surveys and systems to capture the complaints and misgivings of users.[26]

Countries such as Bangladesh, Chad and Niger, are common in conflict and post-conflict areas where health workers have departed and the health infrastructure has been destroyed and needs to be rebuilt from scratch. In other parts of the world, the challenge is in providing health support to widely dispersed populations, for example, in small island states, remote desert or mountainous regions, and among nomadic and some indigenous populations.

Ensuring access to quality care in these settings entails grappling with the diseconomies of scale connected with small, scattered populations; logistical constraints on referral; difficulties linked to limited infrastructure and communications capacities; and, in some cases, more specific technical complications, such as maintaining patient records for nomadic groups.

A different challenge is extending coverage in settings where inequalities do not result from the lack of available health infrastructure, but from the way health care is organized, regulated and, above all, paid for by official or under-the-counter user charges. These are situations where underutilization of available services is concentrated among the poor, whereas users are exposed to the risks of catastrophic expenditure. Such patterns of exclusion occur in countries such as Colombia, Nicaragua and Turkey. It is particularly striking in the many urban areas of low- and middle-income countries where a plethora of assorted, unregulated, commercial health care providers charge users prohibitive fees while providing inadequate services.

Rolling out primary care networks to fill the availability gap In areas where no health services are available for large population groups, or where such services are grossly inadequate or fragmented, the basic health care infrastructure needs to be built or rebuilt, often from the ground up. These areas are always severely resource-constrained and frequently affected by conflicts or complex emergencies, while the scale of under-servicing, also in other sectors, engenders logistical difficulties and problems in deploying health professionals. Health planners in these settings face a fundamental strategic dilemma: whether to prioritize a massive scale-up of a limited set of interventions to the entire population or a progressive roll-out of more comprehensive primary care systems on a district-by-district basis. Some would advocate, in the name of speed and equity, an approach in which a restricted number of priority programmes is rolled out simultaneously to all the inhabitants in the deprived areas. This allows for task shifting to low-skilled personnel, lay workers and volunteers and, consequently, rapid extension of coverage. It is still central to what the global community often prescribes for the rural areas of the poorest countries,[28] and quite a number of countries have chosen this option over the last 30 years.

Ethiopia, for example, is currently deploying 30,000 health extension workers to provide massive numbers of people with a limited package of priority preventive interventions. The poor skills base is often well recognized as a limiting factor,[29] but Ethiopia's extension workers are no longer as low skilled as they once were, and currently benefit from a year of post-Grade 10 training. Nevertheless, skill limitations reinforce the focus on a limited number of effective but simple interventions.

Scaling up a limited number of interventions has the advantage of rapidly covering the entire population and focusing resources on what is known to be cost effective. The downside is that when people experience health problems, they want them to be dealt with, whether or not they fit nicely within the programmatic priorities that are being proposed. Ignoring this dimension of demand too much opens the door to "drug peddlers", "injectors" and other types of providers, who can capitalize on commercial opportunities arising from unmet health needs. They offer patients an appealing alternative, but one that is often exploitative and harmful. Compared with a situation of utter lack of health action, there is an indisputable benefit in scaling up even a very limited package of interventions and the possibility of relying on low-skilled staff makes it an attractive option. However, upgrading often proves more difficult than initially envisaged[30] and, in the meantime, valuable time, resources and credibility are lost which might have allowed for investment in a more ambitious, but also more sustainable and effective primary care infrastructure. The alternative is a progressive roll-out of primary care, district-by-district, of a network of health centres with the necessary hospital support. Such a response obviously includes the priority interventions, but integrated in a comprehensive primary care package. The extension platform is the primary care centre: a professionalized infrastructure where the interface with the community is organized, with a problem-solving capacity and modular expansion of the range of activities. The Islamic Republic of Iran's progressive roll-out of rural coverage is an impressive example of this model. As one of the fathers of the country's PHC strategy put it: "Since it was impossible to launch the project in all provinces at the same time, we decided to focus on a single province each year". (Box 2.3)

The limiting factors for a progressive roll-out of primary care networks are the lack of a stable cadre of mid-level staff with the leadership qualities to organize health districts and with the ability to maintain, over the years, the constant effort required to build sustainable results for the entire population. Where the roll-out has been conducted as an administrative exercise, it has led to disappointment: many health districts exist in name only. But where impatience and pressure for short-term visibility has been managed adequately, a blend of response to need and demand, and participation of the population and key actors has made it possible to build robust primary care networks, even in very difficult and resource-constrained settings of conflict, and post-conflict environments (Box 2.4).

Box 2.3: Closing the urban-rural gap through progressive expansion of PHC coverage in rural areas in the Islamic Republic of Iran[31]

In the 1970s, the Iranian Government's policies emphasized prevention as a long-term investment, allocation of resources to rural and under-privileged areas, and prioritizing ambulatory care over hospitalization. A network of district teams to manage and oversee almost 2500 village-based rural health centers was established. These centers are staffed by a team that includes a general practitioner, midwife, nurse and several health technicians. Each of the rural health centers oversees 1-5 smaller points of care known as "health houses". With 17,000 of these health houses, over 90% of the rural population has access to health care. In remote rural areas, these health houses are staffed by Behvarz (multi-purpose health workers) who are selected by the community, receive between 12 and 18 months training and are then recruited by the Government. The district teams provide training based on problem-solving, as well as ongoing supervision and support. The Government deployed this strategy progressively, extending coverage to one province at a time. Over the years, the PHC network has grown and is now able to provide services to over 24 million people in rural villages and small cities by bringing the points of care closer to where people live and work, as well as by training the necessary auxiliary health staff to provide family planning, preventive care services, and essential curative care for the majority of health problems.

Rural health service utilization rates are now the same as in urban areas. The progressive roll-out of this system has helped to reduce the urban-rural gap in child mortality.

The distinction between rapid deployment of priority interventions and progressive roll-out of primary care networks is, in practice, often not as straightforward as described above. However, for all the convergence, trying to balance speed and sustainability is a real political dilemma.[30] Mali, among others, has shown that, given the choice, people willingly opt for progressive rollout, making community health centres—whose infrastructure is owned and personnel employed by the local community—the basis of functional health districts. Crucially, concern for equity should not be translated into a "lowest common denominator" approach: equal access for all to a set of largely unsatisfactory services. Quality and sustainability are important, particularly since nowadays the multitude of varied and dynamic governmental, not-for-profit and for-profit private providers of various kinds are in dire need of alignment.

Progressive roll-out of health services provides the opportunity to establish welcome leadership coherence in health care provision at district level.

Typical large-scale examples of this approach in developing countries are the contracting out of district health services in Cambodia, or the incorporation of missionary "designated district hospitals" in East Africa. Nevertheless, there is no getting away from the need for massive and sustained investment to expand and maintain health districts in the long term and from the fact that this represents a considerable challenge in a context of sluggish economic growth and stagnating health expenditure. Extending health care networks to underserved areas depends on public initiative and incentives. One way to accelerate the extension of coverage is to adjust budget allocation formulae (or contract specifications) to reflect the extra efforts required to contact hard-to-reach populations. Several countries have taken steps in this direction. In January 2004, for example, the United Republic of Tanzania adopted a revised formula for the allocation of basket funds to districts that includes population size and under five mortality as a proxy for disease burden and poverty level, while adjusting for the differential costs of providing health services in rural and low-density areas. Similarly, allocations to districts under Uganda's PHC budget factor in the districts' Human Development Index and levels of external health funding, in addition to population size. Supplements are paid to districts with difficult security situations or lacking a district hospital.[20] In Chile, budgets are allocated on a capitation basis but, as part of the PHC reforms, these were adjusted using municipal human development indices and a factor to reflect the isolation of underserved areas.

Overcoming the isolation of dispersed populations

Although providing access to services for dispersed populations is often a daunting logistical challenge, some countries have dealt with it by developing creative approaches. Devising mechanisms to share innovative experiences and results has clearly been a key step, for example, through the "Healthy Islands" initiative, launched at the meeting of Ministers and Heads of Health in Yanuca, Fiji, in 199534. The initiative brings together health policy-makers and practitioners to address challenges to islanders' health and well-being from an explicitly multi-sectoral perspective, with a focus on expanding coverage of curative health care services, but also reinforcing promotive strategies and cross-sectoral action on the determinants of health and health equity. Through the Healthy Islands initiative and related experiences, a number of principles have emerged as crucial to the advancement of universal coverage in these settings. The first concerns collaboration in organizing infrastructure that maximizes scales of efficiency. An isolated community may be unable to afford key inputs to expand coverage, which includes infrastructure, technologies and human resources (particularly the training of personnel). However, when communities join forces, they can secure such inputs at manageable costs.[35] A second strategic focus is on "mobile resources" or those that can overcome distance and geographical obstacles efficiently and affordably. Depending on the setting, this strategic focus may include transportation, radio communications, and other information and communications technologies.

In the long-run, PHC-led health districts are an organizational model that has the robustness to resist extremely adverse conditions. Maintaining minimal financial support and supervision to such districts can yield very significant results, while empowering and retaining national health professionals.

Box 2.4: Local health services have a considerable potential for coping with crises[33]

Providing alternatives to unregulated commercial services In urban and peri-urban contexts, health services are physically within reach of the poor and other vulnerable populations. The presence of multiple health care providers does not mean, however, that these groups are protected from diseases, nor that they can get quality care when they need it: the more privileged tend to get better access to the best services, public and private, easily coming out on top in a *de facto* competition for scarce resources. In the urban and increasingly in the rural areas of many low- and middle-income countries - from India and Viet Nam to sub-Saharan Africa - much health care for the poor is provided by small-scale, largely unregulated and often unlicensed providers, both commercial and not-for-profit. Often, they work alongside dysfunctional public services and capture an overwhelmingly large part of the health care market, while the health promotion and prevention agenda is totally ignored. Vested interests make the promotion of universal coverage paradoxically more difficult in these circumstances than in areas where the challenge is to build health care delivery networks from scratch. These contexts often combine problems of financial exploitation, bad quality and unsafe care, and exclusion from needed services.[37,38,39,40,41,42,43,44,45,46]

The Pan American Health Organization (PAHO) has estimated that 47% of Latin America's population is excluded from needed services47. This may be for broader reasons of poverty, ethnicity or gender, or because the resources of the health system are not correctly targeted. It may be because there are no adequate systems to protect people against catastrophic expenditure or from financial exploitation by unscrupulous or insensitive providers. It may have to do with the way people, rightly or wrongly, perceive health services: lack of trust, the expectation of ill-treatment or discrimination, uncertainty about the cost-of-care, or the anticipation that the cost will be unaffordable or catastrophic. Services may also be untimely, ineffective, unresponsive or plain discriminatory, providing poorer patients with inferior treatment.[48,49,21] As a result, health outcomes vary considerably by social class, even in well-regulated and well-funded health care systems.

In addressing these patterns of exclusion within the health care sector, the starting point is to create or strengthen networks of accessible quality primary care services that rely on pooled pre-payment or public resources for their funding. Whether these networks are expanded by contracting commercial or not-for-profit providers, or by revitalizing dysfunctional public facilities is not the critical issue. The point is to ensure that they offer care of an acceptable standard. A critical mass of primary care centres that provide an essential package of quality services free-of charge, provides an important alternative to substandard, exploitative commercial care. Furthermore, peer pressure and consumer demand can help to create an environment in which regulation of the commercial sector becomes possible. More active involvement of municipal authorities in pre-payment and pooling schemes to improve the supply of quality care is probably one of the avenues to follow, particularly where ministries of health with budgetary constraints also have to extend services to underserved rural areas.

Targeted interventions to complement universal coverage mechanisms

Rising average national income, a growing supply of health care providers and accelerated progress towards universal coverage are, unfortunately, not sufficient to eliminate health inequities. Socially determined health differences among population groups persist in high-income countries with robust, universal health care and social-service systems, such as Finland and France.[11,50] Health inequalities do not just exist between the poor and the non-poor, but across the entire socioeconomic gradient. There are circumstances where other forms of exclusion are of prime concern, including the exclusion of adolescents, ethnic groups, drug users and those affected by stigmatizing diseases.[51] In Australia, Canada and New Zealand, among others, health equity gaps between

Aboriginal and non-Aboriginal populations have emerged as national political issues.[52,53,54] In other settings, inequalities in women's access to health care merit attention.[55] In the United States, for example, declines in female life expectancy of up to five years in over 1000 counties point to differential exposure and clustering of risks to health even as the country's economy and health sector continues to grow.[56] For a variety of reasons, some groups within these societies are either not reached or insufficiently reached by opportunities for health or services and continue to experience health outcomes systematically inferior to those of more advantaged groups.

Thus, it is necessary to embed universal coverage in wider social protection schemes and to complement it with specially designed, targeted forms of outreach to vulnerable and excluded groups.[57] Established health care networks often do not make all possible efforts to ensure that everyone in their target population has access to the full range of health benefits they need, as this requires extra efforts, such as home visits, outreach services, specialized language and cultural facilitation, evening consultations, etc.

These may, however, mitigate the effect of social stratification and inequalities in the uptake of services.[58] They may also offer the opportunity to construct comprehensive support packages to foster social inclusion of historically marginalized populations, in collaboration with other government sectors and with affected communities.

Chile's Chile Solidario (Chilean Solidarity) model of outreach to families in long-term poverty is one example (Box 2.5).[59] Such targeted measures may include subsidizing people—not services—to take up specific health services, for example, through vouchers60,61 for maternal care as in India and Yemen, for bed nets as in the United Republic of Tanzania62,63, for contraceptive uptake by adolescents[64] or care for the elderly uninsured as in the United States.[65] Conditional cash transfers, where the beneficiary is not only enabled, but compelled to take up services is another model, which has been introduced in several countries in Latin America. A recent systematic review of six such programmes suggests that conditional cash transfers can be effective in increasing the use of preventive services and improving nutritional and anthropometric outcomes, sometimes improving health status.[66] However, their overall effect on health status remains less clear and so does their comparative advantage over traditional, unconditional, income maintenance, through universal entitlements, social insurance or—less-effective—means-tested social assistance. Targeted measures are not substitutes for the long-term drive towards universal coverage. They can be useful and necessary complements, but without simultaneous institutionalization of the financing models and system structures that support universal coverage, targeted approaches are unlikely to overcome the inequalities generated by socio-economic stratification and exclusion.

Box 2.5: Targeting Social Protection in Chile[59]

Established by law, the Chilean social protection programme (Chile Solidario) involves three main components to improve conditions for people living in extreme poverty: direct psycho-social support, financial support and priority access to social programmes. The direct psycho-social support component involves families in extreme poverty being identified according to pre-defined criteria and invited to enter into an agreement with a designated social worker. The social worker assists them to build individual and family capacities that help them to strengthen their links with social networks and to gain access to the social benefits to which they are entitled. In addition to psycho-social support, there is also financial support in terms of cash transfers and pensions, as well as subsidies for raising families or covering water and sanitation costs. Finally, the social protection programme also provides preferential access to pre-school programmes, adult literacy courses, employment programmes and preventive health visits for women and children. This social protection programme complements a multisectoral effort targeting all children aged 0-18 years (Chile Crece Contigo—Chile Grows with You). The aim is to promote early childhood development through pre-school education programmes, preventive health checks, improved parental leave and increased child benefits. Better access to child-care services is also included as is enforcing the right of working mothers to nurse their babies, which is designed to stimulate women's insertion into the employment market.

Health systems are invariably inequitable. More and higher quality services gravitate to the well-off who need them less than the poor and marginalized.[8] The universal coverage reforms required to move towards greater equity demand the enduring commitment of the highest political levels of society. Two levers may be especially important in accelerating action on health equity and maintaining momentum over time. The first is raising the visibility of health inequities in public awareness and policy debates: the history of progress in the health of populations is intimately linked to the measurement of health inequalities. It was the observation of excess mortality among the working class that informed the "Great Sanitary Awakening" reforms of the Poor Laws Commission in the United Kingdom in the 1830s.[68] The second is the creation of space for civil society participation in shaping the PHC reforms that are to advance health equity: the history of progress in universal coverage is intimately linked to that of social movements. Increasing the visibility of health inequities.

With the economic optimism of the 1960s and 1970s (and the expansion of social insurance in industrialized countries), poverty ceased being a priority issue for many policy-makers. It took Alma-Ata to put equity back on the political agenda. The lack of systematic measurement and monitoring to translate this agenda into concrete challenges has long been a major constraint in advancing the PHC agenda. In recent years, income-related and other health inequalities have been studied in greater depth. The introduction of composite asset indices has made it possible to reanalyze demographic and health surveys from an equity viewpoint.[69] This has generated a wealth of documentary evidence on socioeconomic differentials in health outcomes and access to care. It took this acceleration of the measurement of poverty and inequalities, particularly since the mid-1990s, to bring first poverty and then, more generally, the challenge of persisting inequalities to the centre of the health policy debate. Measurement of health inequities is paramount when confronting the common misperceptions that strongly infl uence health policy debates.[70,71] Simple population averages are sufficient to assess progress—they are not.

- Health systems designed for universal access are equitable—they are a necessary, but not a sufficient condition.
- In poor countries, everybody is equally poor and equally unhealthy—all societies are stratified.
- The main concern is between countries' differences—inequalities within countries matter most to people.
- Well-intended reforms to improve efficiency will ultimately benefit everybody—they often have unintended inequitable consequences. Measurement matters for a variety of reasons.[2]
- It is important to know the extent and understand the nature of health inequalities and exclusion in a given society, so as to be able to share that information and translate it into objectives for change.
- It is equally important, for the same reasons, to identify and understand the determinants of health inequality not only in general terms, but also within each specific national context. Health authorities must be informed of the extent to which current or planned health policies contribute to inequalities, so as to be able to correct them.
- Progress with reforms designed to reduce health inequalities, i.e. progress in moving towards universal coverage, needs to be monitored, so as to steer and correct these reforms as they unfold.

Despite policy-makers' long-held commitment to the value of equity in health, its definition and measurement represent a more recent public health science. Unless health information systems collect data using standardized social stratifiers, such as socio-economic status, gender, ethnicity and geographical area, it is difficult to identify and locate inequalities and, unless their magnitude and nature are uncovered, it is unlikely that they will be adequately addressed.[72] The now widely available analyses of Demographic and Health Survey (DHS) data by asset quintiles have made a major difference in the awareness of policy-makers about health equity problems in their countries. There are also examples of how domestic capacities and capabilities can be strengthened to better understand and manage equity problems. For example, Chile has recently embarked on integrating health sector information systems in order to have more comprehensive information on determinants and to improve the ability to disaggregate information according to socio-economic groups.

Indonesia has added health modules to household expenditure and demographic surveys. Building in capabilities, across administrative database systems, to link health and socio-economic data through unique identifiers (national insurance numbers or census geo-codes) is key to socio-economic stratification and provides information that is usually inaccessible. However, this is more than a technical challenge. Measuring health systems' progress towards equity requires an explicit deliberative process to identify what constitutes a fair distribution of health against shortfalls and gaps that can be measured.[73] It relies on the development of institutional collaboration between multiple stakeholders to ensure that measurement and monitoring translates into concrete political proposals for better equity and solidarity.

Creating space for civil society participation and empowerment

Knowledge about health inequalities can only be translated into political proposals if there is organized social demand. Demand from the communities that bear the burden of existing inequities and other concerned groups in civil society are among the most powerful motors driving universal coverage reforms and efforts to reach the unreached and the excluded. The amount of grassroots advocacy to improve the health and welfare of populations in need has grown enormously in the last 30 years, mostly within countries, but also globally. There are now thousands of groups around the world, large and small, local and global, calling for action to improve the health of particularly deprived social groups or those suffering from specific health conditions. These groups, which were virtually non-existent in the days of the Alma-Ata, constitute a powerful voice of collective action.

Box 2.6: Social policy in the city of Ghent, Belgium: how local authorities can support intersectoral collaboration between health and welfare organizations[76]

In 2004, a regional government decree in Flanders, Belgium, institutionalized the direct participation of local stakeholders and citizens in intersectoral collaboration on social rights. This now applies at the level of cities and villages in the region. In one of these cities, Ghent, some 450 local actors of the health and welfare sector have been clustered in 11 thematic forums: legal help; support and security of minors; services for young people and adolescents; child care; ethnic cultural minorities; people with a handicap; the elderly; housing; work and employment; people living on a "critical income"; and health.

The local authorities facilitate and support the collaboration of the various organizations and sectors, for example, through the collection and monitoring of data, information and communication, access to services, and efforts to make services more pro-active. They are also responsible for networking between all the sectors with a view to improving coordination. They pick up the signals, bottlenecks, proposals and plans, and are responsible for channeling them, if appropriate, to the province, region, federal state or the European Union for translation into relevant political decisions and legislation. A steering committee reports directly to the city council and integrates the work of the 11 forums. The support of the administration and a permanent working party is critical for the sustainability and quality of the work in the different groups. Participation of all stakeholders is particularly prominent in the health forum: it includes local hospitals, family physicians, primary care services, pharmacists, mental health facilities, self-help groups, home care, health promotion agencies, academia sector, psychiatric home care, and community health centers. This complex web of collaboration is showing results. Intersectoral coordination contributes to a more efficient local social policy. For the period 2008-13, four priority themes have been identified in a bottom-up process: sustainable housing, access to health care, reduced thresholds to social rights, and optimization of growth and development. The yearly action plan operationalizes the policy through improvement projects in areas that include financial access to health care, educational support, care for the homeless, and affordable and flexible child care. Among the concrete realizations is the creation of Ghent's "social house", a network of service entry points situated in the different neighbourhoods of the city, where delivery of primary care is organized with special attention to the most vulnerable groups of people. The participating organizations report that the creation of the sectoral forums, in conjunction with the organization of intersectoral cooperation, has significantly improved the way social determinants of health are tackled in the city.

The mobilization of groups and communities to address what they consider to be their most important health problems and health-related inequalities is a necessary complement to the more technocratic and top-down approach to assessing social inequalities and determining priorities for action. Many of these groups have become capable lobbyists, for example, by gaining access to HIV/AIDS treatment, abolishing user fees and promoting universal coverage. However, these achievements should not mask the contributions that the direct engagement of affected communities and civil society organizations can have in eliminating sources of exclusion within local health services. Costa Rica's "bias-free framework" is one example among many. It has been used successfully to foster dialogue with and among members of vulnerable communities by uncovering local practices of exclusion and barriers to access not readily perceived by providers and by spurring action to address the underlying causes of ill-health.

Concrete results, such as the reorganization of a maternity hospital around the people's needs and expectations can transcend the local dimension, as was the case in Costa Rica when local reorganization was used as a template for a national effort.[74] However, there is much the health system itself can do to mitigate the effects of social inequities and promote fairer access to health services at local level. Social participation in health action becomes a reality at the local level and, at times, it is there that intersectoral action most effectively engages the material and social factors that shape people's health prospects, widening or reducing health equity gaps. One such example is the Health Action Zones in the United Kingdom, which were partner-based entities whose mission was to improve the well-being of disadvantaged groups. Another example is the work of the municipality of Barcelona, in Spain, where a set of interventions, including the reform of primary care, was followed by health improvements in a number of disadvantaged groups, showing that local governments can help reduce health inequities.[75] Local action can also be the starting point for broader structural changes, if it feeds into relevant political decisions and legislation (Box 2.6).

Primary care is the way of organizing health care delivery that is best geared not only to improving health equity, but also to meeting people's other basic needs and expectations.

Sources

1. Houston, S. Matt Anderson's 1939 health plan: how effective and how economical? *Saskatchewan History*, 2005, 57:4-14.
2. Xu, K. *et al*. Protecting households from catastrophic health spending, *Health Affairs*, 2007, 26:972-83.
3. A conceptual framework for action on the social determinants of health; discussion paper for the Commission on Social Determinants for Health. Geneva, World Health Organization, 2007.
4. Whitehead, M., Dahlgren, G. Concepts and principles for tackling social inequities in health: levelling up part 1. Copenhagen, World Health Organization Regional Office for Europe, 2006 (Studies on Social and Economic Determinants of Population Health No. 2.
5. Adler, N., Stewart, J. Reaching for a healthier life. Facts on socioeconomic status and health in the US. Chicago, JD and CT MacArthur Foundation Research Network on Socio-economic Status and Health, 2007.
6. Dans, A. *et al*. Assessing equity in clinical practice guidelines. Journal of Clinical Epidemiology, 2007, 60:540-546.
7. Hart, J.T. The inverse care law. *Lancet*, 1971, 1:405-412.
8. Gwatkin, D.R., Bhuiya, A., Victora, C.G. Making health systems more equitable. *Lancet*, 2004, 364:1273-1280.
9. Gilson, L., McIntyre, D. Post-apartheid challenges: household access and use of care. *International Journal of Health Services*, 2007, 37:673-691.
10. Hanratty, B., Zhang, T., Whitehead, M. How close have universal health systems come to achieving equity in use of curative services? A systematic review. *International Journal of Health Services*, 2007, 37:89-109.
11. Mackenbach, J.P. *et al*. Strategies to reduce socioeconomic inequalities in health. In: Mackenbach, J.P., Bakker, M., eds. Reducing inequalities in health: a European perspective. London, Routledge, 2002.
12. Report No. 20 (2006-2007): National strategy to reduce social inequalities in health. Paper presented to the Storting. Oslo, Norwegian Ministry of Health and Care Services, 2007 (http://www.regjeringen.no/en/dep/hod/Documents/regpubl/stmeld/2006-2007/Report-No-20-2006-2007-to-the-Storting.html?id=466505, accessed 19 July 2008).

13. Diderichsen, F., Hallqvist, J. Social inequalities in health: some methodological considerations for the study of social position and social context. In: Arve-Parès B,ed. Inequality in health - a Swedish perspective. Stockholm, Swedish Council for Social Research, 1998.

14. International Labour Office, Deutsche Gesellschaft für Technische Zusammenarbeit (GTZ) Gmbh and World Health Organization. Extending social protection in health: developing countries, experiences, lessons learnt and recommendations. International Conference on Social Health Insurance in Developing Countries, Berlin, 5-7 December 2005. Eschborn, Deutsche Gesellschaft für Technische Zusammenarbeit

15. Achieving universal health coverage: developing the health financing system. Geneva, World Health Organization, Department of Health Systems Financing, 2005 (Technical Briefs for Policy-makers No. 1).

16. The World Health Report 2000 - Health systems: improving performance. Geneva, World Health Organization, 2000.

17. Busse, R., Schlette, S., eds. Focus on prevention, health and aging and health professions. Gütersloh, Verlag Bertelsmann Stiftung, 2007 (Health Policy Developments 7/8).

18. Carrin, G., Waelkens, M.P., Criel, B. Community-based health insurance in developing countries: a study of its contribution to the performance of health financing systems. *Tropical Medicine and International Health*, 2005, 10:799-811.

19. Jacobs, B. *et al.* Bridging community-based health insurance and social protection for health care—a step in the direction of universal coverage? *Tropical Medicine and International Health*, 2008, 13:140-143.

20. Reclaiming the resources for health. A regional analysis of equity in health in East and Southern Africa. Kampala, Regional Network on Equity in Health in Southern Africa (EQUINET), 2007.

21. Gilson, L. The lessons of user fee experience in Africa. *Health Policy and Planning*, 1997, 12:273-85.

22. Ke, X. *et al.* The elimination of user fees in Uganda: impact on utilization and catastrophic health expenditures. Geneva, World Health Organization, Department of Health System Financing, Evidence, Information and Policy Cluster, 2005 (Discussion Paper No. 4).

23. Hutton, G. Charting the path to the World Bank's "No blanket policy on user fees". A look over the past 25 years at the shifting support for user fees in health and education, and refl ections on the future. London, Department for International Development (DFID) Health Resource Systems Resource Centre, 2004

24. Tarimo, E. Essential health service packages: uses, abuse and future directions. Current concerns. Geneva, World Health Organization, 1997 (ARA Paper No. 15; WHO/ARA/CC/97.7).

26. Moccero, D. Delivering cost-efficient public services in health care, education and housing in Chile. Paris, Organisation for Economic Co-operation and Development, 2008 (Economics Department Working Papers No. 606).

27. Gwatkin, D.R. *et al.* Socio-economic differences in health, nutrition, and population within developing countries. An overview. Washington DC, The World Bank, Human Development Network, Health, Population and Nutrition, and Population Family, 2007 (POPLINE Document Number: 324740).

28. Conway, M.D., Gupta, S., Khajavi, K. Addressing Africa's health workforce crisis. *The Mckinsey Quarterly*, November 2007.

29. Bossyns, P., Van Lerberghe, W. The weakest link: competence and prestige as constraints to referral by isolated nurses in rural Niger. Human Resources for Health, 2004, 2:1.

30. Maiga, Z., Traoré Nafo, F., El Abassi, A. La Réforme du secteur santé au Mali, 1989-96. Studies in Health Services Organisation and Policy, 1999, 12:1-132.

31. Abolhassani, F. Primary health care in the Islamic Republic of Iran. Teheran, Teheran University of Medical Sciences, Health Network Development Centre (unpublished).

32. Naghavi, M. Demographic and health surveys in Iran, 2008 (personal communication).

33. Porignon, D. *et al*. How robust are district health systems? Coping with crisis and disasters in Rutshuru, Democratic Republic of Congo. Tropical Medicine and International Health, 1998, 3:559-65.

34. Gauden, G.I., Powis, B., Tamplin, S.A. Healthy Islands in the Western Pacific-international settings development. Health Promotion International, 2000, 15:169-78.

35. The World Health Report 2006: Working together for health. Geneva, World Health Organization, 2006.

36. Bossyns, P. *et al*. Unaffordable or cost-effective? Introducing an emergency referral system in rural Niger. Tropical Medicine and International Health, 2005, 10:879-887.

37. Tibandebage, P., Mackintosh, M. The market shaping of charges, trust and abuse: health care transactions in Tanzania. *Social Science and Medicine*, 2005, 61:1385-1395.

38. Segall, M. *et al*. Health care seeking by the poor in transitional economies: the case of Vietnam. Brighton, Institute of Development Studies, 2000 (IDS Research Reports No. 43).

39. Baru, R.V. Private health care in India: social characteristics and trends. New Delhi, Sage Publications, 1998.

40. Tu, N.T.H., Huong, N.T.L., Diep, N.B. Globalisation and its effects on health care and occupational health in Viet Nam. Geneva, United Nations Research Institute for Social Development, 2003 (http://www.unrisd.org, accessed 19 July 2008).

41. Narayana, K. The role of the state in the privatisation and corporatisation of medical care in Andhra Pradesh, India. In: Sen K, ed. Restructuring health services: changing contexts and comparative perspectives. London and New Jersey, Zed Books, 2003.

42. Bennett, S., McPake, B., Mills, A. The public/private mix debate in health care. In: Bennett, S., McPake, B., Mills, A., eds. Private health providers in developing countries. Serving the public interest? London and New Jersey, Zed Books, 1997.

43. Ogunbekun, I., Ogunbekun, A., Orobaton, N. Private health care in Nigeria: walking the tightrope. Health Policy and Planning, 1999, 14:174-181.

44. Mills, A., Bennett, S., Russell, S. The challenge of health sector reform: what must governments do? Basingstoke, Palgrave Macmillan, 2001.

45. The unbearable cost of illness: poverty, ill-health and access to health care—evidence from Lindi Rural District, Tanzania, London, Save the Children, 2001.

46. Ferrinho, P., Bugalho, A.M., Van Lerberghe, W. Is there a case for privatising reproductive health? Patchy evidence and much wishful thinking. Studies in Health Services Organisation and Policy, 2001, 17:343-370.

47. Pan American Health Organization and Swedish International Development Agency. Exclusion in health in Latin America and the Caribbean. Washington DC, Pan American Health Organization, 2003 (Extension of Social Protection in Health Series No. 1). The World Health Report

48. Jaffré, Y., Olivier de Sardan, J.-P., eds. Une médecine inhospitalière. Les difficiles relations entre soignants et soignés dans cinq capitales d'Afrique de l'Ouest. Paris, Karthala, 2003.

49. Schellenberg, J.A. *et al*. Inequalities among the very poor: health care for children in rural southern Tanzania. Ifakara, Ifakara Health Research and Development Centre, 2002.

50. Oliver, A., ed. Health care priority setting: implications for health inequalities. Proceedings from a meeting of the Health Equity Network. London, The Nuffield Trust, 2003.

51. Overcoming obstacles to health: report from the Robert Wood Johnson Foundation to the Commission to Build a Healthier America. Princeton NJ, Robert Wood Johnson Foundation, 2008.

52. Franks, A. Self-determination background paper. Aboriginal health promotion project. Lismore NSW, Northern Rivers Area Health Service, Division of Population Health, Health Promotion Unit, 2001

53. Gathering strength—Canada's Aboriginal action plan: a progress report. Ottawa, Ministry of Indian Affairs and Northern Development, 2000.

54. King, A., Turia, T. He korowai orange - Maori Health Strategy. Wellington, Ministry of Health of New Zealand, 2002.

55. Cecile, M.T. *et al.* Gender perspectives and quality of care: towards appropriate and adequate health care for women. *Social Science and Medicine,* 1996, 43:707-20.

56. Murray, C., Kulkarni, S., Ezzati, M. Eight Americas: new perspectives on U.S. health disparities. *American Journal of Preventive Medicine,* 2005, 29:4-10.

57. Paterson, I., Judge, K. Equality of access to health care. In: Mackenbach, J.P., Bakker, M., eds. Reducing inequalities in health: a European perspective. London, Routledge, 2002.

58. Doblin, L., Leake, B.D. Ambulatory health services provided to low-income and homeless adult patients in a major community health center. *Journal of General Internal Medicine,* 1996 11:156-62.

59. Frenz, P. Innovative practices for intersectoral action on health: a case study of four programs for social equity. Chilean case study prepared for the CSDH. Santiago, Ministry of Health, Division of Health Planning, Social Determinants of Health Initiative, 2007.

60. Emanuel, E.J., Fuchs, V.R. Health care vouchers—a proposal for universal coverage. *New England Journal of Medicine,* 2005, 352:1255-60.

61. Morris, S. *et al.* Monetary incentives in primary health care and effects on use and coverage of preventive health care interventions in rural Honduras: cluster randomised trial. *Lancet,* 2004, 364:2030-37.

62. Armstrong, J.R.M. *et al.* KINET: a social marketing programme of treated nets and net treatment for malaria control in Tanzania, with evaluation of child health and long term survival. Transactions of the Royal Society of Tropical Medicine and Hygiene, 1999, 93:225-31.

63. Adiel, K. *et al.* Targeted subsidy for malaria control with treated nets using a discount voucher system in Tanzania. Health Policy and Planning, 2003, 18:163-71.

64. Kirby, D., Waszak, C., Ziegler, J. Six school-based clinics: their reproductive health services and impact on sexual behaviour. Family Planning Perspectives, 1991, 23:6-16.

65. Meng, H. *et al.* Effect of a consumer-directed voucher and a disease-management health-promotion nurse intervention on home care use. The Gerontologist, 2005, 45:167-76.

66. Lagarde, M., Haines, A., Palmer, N. Conditional cash transfers for improving uptake of health interventions in low- and middle-income countries. A systematic review. *Journal of the American Medical Association,* 2007, 298:1900-10.

67. Gwatkin, D.R., Wagstaff, A., Yazbeck, A., eds. Reaching the poor with health, nutrition and population services. What works, what doesn't and why. Washington DC, The World Bank, 2005.

68. Sretzer, S. The importance of social intervention in Britain's mortality decline, c.1850-1914: a reinterpretation of the role of public health. Society for the Social History of Medicine, 1988, 1:1-41.

69. Gwatkin, D.R. 10 best resources on ... health equity. Health Policy and Planning, 2007, 22:348-51.

70. Burström, B. Increasing inequalities in health care utilisation across income groups in Sweden during the 1990s? *Health Policy*, 2002, 62:117-29.

71. Whitehead, M. *et al.* As the health divide widens in Sweden and Britain, what's happening to access to care? *British Medical Journal*, 1997, 315:1006-09.

72. Nolen, L.B. *et al.* Strengthening health information systems to address health equity challenges, *Bulletin of the World Health Organization*, 2005, 83:597-603.

73. Whitehead, M., Dahlgren, G., Evans, T. Equity and health sector reforms: can lowincome countries escape the medical poverty trap. *Lancet*, 2001, 358:833-36.

74. Burke, M.A., Eichler, M. The BIAS FREE framework: a practical tool for identifying and eliminating social biases in health research. Geneva, Global Forum for Health Research, 2006

75. Benach, J., Borell, C., Daponte, A. Spain. In: Mackenbach, J.P., Bakker, M., eds. Reducing inequalities in health: a European perspective. London, Routledge, 2002.

76. Balthazar, T., Versnick, G. Lokaal sociaal beleidsplan, Gent. Strategisch meerjarenplan, 2008-2013. Gent, Lokaal Sociaal Beleid, 2008

Appendix 2

WORLD HEALTH REPORT 2008: PUTTING PEOPLE FIRST

This chapter describes how primary care brings promotion and prevention, cure and care together in a safe, effective and socially productive way at the interface between the population and the health system. In short, what needs to be done to achieve this is "to put people first": to give balanced consideration to health and well-being as well as to the values and capacities of the population and the health workers.[1]

These features are person-centeredness, comprehensiveness and integration, and continuity of care, with a regular point of entry into the health system, so that it becomes possible to build an enduring relationship of trust between people and their health care providers. The chapter then defines what this implies for the organization of health care delivery: the necessary switch from specialized to generalist ambulatory care, with responsibility for a defined population and the ability to coordinate support from hospitals, specialized services and civil society organizations.

Good care is about people

Biomedical science is, and should be, at the heart of modern medicine. Yet, as William Osler, one of its founders, pointed out, "it is much more important to know what sort of patient has a disease than what sort of disease a patient has."[2] Insufficient recognition of the human dimension in health and of the need to tailor the health service's response to the specificity of each community and individual situation represent major shortcomings in contemporary health care, resulting not only in inequity and poor social outcomes, but also diminishing the health outcome returns on the investment in health services. Putting people first, the focus of service delivery reforms is not a trivial principle. It can require significant—even if often simple—departures from business as usual. The reorganization of a medical centre in Alaska in the United States, accommodating 45,000 patient contacts per year, illustrates how far-reaching the effects can be. The centre functioned to no great satisfaction of either staff or clients until it decided to establish a direct relationship between each individual and family in the community and a specific staff member.[3] The staff were then in a position to know "their" patients' medical history and understand their personal and family situation. People were in a position to get to know and trust their health care provider: they no longer had to deal with an institution but with their personal caregiver. Complaints about compartmentalized and fragmented services abated4. Emergency room visits were reduced by approximately 50% and referrals to specialty care by 30%; waiting times shortened significantly. With fewer "rebound" visits for unresolved health problems, the workload actually decreased and staff job satisfaction improved. Most importantly, people felt that they were being listened to and respected—a key aspect of what people value about health care.[5,6] A slow bureaucratic system was thus transformed into one that is customer-responsive, customer owned and customer-driven.[4]

In a very different setting, the health centres of Ouallam, a rural district in Niger, implemented an equally straightforward reorganization of their way of working in order to put people first. Rather than the traditional morning curative care consultation and specialized afternoon clinics (growth monitoring, family planning, etc.), the full range of services was offered at all times, while the nurses were instructed to engage in an active dialogue with their patients. For example, they no longer waited for women to ask for contraceptives, but informed them, at every contact, about the range of services available. Within a few months, the very low uptake of family planning, previously attributed to cultural constraints, was a thing of the past.[7]

People's experiences of care provided by the health system are determined first and foremost by the way they are treated when they experience a problem and look for help: by the responsiveness of the health-worker interface between population and health services. People value some freedom in choosing a health provider because they want one they can trust and who will attend to them promptly and in an adequate environment, with respect and confidentiality.[8]

Health care delivery can be made more effective by making it more considerate and convenient, as in Ouallam district. However, primary care is about more than shortening waiting times, adapting opening hours or getting staff to be more polite. Health workers have to care for people throughout the course of their lives, as individuals and as members of a family and a community whose health must be protected and enhanced9, and not merely as body parts with symptoms or disorders that require treating.[10] The service delivery reforms advocated by the PHC movement aim to put people at the centre of health care, so as to make services more effective, efficient and equitable. Health services that do this start from a close and direct relationship between individuals and communities and their caregivers. This, then, provides the basis for person- centeredness, continuity, comprehensiveness and integration, which constitute the distinctive features of primary care.

Technical and safety parameters are not the only determinants of the outcomes of health care. The disappointingly low success rate in preventing mother-to-child transmission (MTCT) of HIV in a study in the Côte d'Ivoire illustrates that other features of the organization of health care are equally critical.

Box 3.1: Towards a science and culture of improvement: evidence to promote patient safety and better outcomes

The outcome of health care results from the balance between the added value of treatment or intervention, and the harm it causes to the patient.[16] Until recently, the extent of such harm has been underestimated. In industrialized countries, approximately 1 in 10 patients suffers harm caused by avoidable adverse events while receiving care:[17] up to 98,000 deaths per year are caused by such events in the United States alone.[18] Multiple factors contribute to this situation,[19] ranging from systemic faults to problems of competence, social pressure on patients to undergo risky procedures, to incorrect technology usage.[20] For example, almost 40% of the 16 billion injections administered worldwide each year are given with syringes and needles that are reused without sterilization.[14] Each year, unsafe injections thus cause 1.3 million deaths and almost 26 million years of life lost, mainly because of transmission of hepatitis B and C, and HIV.[21] Especially disquieting is the paucity of information on the extent and determinants of unsafe care in low- and middle-income countries. With unregulated commercialization of care, weaker quality control and health resource limitations, health care users in low-income countries may well be even more exposed to the risk of unintended patient harm than patients in high-income countries. The World Alliance for Patient Safety,[22] among others, advocates making patients safer through systemic interventions and a change in organizational culture rather than through the denunciation of individual health care practitioners or administrators.[23]

Box 3.2: When supplier-induced and consumer-driven demand determine medical advice: ambulatory care in India

"Ms. S is a typical patient who lives in urban Delhi. There are over 70 private-sector medical care providers within a 15-minute walk from her house (and virtually any household in her city). She chooses the private clinic run by Dr. SM and his wife. Above the clinic a prominent sign says "Ms. MM, Gold Medalist, MBBS", suggesting that the clinic is staffed by a highly proficient doctor (an MBBS is the basic degree for a medical doctor as in the British 2 system). As it turns out, Ms. MM is rarely at the clinic. We were told that she sometimes comes at 4 a.m. to avoid the long lines that form if people know she is there. We later discover that she has "franchised" her name to a number of different clinics. Therefore, Ms. S sees Dr. SM and his wife, both of whom were trained in traditional Ayurvedic medicine through a six-month long-distance course. The doctor and his wife sit at a small table surrounded, on one side, by a large number of bottles full of pills, and on the other, a bench with patients on them, which extends into the street. Ms. S sits at the end of this bench. Dr. SM and his wife are the most popular medical care providers in the neighbourhood, with more than 200 patients every day. The doctor spends an average of 3.5 minutes with each patient, asks 3.2 questions, and performs an average of 2.5 examinations. Following the diagnosis, the doctor takes two or three different pills, crushes them using a mortar and pestle, and makes small paper packets from the resulting powder which he gives to Ms. S and asks her to take for two or three days. These medicines usually include one antibiotic and one analgesic and anti-inflammatory drug. Dr. SM tells us that he constantly faces unrealistic patient expectations, both because of the high volume of patients and their demands for treatments that even Dr. SM knows are inappropriate. Dr. SM and his wife seem highly motivated to provide care to their patients and even with a very crowded consultation room they spend more time with their patients than a public sector doctor would. However, they are not bound by their knowledge [...] and instead deliver health care like the crushed pills in a paper packet, which will result in more patients willing to pay more for their services"[24] not enough. How services deal with people is also vitally important. Surveys in Australia, Canada,

Germany, New Zealand, the United Kingdom and the United States show that a high number of patients report safety risks, poor care coordination and deficiencies in care for chronic conditions.[25] Communication is often inadequate and lacking in information on treatment schedules. Nearly one in every two patients feels that doctors only rarely or never asked their opinion about treatment. Patients may consult different providers for related or even for the same conditions which, given the lack of coordination among these providers, results in duplication and contradictions.[25] This situation is similar to that reported in other countries, such as Ethiopia,[26] Pakistan[27] and Zimbabwe.[28]

There has, however, been progress in recent years. In high-income countries, confrontation with chronic disease, mental health problems, multi-morbidity and the social dimension of disease has focused attention on the need for more comprehensive and person-centered approaches and continuity of care. This resulted not only from client pressure, but also from professionals who realized the critical importance of such features of care in achieving better outcomes for their patients. Many health professionals have begun to appreciate the limitations of narrow clinical approaches, for example, to cardiovascular disease. As a result there has been a welcome blurring of the traditional boundaries between curative care, preventive medicine and health promotion. In low-income countries, this evolution is also visible. In recent years, many of the programmes targeting infectious disease priorities have given careful consideration to comprehensiveness, continuity and patient-centeredness. Maternal and child health services have often been at the forefront of these attempts, organizing a continuum of care and a comprehensive approach. This process has been consolidated through the joint UNICEF/WHO Integrated Management of Childhood Illness initiatives.[30] Their experience with programmes such as the WHO's Extended Programme for Immunization has put health professionals in many developing countries a step ahead compared to their high-income country colleagues, as they more readily see themselves responsible not just for patients, but also for population coverage. More recently, HIV/AIDS programmes have drawn the attention of providers and policy-makers to the importance of counseling, continuity of care, the complementarity of prevention, treatment and palliation and critically, to the value of empathy and listening to patients.

Understanding people: person-centred care: When people are sick they are a great dealless concerned about managerial considerations of productivity, health targets, cost-effectiveness and rational organization than about their own predicament. Each individual has his or her own way of experiencing and coping with health problems within their specific life circumstances.[31] Health workers have to be able to handle that diversity. For health workers at the interface between the population and the health services, the challenge is much more complicated than for a specialized referral service: managing a well-defined disease is a relatively straightforward technical challenge. Dealing with health problems, however, is complicated as people need to be understood holistically: their physical, emotional and social concerns, their past and their future, and the realities of the world in which they live. Failure to deal with the whole person in their specific familial and community contexts misses out on important aspects of health that do not immediately fit into disease categories. Partner violence against women (Box 3.3), for example, can be detected, prevented or mitigated by health services that are sufficiently close to the communities they serve and by health workers who know the people in their community.

People want to know that their health worker understands them, their suffering and the constraints they face. Unfortunately, many providers neglect this aspect of the therapeutic relation, particularly when they are dealing with disadvantaged groups. In many health services, responsiveness and person-centeredness are treated as luxury goods to be handed out only to a selected few.

Over the last 30 years, a considerable body of research evidence has shown that person centeredness is not only important to relieve the patient's anxiety but also to improve the provider's job satisfaction.[50] The response to a health problem is more likely to be effective if the provider understands its various dimensions.[51]

For a start, simply asking patients how they feel about their illness, how it affects their lives, rather than focusing only on the disease, results in measurably increased trust and compliance[52] that allows patient and provider to find a common ground on clinical management, and facilitates the integration of prevention and health promotion in the therapeutic response.[50,51]

Thus, person-centeredness becomes the "clinical method of participatory democracy",[53] measurably improving the quality of care, the success of treatment and the quality of life of those benefiting from such care.

In practice, clinicians rarely address their patients' concerns, beliefs and understanding of illness, and seldom share problem management options with them.[58] They limit themselves to simple technical prescriptions, ignoring the complex human dimensions that are critical to the appropriateness and effectiveness of the care they provide.[59] Thus, technical advice on lifestyle, treatment schedule or referral all too often neglects not only the constraints of the environment in which people live, but also their potential for self-help in dealing with a host of health problems ranging from diarrheal disease[60] to diabetes management.[61] Yet, neither the nurse in Niger's rural health centre nor the general practitioner in Belgium can, for example, refer a patient to hospital without negotiating:[62,63] along with medical criteria, they have to take into account the patient's values, the family's values, and their lifestyle and life perspective.[64]

Few health providers have been trained for person-centered care. Lack of proper preparation is compounded by cross-cultural conflicts, social stratification, discrimination and stigma.[63] As a consequence, the considerable potential of people to contribute to their own health through lifestyle, behaviour and self-care, and by adapting better integration of preventive and promotive care? Mead (1982)[50]

Box 3.3: The health care response to partner violence against women

Intimate partner violence has numerous well-documented consequences for women's health (and for the health of their children), including injuries, chronic pain syndromes, unintended and unwanted pregnancies, pregnancy complications, sexually transmitted infections and a wide range of mental health problems.[32,33,34,35,36,37] Women suffering from violence are frequent health care users 38,39. Health workers are, therefore, well placed to identify and provide care to the victims of violence, including referral for psychosocial, legal and other support. Their interventions can reduce the impact of violence on a woman's health and well-being, and that of her children, and can also help prevent further violence. Research has shown that most women think health care providers should ask about violence.[40] While they do not expect them to solve their problem, they would like to be listened to and treated in a non-judgemental way and get the support they need to take control over their decisions. Health care providers often find it difficult to ask women about violence. They lack the time and the training and skills to do it properly, and are reluctant to be involved in judicial proceedings.

The most effective approach for health providers to use when responding to violence is still a matter of debate.[41] They are generally advised to ask all women about intimate partner abuse as a routine part of any health assessment, usually referred to as "screening" or routine enquiry.[42] Several reviews found that this technique increased the rate of identification of women experiencing violence in antenatal and primary care clinics, but there was little evidence that this was sustained,[40] or was effective in terms of health outcomes.[43]

Among women who have stayed in shelters, there is evidence that those who received a specific counseling and advocacy service reported a lower rate of re-abuse and an improved quality of life.[44] Similarly, among women experiencing violence during pregnancy, those who received "empowerment counseling" reported improved functioning and less psychological and non-severe physical abuse, and had lower postnatal depression scores.[45] While there is still no consensus on the most effective strategy, there is growing agreement that health services should aim to identify and support women experiencing violence,[46] and that health care providers should be well educated about these issues, as they are essential in building capacity and skills. Health care providers should, as a minimum, be informed about violence against women, its prevalence and impact on health, when to suspect it and how to best respond. Clearly, there are technical dimensions to this. For example, in the case of sexual assault, providers need to be able to provide the necessary treatment and care, including provision of emergency contraception and prophylaxis for sexually transmitted infections, including HIV where relevant, as well as psycho-social support. There are other dimensions too: health workers need to be able to document any injuries as completely and carefully as possible[47,48,49] and they need to know how to work with communities—in particular with men and boys—on changing attitudes and practices related to gender inequality and violence.

There are numerous, albeit often missed, opportunities to empower people to participate in decisions that affect their own health and that of their families (Box 3.4). They require health care providers who can relate to people and assist them in making informed choices. The current payment systems and incentives in community health care delivery often work against establishing this type of dialogue.[65] Conflicts of interest between provider and patient, particularly in unregulated commercial settings, are a major disincentive to person centered care. Commercial providers may be more courteous and client-friendly than in the average health centre, but this is no substitute for person centeredness.

Comprehensive and integrated responses

The diversity of health needs and challenges that people face does not fit neatly into the discrete diagnostic categories of textbook promotive, preventive, curative or rehabilitative care.[78,79] They call for the mobilization of a comprehensive range of resources that may include health promotion and prevention interventions as well as diagnosis and treatment or referral, chronic or long-term home care, and, in some models, social services.[80] It is at the entry point of the system, where people first present their problem, that the need for a comprehensive and integrated offer of care is most critical. Comprehensiveness makes managerial and operational sense and adds value. People take up services more readily if they know a comprehensive spectrum of care is on offer.

Moreover, it maximizes opportunities for preventive care and health promotion while reducing unnecessary reliance on specialized or hospital care.[81] Specialization has its comforts, but the fragmentation it induces is often visibly counterproductive and inefficient: it makes no sense to monitor the growth of children and neglect the health of their mothers (and *vice versa*), or to treat someone's tuberculosis without considering their HIV status or whether they smoke.

Box 3.4: Empowering users to contribute to their own health

Families can be empowered to make choices that are relevant to their health. Birth and emergency plans,[66] for example, are based on a joint examination between the expectant mother and health staff—well before the birth—of her expectations regarding childbirth. Issues discussed include where the birth will take place, and how support for care of the home and any other children will be organized while the woman is giving birth. The discussion can cover planning for expenses, arrangements for transport and medical supplies, as well as identification of a compatible blood donor in case of hemorrhage. Such birth plans are being implemented in countries as diverse as Egypt, Guatemala, Indonesia, the Netherlands and the United Republic of Tanzania. They constitute one example of how people can participate in decisions relating to their health in a way that empowers them.[67] Empowerment strategies can improve health and social outcomes through several pathways; the condition for success is that they are embedded in local contexts and based on a strong and direct relationship between people and their health workers.[68] The strategies can relate to a variety of areas, as shown below:

- Developing household capacities to stay healthy, make healthy decisions and respond to emergencies;
- France's self-help organization of diabetics,[69] South Africa's family empowerment and parent training programmes,[70] the United Republic of Tanzania's negotiated treatment plans for safe motherhood,[71] and Mexico's active ageing programme;[72]
- increasing citizens' awareness of their rights, needs and potential problems—Chile's information on entitlements[73] and Thailand's Declaration of Patients' Rights;[74] and
- strengthening linkages for social support within communities and with the health system—support and advice to family caregivers dealing with dementia in developing country settings,[75] Bangladesh's rural credit programmes and their impact on care-seeking behaviour,[76] and Lebanon's neighbourhood environment initiatives.[77]

That does not mean that entry-point health workers should solve all the health problems that are presented there, nor that all health programmes always need to be delivered through a single integrated service-delivery point. Nevertheless, the primary care team has to be able to respond to the bulk of health problems in the community. When it cannot do so, it has to be able to mobilize other resources, by referring or by calling for support from specialists, hospitals, specialized diagnostic and treatment centres, public-health programmes, long-term care services, home-care or social services, or self-help and other community organizations. This cannot mean giving up responsibility: the primary care team remains responsible for helping people to navigate this complex environment.

Comprehensive and integrated care for the bulk of the assorted health problems in the community is more efficient than relying on separate services for selected problems, partly because it leads to a better knowledge of the population and builds greater trust. One activity reinforces the other. Health services that offer a comprehensive range of services increase the uptake and coverage of, for example, preventive programmes, such as cancer screening or vaccination.

They prevent complications and improve health outcomes. Comprehesive services also facilitate early detection and prevention of problems, even in the absence of explicit demand. There are individuals and groups who could benefit from care even if they express no explicit spontaneous demand, as in the case of women attending the health centres in Ouallam district, Niger, or people with undiagnosed high blood pressure or depression. Early detection of disease, preventive care to reduce the incidence of poor health, health promotion to reduce risky behaviour, and addressing social and other determinants of health all require the health service to take the initiative. For many problems, local health workers are the only ones who are in a position to effectively address problems in the community: they are the only ones, for example, in a position to assist parents with care in early childhood development, itself an important determinant of later health, well-being and productivity.[87] Such interventions require proactive health teams offering a comprehensive range of services. They depend on a close and trusting relationship between the health services and the communities they serve, and, thus, on health workers who know the people in their community.[88]

Continuity of care

Understanding people and the context in which they live is not only important in order to provide a comprehensive, person-centred response, it also conditions continuity of care. Providers often behave as if their responsibility starts when a patient walks in and ends when they leave the premises. Care should not, however, be limited to the moment a patient consults nor be confined to the four walls of the consultation room. Concern for outcomes mandates a consistent and coherent approach to the management of the patient's problem, until the problem is resolved or the risk that justified follow-up has disappeared. Continuity of care is an important determinant of effectiveness, whether for chronic disease management, reproductive health, mental health or for making sure children grow up healthily.

In Singapore, for example, patients were formerly not allowed to use their health savings account (Medisave) for outpatient treatment, resulting in patient delays and lack of treatment compliance for the chronically ill. This had become so problematic that regulations were changed. Hospitals are now encouraged to transfer patients with diabetes, high blood pressure, lipid disorder and stroke to registered general practitioners, with Medisave accounts covering ambulatory care.[108]

Other barriers to continuity include treatment schedules requiring frequent clinic attendance that carry a heavy cost in time, travel expenses or lost wages. They may be ill-understood and patient motivation may be lacking. Patients may get lost in the complicated institutional environment of referral hospitals or social services. Such problems need to be anticipated and recognized at an early stage. The effort required from health workers is not negligible: negotiating the modalities of the treatment schedule with the patients so as to maximize the chances that it can be completed; keeping registries of clients with chronic conditions; and creating communication channels through home visits, liaison with community workers, telephonic reminders and text messages to re-establish interrupted continuity. These mundane tasks often make the difference between a successful outcome and a treatment failure, but are rarely rewarded. They are much easier to implement when patient and caregiver have clearly identified how and by whom follow up will be organized. A regular and trusted provider as entry point comprehensiveness, continuity and person-centredness are critical to better health outcomes. They all depend on a stable, long-term, personal relationship (a feature also called "longitudinality"[84]) between the population and the professionals who are their entry point to the health system.

Most ambulatory care in conventional settings is not organized to build such relationships. The Continuity of care: evidence of its contribution to quality of care and better outcomes Lower all-cause mortality—Shi (2003)90, Franks (1998),[91] Villalbi (1999),[92] PAHO (2005)[93] Better access to care—Weinick (2000),[94] Forrest (1998),[95] Less re-hospitalization—Weinberger (1996),[96] Fewer consultations with specialists—Woodward (2004),[97] Less use of emergency services—Gill (2000),[98] Better detection of adverse effects of medical interventions—Rothwell (2005),[99] Kravitz (2004).[100]

Continuity of care depends on ensuring continuity of information as people get older, when they move from one residence to another, or when different professionals interact with one particular individual or household. Access to medical records and discharge summaries, electronic, conventional or client-held, improves the choice of the course of treatment and of coordination of care. In Canada, for example, one in seven people attending an emergency department had medical information missing that was very likely to result in patient harm.[101] Missing information is a common cause of delayed care and uptake of unnecessary services.[102] In the United States, it is associated with 15.6% of all reported errors in ambulatory care.[103] Today's information and communication technologies, albeit underutilized, gives unprecedented possibilities to improve the circulation of medical information at an affordable cost104, thus enhancing continuity, safety and learning (Box 3.5). Moreover, it is no longer the exclusive privilege of high-resource environments, as the Open Medical Record System demonstrates: electronic health records developed through communities of practice and open-source software are facilitating continuity and quality of care for patients with HIV/AIDS in many low-income countries.[105] Better patient records are necessary but not sufficient. Health services need to make active efforts to minimize the numerous obstacles to continuity of care. Compared to payment by busy, anonymous and technical environment of hospital outpatient departments, with their many specialists and sub-specialists, produce mechanical interactions between nameless individuals and an institution—not people-centered care. Smaller clinics are less anonymous, but the care they provide is often more akin to a commercial or administrative transaction that starts and ends with the consultation than to a responsive problem-solving exercise. In this regard, private clinics do not perform differently than public health centres.[64] In the rural areas of low-income countries, governmental health centers are usually designed to work in close relationship with the community they serve. The reality is often different. Earmarking of resources and staff for selected programmes is increasingly leading to fragmentation,[109] while the lack of funds, the pauperization of the health staff and rampant commercialization makes building such relationships difficult.[110] There are many examples to the contrary, but the relationship between providers and their clients, particularly the poorer ones, is often not conducive to building relationships of understanding, empathy and trust.[62]

Building enduring relationships requires time

Studies indicate that it takes two to five years before its full potential is achieved[84] but, as the Alaska health centre mentioned at the beginning of this chapter shows, it drastically changes the way care is being provided. Access to the same team of health care providers over time fosters the development of a relationship of trust between the individual and their health care provider.[97,111,112] Health professionals are more likely to respect and understand patients they know.

Box 3.5: Using information and communication technologies to improve access, quality and efficiency in primary care

Information and communication technologies enable people in remote and underserved areas to have access to services and expertise otherwise unavailable to them, especially in countries with uneven distribution or chronic shortages of physicians, nurses and health technicians or where access to facilities and expert advice requires travel over long distances. In such contexts, the goal of improved access to health care has stimulated the adoption of technology for remote diagnosis, monitoring and consultation. Experience in Chile of immediate transmission of electrocardiograms in cases of suspected myocardial infarction is a noteworthy example: examination is carried out in an ambulatory setting and the data are sent to a national centre where specialists confirm the diagnosis via fax or e-mail. This technology-facilitated consultation with experts allows rapid response and appropriate treatment where previously it was unavailable. The Internet is a key factor in its success, as is the telephone connectivity that has been made available to all health facilities in the country.

A further benefit of using information and communication technologies in primary care services is the improved quality of care. Health care providers are not only striving to deliver more effective care, they are also striving to deliver safer care. Tools, such as electronic health records, computerized prescribing systems and clinical decision aids, support practitioners in providing safer care in a range of settings. For example, in a village in western Kenya, electronic health records integrated with laboratory, drug procurement and reporting systems have drastically reduced clerical labour and errors, and have improved follow-up care.

As the costs of delivering health care continue to rise, information and communication technologies provide new avenues for personalized, Citizen-centered and home-centered care. Towards this end, there has been significant investment in research and development of consumer-friendly applications. In Cape Town, South Africa, an "on cue compliance service" takes the names and mobile telephone numbers of patients with tuberculosis (supplied by a clinic) and enters them into a database. Every half an hour, the on cue server reads the database and sends personalized SMS messages to the patients, reminding them to take their medication. The technology is low-cost and robust. Cure and completion rates are similar to those of patients receiving clinic-based DOTS, but at lower cost to both clinic and patient, and in a way that interferes much less with everyday life than the visits to the clinic106. In the same concept of supporting lifestyles linked to primary care, network devices have become a key element of an innovative community programme in the Netherlands, where monitoring and communication devices are built into smart apartments for senior citizens. This system reduces clinic visits and facilitates living independently with chronic diseases that require frequent checks and adjustment of medications.

Many clinicians who want to promote health and prevent illness are placing high hopes in the Internet as the place to go for health advice to complement or replace the need to seek the advice of a health professional. New applications, services and access to information have permanently altered the relationships between consumers and health professionals, putting knowledge directly into people's own hands.

More mindful of the circumstances in which people live, they can tailor care to the specific needs of the person and recognize health problems at earlier stages. This is not merely a question of building trust and patient satisfaction, however important these may be.[114,115] It is worthwhile because it leads to better quality and better outcomes. People who use the same source of care for most of their health care needs tend to comply better with advice given, rely less on emergency services, require less hospitalization and are more satisfied with care.[98 116,117,118] Providers save consultation time, reduce the use of laboratory tests and costs,[95,119,120] and increase uptake of preventive care.[121] Motivation improves through the social recognition built up by such relationships.

Still, even dedicated health professionals will not seize all these opportunities spontaneously.[122,123] The interface between the population and their health services needs to be designed in a way that not only makes this possible, but also the most likely course of action.

Organizing primary care networks

A health service that provides entry point ambulatorycare for health- and health-related problems should, thus, offer a comprehensive range of integrated diagnostic, curative, rehabilitative and palliative services. In contrast to most conventional health care delivery models, the offer of services should include prevention and promotion as well as efforts to tackle determinants of ill-health locally. A direct and enduring relationship between the provider and the people in the community served is essential to be able to take into account the personal and social context of patients and their families, ensuring continuity of care over time as well as across services. In order for conventional health services to be transformed into primary care, i.e. to ensure that these distinctive features get due prominence, they must reorganized. A precondition is to ensure that they become directly and permanently accessible, without undue reliance on out-of-pocket payments and with social protection offered by universal coverage schemes. But another set of arrangements is critical for the transformation of conventional care—ambulatory- and institution-based, generalist and specialist—into local networks of primary care centres:[135,136,137,138,139,140] bringing care closer to people, in settings in close proximity and direct relationship with the community, relocating the entry point to the health system from hospitals and specialists to close-to-client generalist primary care centres:

- giving primary care providers the responsibility for the health of a defined population, in its entirety: the sick and the healthy, those who choose to consult the services and those who choose not to do so; and
- strengthening primary care providers' role as coordinators of the inputs of other levels of care by giving them administrative authority and purchasing power.

Regular entry point: evidence of its contribution to quality of care and better outcomes Increased satisfaction with services—Weiss (1996)116, Rosenblatt (1998),[117] Freeman (1997),[124] Miller (2000),[125] Better compliance and lower hospitalization rate—Weiss (1996),[116] Rosenblatt (1998),[117] Freeman (1997),[124] Mainous (1998),[126] Less use of specialists and emergency services—Starfield (1998),[82] Parchman (1994),[127] Hurley (1989),[128] Martin

(1989),[129] Gadomski (1998),[130] Fewer consultations with specialists—Hurley (1989),[128] Martin (1989).[129] More efficient use of resources—Forrest (1996),[82] Forrest (1998),[95] Hjortdahl (1991),[131] Roos (1998).[132] Better understanding of the psychological aspects of a patient's problem—Gulbrandsen (1997).[55] Better uptake of preventive care by adolescents—Ryan (2001).[133] Protection against over-treatment—Schoen (2007).[134]

Bringing care closer to the people

A first step is to relocate the entry point to the health system from specialized clinics, hospital outpatient departments and emergency services, to generalist ambulatory care in close-to-client settings. Evidence has been accumulating that this transfer carries measurable benefits in terms of relief from suffering, prevention of illness and death, and improved health equity. These findings hold true in both national and cross-national studies, even if all of the distinguishing features of primary care are not fully realized.[31] Generalist ambulatory care is more likely or as likely to identify common life-threatening conditions as specialist care.[141,142] Generalists adhere to clinical practice guidelines to the same extent as specialists,[143] although they are slower to adopt them.[144,145] They prescribe fewer invasive interventions,[146,147,148,149] fewer and shorter hospitalizations[127,133,149] and have a greater focus on preventive care.[133,150] This results in lower overall health care costs[82] for similar health outcomes[146,151,152,153,154,155] and greater patient satisfaction.[125,150,156] Evidence from comparisons between high-income countries shows that higher proportions of generalist professionals working in ambulatory settings are associated with lower overall costs and higher quality rankings.[157] Conversely, countries that increase reliance on specialists have stagnating or declining health outcomes when measured at the population level, while fragmentation of care exacerbates user dissatisfaction and contributes to a growing divide between health and social services.[157,158,159] Information on low- and middle-income countries is harder to obtain,[160] but there are indications that patterns are similar. Some studies estimate that in Latin America and the Caribbean more reliance on generalist care could avoid one out of two hospital admissions.[161] In Thailand, generalist ambulatory care outside a hospital context has been shown to be more patient-centered and responsive as well as cheaper and less inclined to over-medicalization.[162] The relocation of the entry point into the system from specialist hospital to generalist ambulatory care creates the conditions for more comprehensiveness, continuity and person-centeredness. This amplifies the benefits of the relocation. It is particularly the case when services are organized as a dense network of small, close-to-client service delivery points. This makes it easier to have teams that are small enough to know their communities and be known by them, and stable enough to establish an enduring relationship. These teams require relational and organizational capacities as much as the technical competencies to solve the bulk of health problems locally. Responsibility for a well-identified population.

In conventional ambulatory care, the provider assumes responsibility for the person attending the consultation for the duration of the consultation and, in the best of circumstances, that responsibility extends to ensuring continuity of care. This passive, response-to-demand approach fails to help a considerable number of people who could benefit from care. There are people who, for various reasons, are or feel, excluded from access to services and do not take up care even when they are in need. There are people who suffer illness but delay seeking care. Others present risk factors and could benefit from screening or prevention programmes (e.g. for cervical cancer or for childhood obesity), but are left out because they do not consult: preventive services that are limited to service users often leave out those most in need.[163] A passive, response-to-demand approach has a second untoward consequence: it lacks the ambition to deal with local determinants of ill-health—whether social, environmental or work-related. All this represents lost opportunities for generating health: providers that only assume responsibility for their customers concentrate on repairing rather than on maintaining and promoting health. The alternative is to entrust each primary care team with the explicit responsibility for a well defined community or population. They can then be held accountable, through administrative measures or contractual arrangements, for providing comprehensive, continuous and person-centered care to that population, and for mobilizing a comprehensive range of support services—from promotive through to palliative. The simplest way of assigning responsibility is to identify the community served on the basis of geographical criteria—the classic approach in rural areas. The simplicity of geographical assignment, however, is deceptive. It follows an administrative, public sector logic that often has problems adapting to the emergence of a multitude of other providers.

Furthermore, administrative geography may not coincide with sociological reality, especially in urban areas. People move around and may work in a different area than where they live, making the health unit closest to home actually an inconvenient source of care. More importantly, people value choice and may resent an administrative assignment to a particular health unit. Some countries find geographical criteria of proximity the most appropriate to define who fits in the population of responsibility, others rely on active registration or patient lists. The important point is not how but whether the population is well identified and mechanisms exist to ensure that nobody is left out. Once such explicit comprehensive responsibilities for the health of a well-identified and defined population are assigned, with the related financial and administrative accountability mechanisms, the rules change. The primary care team has to broaden the portfolio of care it offers, developing activities and programmes that can improve outcomes, but which they might otherwise neglect.[164] This sets the stage for investment in prevention and promotion activities, and for venturing into workers, self-help groups, etc.

It forces the team to move out of the four walls of their consultation room and reach out to the people in the community. This can bring significant health benefits. For example, large scale programmes, based on home-visits and community animation, have been shown to be effective in reducing risk factors for neonatal mortality and actual mortality rates. In the United States, such programmes have reduced neonatal mortality by 60% in some settings.[165]

Part of the benefit is due to better uptake of effective care by people who would otherwise remain deprived. In Nepal, for example, the community dynamics of women's groups led to the better uptake of care, with neonatal and maternal mortality lower than in control communities by 29% and 80%, respectively.[166]

It forces the team to take targeted initiatives, in collaboration with other sectors, to reach the excluded and the unreached and tackle broader determinants of ill-health. This is a necessary complement to establishing universal coverage and one where local health services play a vital role. The 2003 heatwave in western Europe, for example, highlighted the importance of reaching out to the isolated elderly and the dramatic consequences of failing to do so: an excess mortality of more than 50,000 people.[167] For people and communities, formal links with an identifiable source of care enhance the likelihood that long-term relationships will develop; that services are encouraged to pay more attention to the defining features of primary care; and that lines of communication are more intelligible.

At the same time, coordination linkages can be formalized with other levels of care—specialists, hospitals or other technical services—and with social services.

The primary care team as a hub of coordination

Primary care teams cannot ensure comprehensive responsibility for their population without support from specialized services, organizations and institutions that are based outside the community served. In resource-constrained circumstances, these sources of support will typically be concentrated in a "first referral level district hospital". Indeed, the classic image of a health care system based on PHC is that of a pyramid with the district hospital at the top and a set of (public) health centres that refer to the higher authority.

In conventional settings, ambulatory care professionals have little say in how hospitals and specialized services contribute—or fail to contribute—to the health of their patients, and feel little inclination to reach out to other institutions and stakeholders that are relevant to the health of the local community. This changes if they are entrusted with responsibility for a defined population and are recognized as the regular point of entry for that population. As health care networks expand, the health care landscape becomes far more crowded and pluralistic. More resources allow for diversification: the range of specialized services that comes within reach may include emergency services, specialists, diagnostic infrastructure, dialysis centres, cancer screening, environmental technicians, long-term care institutions, pharmacies, etc. This represents new opportunities, provided the primary care teams can assist their community in making the best use of that potential, which is particularly critical to public health, mental health and long term care.[168] The coordination (or gate-keeping) role this entails effectively transforms the primary care pyramid into a network, where the relations between the primary care team and the other institutions and services are no longer based only on top-down hierarchy and bottom-up referral, but on cooperation and coordination. The primary care team then becomes the mediator between the community and the other levels Surgery or Maternity.

Independent ombudsman structures or consumer organizations can help users handle complaints. Most importantly, there is a wealth of self-help and mutual support associations for diabetics, people living with handicaps and chronic diseases that can help people to help themselves.[171] In the United States alone, more than five million people belong to mutual help groups while, in recent years, civil society organizations dealing with health and health-related issues, from self-help to patient's rights, have been mushrooming in many low- and middle-income countries. These groups do much more than just inform patients.

They help people take charge of their own situation, improve their health, cope better with ill-health, increase self-confidence and diminish-over-medicalization.[172] Primary care teams can only be strengthened by reinforcing their linkages with such groups. Where primary care teams are in a position to take on this coordinator role, their work becomes more rewarding and attractive, while the overall effects on health are positive. Reliance on specialists and hospitalization is reduced by filtering out unnecessary uptake, whereas patient delay is reduced for those who do need referral care, the duration of their hospitalization is shortened, and post-hospitalization follow-up is improved.[83,128,129] The coordination function provides the institutional framework for mobilizing across sectors to secure the health of local communities. It is not an optional extra but an essential part of the remit of primary care teams. This has policy implications: coordination will remain wishful thinking unless the primary care team has some form of either administrative or financial leverage. Coordination also depends on the different institutions' recognition of the key role of the primary care teams. Current professional education systems, career structure and remuneration mechanisms most often give signals to the contrary. Reversing these well-entrenched disincentives to primary care requires strong leadership.

Monitoring progress

The switch from conventional to primary care is a complex process that cannot be captured in a single, universal metric. Only in recent years has it been possible to start disentangling the effects of the various features that define primary care. In part, this is because the identification of the features that make the difference between primary care and conventional health care delivery has taken years of trial and error, and the instruments to measure them have not been generalized. This is because these features are never all put into place as a single package of reforms, but are the result of a gradual shaping and transformation of the health system. Yet, for all this complexity, it is possible to measure progress, as a complement to the follow-up required for measuring progress towards universal coverage.

The first dimension to consider is the extent to which the organizational measures required to switch to primary care are being put into place.

Is the predominant type of first-contact provider being shifted from specialists and hospitals to generalist primary care teams in close proximity to where the people live?

- Are primary care providers being made responsible for the health of all the members of a well-identified population: those who attend health services and those who do not?
- Are primary care providers being empowered to coordinate the various inputs of specialized, hospital and social services, by strengthening their administrative authority and purchasing power?

The second dimension to consider is the extent to which the distinctive features of primary care are gaining prominence.

- *Person-centredness*: is there evidence of improvement, as shown by direct observation and user surveys?
- *Comprehensiveness*: is the portfolio of primary care services expanding and becoming more comprehensive, reaching the full essential benefits package, from promotion through to palliation, for all age groups?
- *Continuity*: is information for individuals being recorded over the life-course, and transferred between levels of care in cases of referral and to a primary care unit elsewhere when people relocate?
- *Regular entry point*: are measures taken to ensure that providers know their clients and *vice versa*? This should provide the guidance to policy-makers as to the progress they are making with the transformation of health care delivery. However, they do not immediately make it possible to attribute

Sources

1. People at the centre of health care: harmonizing mind and body, people and systems. New Delhi, World Health Organization Regional Office for South-East Asia, Manila, World Health Organization Regional Office for the Western Pacific, 2007.

2. Osler, W. Aequanimitas. Philadelphia PA, Blakiston, 1904.
3. Eby, D. Primary care at the Alaska Native Medical Centre: a fully deployed "new model" of primary care. *International Journal of Circumpolar Health*, 2007, 66 (Suppl. 1):4-13.
4. Eby. D. Integrated primary care. *International Journal of Circumpolar Health*, 1998, 57(Suppl. 1):665-67.
5. Gottlieb, K, Sylvester I, Eby D. Transforming your practice: what matters most. *Family Practice Management*, 2008, 15:32-38.
6. Kerssens, J.J. *et al*. Comparison of patient evaluations of health care quality in relation to WHO measures of achievement in 12 European countries. *Bulletin of the World Health Organization*, 2004 82:106-114.
7. Bossyns, P., Miye, M., Van Lerberghe, W. Supply-level measures to increase uptake of family planning services in Niger: the effectiveness of improving responsiveness. *Tropical Medicine and International Health*, 2002, 7:383-390.
8. The World Health Report 2000—Health systems: improving performance. Geneva, World Health Organization, 2000.
9. Mercer, S.W., Cawston, P.G., Bikker, A.P. Quality in general practice consultations: a qualitative study of the views of patients living in an area of high socio-economic deprivation in Scotland. *BMC Family Practice*, 2007, 8:22.
10. Scherger, J.E. What patients want. *Journal of Family Practice*, 2001, 50:137.
11. Sackett, D.L *et al*. Evidence based medicine: what it is and what it isn't. *British Medical Journal*, 1996, 312:71-72.
12. Guyatt, G., Cook, D., Haynes, B. Evidence based medicine has come a long way: The second decade will be as exciting as the first. *BMJ*, 2004, 329:990-991.
13. Cochrane database of systematic reviews. The Cochrane Library, 2008 (http:// www. cochrane.org, accessed 27 July 2008).
14. Iha, A., ed. Summary of the evidence on patient safety: implications for research. Geneva, World Health Organization, The Research Priority Setting Working Group of the World Alliance for Patient Safety, 2008.
15. Smith, G.D., Mertens, T. What's said and what's done: the reality of sexually transmitted disease consultations. *Public Health*, 2004, 118:96-103.
16. Berwick, D.M. The science of improvement. *JAMA*, 2008, 299:1182-1184.
17. Donaldson, L., Philip, P. Patient safety: a global priority. *Bulletin of the World Health Organization*, 2004, 82:892-893
18. Kohn, L.T., Corrigan, J.M., Donaldson, M.S., eds. To err is human: building a safer health system. Washington, DC, National Academy Press, Committee on Quality of Health Care in America, Institute of Medicine, 1999.
19. Reason, J. Human error: models and management. *BMJ*, 2000, 320:768-770.
20. Kripalani, S. *et al*. Deficits in communication and information transfer between hospital-based and primary care physicians: implications for patient safety and continuity of care. *JAMA*, 2007, 297:831-841.
21. Miller, M.A., Pisani, E. The cost of unsafe injections. *Bulletin of the World Health Organization*, 1999, 77:808-811.
22. The purpose of a world alliance. Geneva, World Health Organization, *World Alliance for Patient Safety*, 2008
23. Shortell, S.M., Singer, S.J. Improving patient safety by taking systems seriously. *JAMA*, 2008, 299:445-447.
24. Das, J., Hammer, J.S., Kenneth, L.L. The quality of medical advice in low-income countries. Washington DC, The World Bank, 2008 (World Bank Policy Research Working Paper No. 4501; http://ssrn.com/abstract=1089272, accessed 28 July 2008).
25. Schoen, C. *et al*. Taking the pulse of health care systems: experiences of patients with health problems in six countries. *Health Affairs*, 2005 (webexclusive W5-509 DOI 10.1377/hlthaff.W5.509).

26. Mekbib, T.A., Teferi, B. Caesarean section and foetal outcome at Yekatit 12 hospital, Addis Abba, Ethiopia, 1987-1992. *Ethiopian Medical Journal,* 1994, 32:173-179.
27. Siddiqi, S. *et al.* The effectiveness of patient referral in Pakistan. *Health Policy and Planning,* 2001, 16:193-198.
28. Sanders, D. *et al.* Zimbabwe's hospital referral system: does it work? *Health Policy and Planning,* 1998, 13:359-370.
29. Data reported at World Aids Day Meeting, Antwerp, Belgium, 2000.
30. The World Health Report 2005—Make every mother and child count. Geneva, World Health Organization, 2005.
31. Starfield, B., Shi, L., Macinko, J. Contributions of primary care to health systems and health. *The Milbank Quarterly,* 2005, 83:457-502.
32. Heise, L., Garcia-Moreno, C. Intimate partner violence. In: Krug EG *et al,* eds. World report on violence and health. Geneva, World Health Organization, 2002.
33. Ellsberg, M. *et al.* Intimate partner violence and women's physical and mental healthin the WHO multi-country study on women's health and domestic violence: an observational study. *Lancet,* 2008, 371:1165-1172.
34. Campbell, J.C. Health consequences of intimate 34. partner violence. *Lancet,* 2002, 359:1331-1336.
35. Edleson, J.L. Children's witnessing of domestic violence. *Journal of Interpersonal Violence,* 1996, 14: 839-870.
36. Dube, S.R. *et al.* Exposure to abuse, neglect, and household dysfunction among adults who witnessed intimate partner violence as children: implications for health and social services. *Violence and Victims,* 2002, 17: 3-17.
37. Åsling-Monemi, K. *et al.* Violence against women increases the risk of infant and child mortality: a case-referent study in Nicaragua. *Bulletin of the World Health Organization,* 2003, 81:10-18.
38. Bonomi, A. *et al.* Intimate partner violence and women's physical, mental and social functioning. *American Journal of Preventive Medicine,* 2006, 30:458-466.
39. National Centre for Injury Prevention and Control. Costs of intimate partner violence against women in the United States. Atlanta GA, Centres for Disease Control and Prevention, 2003.
40. Ramsay, J. *et al.* Should health professionals screen women for domestic violence? Systematic review. *BMJ,* 2002, 325:314-318.
41. Nelson, H.D. *et al.* Screening women and elderly adults for family and intimate partner violence: a review of the evidence for the U.S. Preventive Services Task force. *Annals of Internal Medicine,* 2004, 140:387-403.
42. Garcia-Moreno, C. Dilemmas and opportunities for an appropriate health-service response to violence against women. *Lancet,* 2002, 359:1509-1514.
43. Wathan, N.C., MacMillan, H.L. Interventions for violence against women. Scientific review. *JAMA,* 2003, 289:589-600.
44. Sullivan, C.M., Bybee, D.I. Reducing violence using community-based advocacy for women with abusive partners. *Journal of Consulting and Clinical Psychology,* 1999, 67:43-53.
45. Tiwari, A. *et al.* A randomized controlled trial of empowerment training for Chinese abused pregnant women in Hong Kong. British Journal of Obstetrics and Gynaecology, 2005, 112:1249-1256.
46. Taket, A. *et al.* Routinely asking women about domestic violence in health settings. *BMJ,* 2003, 327:673-676.
47. MacDonald, R. Time to talk about rape. BMJ, 2000, 321:1034-1035.
48. Basile, K.C., Hertz FM, Back SE. Intimate partner and sexual violence victimization instruments for use in health care settings. 2008. Atlanta GA, Centers for Disease Control and Prevention, 2008.
49. Guidelines for the medico-legal care of victims of sexual violence. Geneva, World Health Organization, 2003.

50. Mead, N., Bower, P. Patient-centredness: a conceptual framework and review of the empirical literature. *Social Science and Medicine,* 51:1087-1110.

51. Stewart M. Towards a global definition of patient centred care. BMJ, 2001, 322:444-445.

52. Fiscella, K. *et al.* Patient trust: is it related to patient-centred behaviour of primary care physicians? Medical, Care, 2004, 42:1049-1055.

53. Marincowitz GJO, Fehrsen GS. Caring, learning, improving quality and doing research: Different faces of the same process. Paper presented at: 11th South African Family Practice Congress, Sun City, South Africa, August 1998.

54. Ferrer, R.L., Hambidge, S.J., Maly, R.C. The essential role of generalists in health care systems. *Annals of Internal Medicine,* 2005, 142:691-699.

55. Gulbrandsen, P., Hjortdahl, P., Fugelli, P. General practitioners' knowledge of their patients' psychosocial problems: multipractice questionnaire survey. *British Medical Journal,* 1997, 314:1014-1018.

56. Jaturapatporn, D., Dellow, A. Does family medicine training in Thailand affect patient satisfaction with primary care doctors? BMC Family Practice, 2007, 8:14.

57. Kovess-Masféty, V. *et al.* What makes people decide who to turn to when faced with a mental health problem? Results from a French survey. *BMC Public Health,* 2007, 7:188.

58. Bergeson, D. A systems approach to patient-centred care. JAMA, 2006, 296:23.

59. Kravitz, R.L *et al.* Recall of recommendations and adherence to advice among patients with chronic medical conditions. *Archives of Internal Medicine,* 1993, 153:1869-1878.

60. Werner, D. *et al.* Questioning the solution: the politics of primary health care and child survival, with an in-depth critique of oral rehydration therapy. Palo Alto CA, *Health Wrights,* 1997.

61. Norris, *et al.* Increasing diabetes self-management education in community settings. A systematic review. *American Journal of Preventive Medicine,* 2002, 22:39-66.

62. Bossyns, P., Van Lerberghe, W. The weakest link: competence and prestige as constraints to referral by isolated nurses in rural Niger. Human Resources for Health, 2004, 2:1.

63. Willems, S. *et al.* Socio-economic status of the patient and doctor-patient communication: does it make a difference. Patient Eucation and Counseling, 2005, 56:139-146.

64. Pongsupap, Y. Introducing a human dimension to Thai health care: the case for family practice. Brussels, Vrije Universiteit Brussel Press. 2007.

65. Renewing primary health care in the Americas. A Position paper of the Pan American Health Organization. Washington DC, Pan American Health Organization, 2007.

66. Penny Simkin, P.T. Birth plans: after 25 years, women still want to be heard. Birth, 34:49-51.

67. Portela, A., Santarelli, C. Empowerment of women, men, families and communities:true partners for improving maternal and newborn health. *British Medical Bulletin,* 2003, 67:59-72.

68. Wallerstein, N. What is the evidence on effectiveness of empowerment to improve health? Copenhagen, World Health Organization Regional Office for Europe 2006.

69. Barlow, J., Cohen, E., Stewart-Brown, S.S.B. Parent training for improving maternal psychosocial health. *Cochrane Database of Systematic Reviews,* 2003, (4) :CD002020.

70. Ahluwalia, I. An evaluation of a community-based approach to safe motherhood in northwestern Tanzania. *International Journal of Gynecology and Obstetrics,* 2003,82:231.

71. De la Luz Martínez-Maldonado, M., Correa-Muñoz E, Mendoza-Núñez VM. Program of active aging in a rural Mexican community: a qualitative approach. *BMC Public Health*, 2007, 7:276 (DOI:10.1186/1471-2458-7-276).

72. Frenz, P. Innovative practices for intersectoral action on health: a case study of four programs for social equity. Chilean case study prepared for the CSDH. Santiago, Ministry of Health, Division of Health Planning, *Social Determinants of Health Initiative*, 2007.

73. Paetthayasapaa. Kam Prakard Sitti Pu Paui, 2003? (http://www.tmc.or.th/, accessed 30 July 2008).

74. Prince, M., Livingston, G., Katona, C. Mental health care for the elderly in low-income countries: a health systems approach. *World Psychiatry*, 2007, 6:5-13.

75. Nanda, P. Women's participation in rural credit programmes in Bangladesh and their demand for formal health care: is there a positive impact? *Health Economics*, 1999, 8:415-428.

76. Nakkash, R. *et al.* The development of a feasible community-specific cardiovascular disease prevention program: triangulation of methods and sources. *Health Education and Behaviour*, 2003, 30:723-739.

77. Stange, K.C. The paradox of the parts and the whole in understanding and improving general practice. *International Journal for Quality in Health Care*, 2002, 14:267-268.

78. Gill, J.M. The structure of primary care: framing a big picture. *Family Medicine*, 2004,36:65-68.

79. Pan-Canadian Primary Health Care Indicator Development Project. Pan-Canadian primary health care indicators, Report 1, Volume 1. Ottawa, *Canadian Institute for Health Information*, 2008 (http:\www.cihi.ca).

80. Bindman, A.B. *et al.* Primary care and receipt of preventive services. *Journal of General Internal Medicine*, 1996, 11:269-276.

81. Forrest, C.B., Starfield B. The effect of fi rst-contact care with primary care clinicians on ambulatory health care expenditures. *Journal of Family Practice*, 1996, 43:40-48.

82. Chande, V.T., Kinane, J.M. Role of the primary care provider in expediting children with acute appendicitis. *Achives of Pediatrics and Adolescent Medicine*, 1996, 150:703-706.

83. Starfield, B. Primary care: balancing health needs, services, and technology. New York, Oxford University Press 1998.

84. Bindman, A.B. *et al.* Primary care and receipt of preventive services. *Journal of General Internal Medicine*, 1996, 11:269-276.

85. Shea, S. *et al.* Predisposing factors for severe, uncontrolled hypertension in an innercity minority population. *New England Journal of Medicine*, 1992, 327:776-781.

86. Galobardes, B., Lynch, J.W., Davey Smith, G. Is the association between childhood socioeconomic circumstances and cause-specific mortality established? Update of a systematic review. *Journal of Epidemiology and Community Health*, 2008, 62:387-390.

87. Guide to clinical preventive services, 2007. Rockville, M.D., Agency for Health Care Research and Quality, 2007 (AHRQ Publication No. 07-05100;

88. Porignon, D. *et al.* Comprehensive is effective: vaccination coverage and health system performance in Sub-Saharan Africa, 2008 (forthcoming).

89. Shi, L. *et al.* The relationship between primary care, income inequality, and mortality in the United States, 1980-1995. *Journal of the American Board of Family Practice*, 2003, 16:412-422.

90. Franks, P., Fiscella, K. Primary care physicians and specialists as personal physicians. Health care expenditures and mortality experience. *Journal of Family Practice*, 1998, 47:105-109.

91. Villalbi, J.R. *et al.* An evaluation of the impact of primary care reform on health. *Atenci'on Primaria,* 1999, 24:468-474.
92. Regional core health data initiative. Washington DC, Pan American Health Organization, 2005
93. Weinick, R.M., Krauss NA. Racial/ethnic differences in children's access to care. *American Journal of Public Health,* 2000, 90:1771-1774.
94. Forrest, C.B., Starfield B. Entry into primary care and continuity: the effects of access. *American Journal of Public Health,* 1998, 88:1330-1336.
95. Weinberger, M., Oddone, E.Z., Henderson, W.G. Does increased access to primary care reduce hospital readmissions? For The Veterans' Affairs Cooperative Study Group on Primary Care and Hospital Readmission. *New England Journal of Medicine,* 1996, 334:1441-1447.
96. Woodward, C.A. *et al.* What is important to continuity in home care? Perspectives of key stakeholders. *Social Science and Medicine,* 2004, 58:177-192.
97. Gill, J.M., Mainous, A.G.I., Nsereko, M. The effect of continuity of care on emergency department use. *Archives of Family Medicine,* 2000, 9:333-338.
98. Rothwell, P. Subgroup analysis in randomised controlled trials: importance, indications, and interpretation, *Lancet,* 2005, 365:176-186.
99. Kravitz, R.L., Duan, N., Braslow, J. Evidence-based medicine, heterogeneity of treatment effects, and the trouble with averages. *The Milbank Quarterly,* 2004, 82:661-687.
100. Stiell, A. *et al.* Prevalence of information gaps in the emergency department and the effect on patient outcomes. *Canadian Medical Association Journal,* 2003, 169:1023-1028.
101. Smith, P.C. *et al.* Missing clinical information during primary care visits. *JAMA,* 2005, 293:565-571.
102. Elder, N.C., Vonder Meulen, M.B., Cassedy, A. The identification of medical errors by family physicians during outpatient visits. *Annals of Family Medicine,* 2004, 2:125-129.
103. Elwyn, G. Safety from numbers: identifying drug related morbidity using electronic records in primary care. *Quality and Safety in Health Care,* 2004, 13:170-171.
104. Open Medical Records System (OpenMRS) [online database]. Cape Town, South African Medical Research Council, 2008.
105. Hüsler, J., Peters, T. Evaluation of the On Cue Compliance Service pilot: testing the use of SMS reminders in the treatment of tuberculosis in Cape Town, South Africa. Prepared for the City of Cape Town Health Directorate and the International Development Research Council (IDRC). Cape Town, Bridges Organization, 2005.
106. Smith-Rohrberg Maru, D. *et al.* Poor follow-up rates at a self-pay northern Indian tertiary AIDS clinic. *International Journal for Equity in Health,* 2007, 6:14.
107. Busse, R., Schlette, S., eds. Focus on prevention, health and aging, and health professions. Gütersloh, Verlag Bertelsmann Stiftung, 2007 (Health policy developments 7/8).
108. James Pfeiffer International. NGOs and primary health care in Mozambique: the need for a new model of collaboration. *Social Science and Medicine,* 2003, 56:725-738.
109. *Ibid.*
110. Naithani, S., Gulliford, M., Morgan, M. Patients' perceptions and experiences of "continuity of care" in diabetes. Health Expectations, 2006, 9:118-129.
111. Schoenbaum, S.C. The medical home: a practical way to improve care and cut costs. *Medscape Journal of Medicine,* 2007, 9:28.
112. Beach, M.C. Are physicians' attitudes of respect accurately perceived by patients and associated with more positive communication behaviours? Patient Education and Counselling, 2006, 62:347-354 (Epub 2006 Jul 21).

113. Farmer, J.E. *et al.* Comprehensive primary care for children with special health care needs in rural areas. *Pediatrics,* 2005, 116:649-656.
114. Pongsupap, Y., Van Lerberghe W. Patient experience with self-styled family practices and conventional primary care in Thailand. *Asia Pacific Family Medicine Journal,* 2006, Vol 5.
115. Weiss, L.J., Blustein, J. Faithful patients: the effect of long term physician-patient relationships on the costs and use of health care by older Americans. *American Journal of Public Health,* 1996, 86:1742-1747.
116. Rosenblatt, R.L. *et al.* The generalist role of specialty physicians: is there a hidden system of primary care? *JAMA,* 1998, 279:1364-1370.
117. Kempe, A. *et al.* Quality of care and use of the medical home in a state-funded capitated primary care plan for low-income children. *Pediatrics,* 2000, 105:1020-1028.
118. Raddish, M.S. *et al.* Continuity of care: is it cost effective? *American Journal of Managed Care,* 1999, 5:727-734.
119. De Maeseneer, J.M. *et al.* Provider continuity in family medicine: does it make a difference for total health care costs? *Annals of Family Medicine,* 2003, 1:131-133.
120. Saver, B. Financing and organization findings brief. Academy for Research and Health Care Policy, 2002, 5:1-2.
121. Tudiver, F., Herbert, C., Goel, V. Why don't family physicians follow clinical practice guidelines for cancer screening? *Canadian Medical Association Journal,* 1998, 159:797-798.
122. Oxman, A.D. *et al.* No magic bullets: a systematic review of 102 trials of interventions to improve professional practice. *Canadian Medical Association Journal,* 1995, 153:1423-1431.
123. Freeman, G., Hjortdahl, P. What future for continuity of care in general practice? *British Medical Journal,* 1997, 314: 1870-1873.
124. Miller, M.R. *et al.* Parental preferences for primary and specialty care collaboration in the management of teenagers with congenital heart disease. *Pediatrics,* 2000, 106:264-269.
125. Mainous, A.G. III, Gill, J.M. The importance of continuity of care in the likelihood of future hospitalization: is site of care equivalent to a primary clinician? *American Journal of Public Health,* 1998, 88:1539-1541.
126. Parchman, M.L., Culler, S.D. Primary care physicians and avoidable hospitalizations. *Journal of Family Practice,* 1994, 39:123-128.
127. Hurley, R.E., Freund, D.A., Taylor, D.E. Emergency room use and primary care case management: evidence from four medicaid demonstration programs. *American Journal of Public Health,* 1989, 79: 834-836.
128. Martin, D.P. *et al.* Effect of a gatekeeper plan on health services use and charges: a randomized trial. *American Journal of Public Health,* 1989, 79:1628-1632.
129. Gadomski, A., Jenkins, P., Nichols, M. Impact of a Medicaid Primary Care Provider and Preventive Care on pediatric hospitalization. *Pediatrics,* 1998,
130. Hjortdahl, P., Borchgrevink, C.F. Continuity of care: infl uence of general practitioners' knowledge about their patients on use of resources in consultations. *British Medical Journal,* 1991, 303:1181-1184.
131. Roos, N.P., Carriere, K.C., Friesen, D. Factors infl uencing the frequency of visits by hypertensive patients to primary care physicians in Winnipeg. *Canadian Medical Association Journal,* 1998, 159:777-783.
132. Ryan, S. *et al.* The effects of regular source of care and health need on medical care use among rural adolescents. *Archives of Pediatric and Adolescent Medicine,* 2001,155:184-190.
133. Schoen, C. *et al.* Towards higher-performance health systems: adults' health care experiences in seven countries, 2007. *Health Affairs,* 2007, 26:w717-w734.

134. Saltman, R., Rico, A., Boerma, W., eds. Primary care in the driver's seat? Organizational reform in European primary care. Maidenhead, England, Open University Press, 2006 (European Observatory on Health Systems and Policies Series).

135. Nutting, P.A. Population-based family practice: the next challenge of primary care. *Journal of Family Practice,* 1987, 24:83-88.

136. Strategies for population health: investing in the health of Canadians. Ottawa, Health Canada, Advisory Committee on Population Health, 1994.

137. Lasker, R. Medicine and public health: the power of collaboration. New York, *New York Academy of Medicine,* 1997.

138. Longlett, S.K., Kruse, J.E., Wesley, R.M. Community-oriented primary care: historical perspective. *Journal of the American Board of Family Practice,* 2001,14:54-563.

139. Improving health for New Zealanders by investing in primary health care. Wellington, National Health Committee, 2000.

140. Provenzale, D. *et al.* Gastroenterologist specialist care and care provided by generalists—an evaluation of effectiveness and efficiency. *American Journal of Gastroenterology,* 2003, 98:21-8.

141. Smetana, G.W. *et al.* A comparison of outcomes resulting from generalist vs specialist care for a single discrete medical condition: a systematic review and methodologic critique. *Archives of Internal Medicine,* 2007, 167:10-20.

142. Beck, C.A. *et al.* Discharge prescriptions following admission for acute myocardial infarction at tertiary care and community hospitals in Quebec. Canadian *Journal of Cardiology,* 2001, 17:33-40.

143. Fendrick, A.M., Hirth, R.A., Chernew, M.E. Differences between generalist and specialist physicians regarding Helicobacter pylori and peptic ulcer disease. *American Journal of Gastroenterology,* 1996, 91:1544-1548.

144. Zoorob, R.J. *et al.* Practice patterns for peptic ulcer disease: are family physicians testing for H. pylori? *Helicobacter,* 1999, 4:243-248.

145. Rose, J.H. *et al.* Generalists and oncologists show similar care practices and outcomes for hospitalized late-stage cancer patients. For SUPPORT Investigators (Study to Understand Prognoses and Preferences for Outcomes and Risks for Treatment). *Medical Care,* 2000, 38:1103-1118.

146. Krikke, E.H., Bell, N.R. Relation of family physician or specialist care to obstetric interventions and outcomes in patients at low risk: a western Canadian cohort study. *Canadian Medical Association Journal,* 1989, 140:637-643.

147. MacDonald, S.E., Voaklander, K., Birtwhistle, R.V. A comparison of family physicians' and obstetricians' intrapartum management of low-risk pregnancies. *Journal of Family Practice,* 1993, 37:457-462.

148. Abyad, A., Homsi, R. A comparison of pregnancy care delivered by family physicians *versus* obstetricians in Lebanon. *Family Medicine,* 1993 25:465-470. The World Health Report.

149. Grunfeld, E. *et al.* Comparison of breast cancer patient satisfaction with follow-up in primary care versus specialist care: results from a randomized controlled trial. *British Journal of General Practice,* 1999, 49:705-710.

150. Grunfeld, E. *et al.* Randomized trial of long-term follow-up for early-stage breast cancer: a comparison of family physician versus specialist care. *Journal of Clinical Oncology,* 2006, 24:848-855.

151. Scott, I.A. *et al.* An Australian comparison of specialist care of acute myocardial infarction. *International Journal for Quality in Health Care,* 2003, 15:155-161..

152. Regueiro, C.R. *et al.* A comparison of generalist and pulmonologist care for patients hospitalized with severe chronic obstructive pulmonary disease: resource intensity, hospital costs, and survival. For SUPPORT Investigators (Study to Understand Prognoses and Preferences for Outcomes and Risks of Treatment). *American Journal of Medicine,* 1998, 105:366-372.

153. McAlister, F.A. *et al.* The effect of specialist care within the fi rst year on subsequent outcomes in 24,232 adults with new-onset diabetes mellitus: population-based cohort study. *Quality and Safety in Health Care,* 2007, 16:6-11.

154. Greenfield, S. *et al.* Outcomes of patients with hypertension and non-insulin dependent diabetes mellitus treated by different systems and specialties. Results from the medical outcomes study. *Journal of the American Medical Association,* 1995, 274:1436-1444.

155. Pongsupap, Y., Boonyapaisarnchoaroen, T., Van Lerberghe, W. The perception of patients using primary care units in comparison with conventional public hospital outpatient departments and "prime mover family practices": an exit survey. *Journal of Health Science,* 2005, 14:3.

156. Baicker, K., Chandra, A. Medicare spending, the physician workforce, and beneficiaries' quality of care. *Health Affairs,* 2004 (Suppl. web exclusive: W4-184-197).

157. Shi, L. Primary care, specialty care, and life chances. *International Journal of Health Services,* 1994, 24:431-458.

158. Baicker, K. *et al.* Who you are and where you live: how race and geography affect the treatment of Medicare beneficiaries. *Health Affairs,* 2004 (web exclusive: VAR33-V44).

159. Briggs, C.J., Garner, P. Strategies for integrating primary health services in middle and low-income countries at the point of delivery. *Cochrane Database of Systematic Reviews,* 2006, (3):CD003318.

160. *Ibid.*

161. Pongsupap Y, Van Lerberghe W. Choosing between public and private or between hospital and primary care? Responsiveness, patient-centeredness and prescribing patterns in outpatient consultations in Bangkok. *Tropical Medicine and International Health,* 2006, 11:81-89.

162. Guide to clinical preventive services, 2007. Rockville, M.D., *Agency for Health Care Research and Quality,* 2007 (AHRQ Publication No. 07-05100;

163. Margolis, P.A. *et al.* From concept to application: the impact of a community-wide intervention to improve the delivery of preventive services to children. *Pediatrics,* 2001, 108:E42.

164. Donovan, E.F. *et al.* Intensive home visiting is associated with decreased risk of infant death. *Pediatrics,* 2007, 119:1145-1151.

165. Manandhar, D. *et al.* Effect of a participatory intervention with women's groups on birth outcomes in Nepal: cluster-randomised controlled trial. *Lancet,* 364:970-979.

166. Rockenschaub, G., Pukkila, J., Prolific MC, eds. Towards health security. A discussion paper on recent health crises in the WHO European Region. Copenhagen, World Health Organization Regional Office for Europe, 2007

167. Primary care. America's health in a new era. Washington DC, National Academy Press Institute of Medicine, 1996.

168. Tableau d'honneur des 50 meilleurs hôpitaux de France. Palmarès des Hôpitaux. Le Point, 2008 (http://hopitaux.lepoint.fr/tableau-honneur.php, accessed 29 July 2008).

169. Davidson, B.N., Sofaer, S., Gertler, P. Consumer information and biased selection in the demand for coverage supplementing Medicare. *Social Science and Medicine,* 1992,34:1023-1034.

170. Davison, K.P., Pennebaker, J.W., Dickerson SS. Who talks? The social psychology of illness support groups. *American Psychology,* 2000, 55:205-217.

171. Segal, S.P., Redman, D., Silverman, C. Measuring clients' satisfaction with self-help agencies. *Psychiatric Services,* 51:1148-1152.

172. Criel, B., De Brouwere, V., Dugas, S. Integration of vertical programmes in multi-function health services. Antwerp, ITG Press, 1997 (Studies in Health Services Organization and Policy 3).

APPENDIX 3

HEALTH CARE IN INDIA—VISION 2020

ISSUES AND PROSPECTS

R. SRINIVASAN

INTRODUCTION

Key Linkages in Health

Health and health care need to be distinguished from each other for no better reason than that the former is often incorrectly seen as a direct function of the latter. Heath is clearly not the mere absence of disease. Good Health confers on a person or groups freedom from illness—and the ability to realize one's potential. Health is therefore best understood as the indispensable basis for defining a person's sense of well-being. The health of populations is a distinct key issue in public policy discourse in every mature society often determining the deployment of huge society. They include its cultural understanding of ill-health and well-being, extent of socio-economic disparities, reach of health services and quality and costs of care and current bio-medical understanding about health and illness.

Health care covers not merely medical care but also all aspects of preventive care too. Nor can it be limited to care rendered by or financed out of public expenditure—within the government sector alone.but must include incentives and disincentives for self-care and care paid for by private citizens to get over ill-health. Where, as in India, private out-of-pocket expenditure dominates the cost financing health care, the effects are bound to be regressive. Heath care at its essential core is widely recognized to be a public good. Its demand and supply cannot therefore, be left to be regulated solely by the invisible had of the market. Nor can it be established on considerations of utility maximizing conduct alone.

What makes for a just health care system even as an ideal? Four criteria could be suggested—First, universal access, and access to an adequate level, and access without excessive burden. Second, fair distribution of financial costs for access and fair distribution of burden in rationing care and capacity and a constant search for improvement to a more just system. Third, training providers for competence, empathy and accountability, pursuit of quality care and cost effective use of the results of relevant research. Last special attention to vulnerable groups such as children, women, disabled and the aged.

Forecasting in Health Sector

In general predictions about future health—of individuals and populations—can be notoriously uncertain. However, all projections of health care in India must in the end rest on the overall changes in its political economy—on progress made in poverty mitigation (health care to the poor) in reduction of inequalities (health inequalities affecting access/ quality'), in generation of employment/income streams (to facilitate capacity to pay and to accept individual responsibility for one's health). in public information and development communication (to promote preventive self care and risk reduction by conducive lifestyles) and in personal lifestyle changes (often directly resulting from social changes and global influences). Of course it will also depend on progress in reducing mortality and the likely disease load, efficient and fair delivery and financing systems in private and public sectors and attention to vulnerable sections—family planning and nutritional services and women's empowerment. To list them is to recall that Indian planning had at its best attempted to capture this synergistic approach within a democratic structure. It is another matter that it is now remembered only for its mixed success.

Available Health Forecasts

There is a forecast on the new health challenges likely to emerge in India over the next few decades. Murry and Lopez <World Bank B 2000> have provided a possible scenario of the burden of disease (BOD) for India in the year 2020, based on a statistical model calculating the change in DALYs are applied to the population projections for 2020 and conversely. The key conclusions must be understood keeping in the mind the tact that the concept of DALYs incorporates not only mortality but disability viewed in terms of healthy years of life lost. In this forecast, DALYs are expected to dramatically decrease in respect of diarrhoeal diseases and respiratory infections and less dramatically for maternal conditions. TB is expected to plateau by 2000, and HIV infections are expected to rise significantly up to 2010. Injuries may increase less significantly, the proportion of people above 65 will increase and as a result the burden of non-communicable disease will rise. Finally cardiovascular diseases resulting any from the risk associated with smoking urban stress and improper diet are expected to increase dramatically.

Under the same BOD methodology another view is available from a four-state analysis done in 1996 <World Bank B 2000> these four states—AP, Karnataka, W. Bengal and Punjab—represent different stages in the Indian health transition. West Bengal, will still face a large incidence of communicable diseases. More prosperous states, such as Punjab further along the health transiting will witness sharply increasing incidence of non-communicable diseases especially, in urban areas. The projections highlight that we still operating on unreliable or incomplete base data on mortality and causes of death in the absence of vital registration statistics and know as yet little about how they differ between social classes and regions or about the dynamic patterns of change at work. It also highlights the policy dilemma of how to balance between the articulate middle upper class demand for more access to technologically advanced and subsidized clinical services and the more pressing needs of the poor for coverage of basic disease control interventions. This conflict over deployment of public resources will only get exacerbated in future. What matters most in such estimates are not societal averages with respect to health but sound data illumining specifically the health conditions of the disadvantaged in local areas <Gwatkin A 2000> that long tradition of health sector analysis looking at unequal access, income poverty and unjustly distributed resources as the trigger to meet health needs of the poor. That tradition has been totally replaced by the currently dominant school of international thought about health which is concerned primarily with efficiency of systems measured by cost effectiveness criteria.

Future of State Provided Health Care

Historically the Indian commitment to health development has been guided by two principles with three consequences. The first principle was State responsibility for health care and the second (after independence) was free medical care for all (and not merely to those unable to pay).

The first set of consequences was inadequate priority to public health, poor investment in safe water and sanitation and to the neglect of the key role of personal hygiene in good health, culminating in the persistence of diseases like Cholera.

The second set of consequences pertains to substantially unrealized goals of NHP 1983 due to funding difficulties from compression of public expenditures and from organizational inadequacies. The ambitious and far reaching NPP-2000 goals and strategies have however been formulated on that edifice in the hope that the gaps and the inadequate would be removed by purposeful action. Without being too defensive or critical about its past failures, the rural health structure should be strengthened and funded and managed efficiently in all States by 2005. This can trigger many dramatically changes over the next twenty years in neglected aspects or rural health and of vulnerable segments.

The third set of consequences appears to be the inability to develop and integrate plural systems of medicine and the failure to assign practical roles to the private sector and to assign public duties for private professionals.

To set right these gaps demanded patient redefinition of the state's role keeping the focus on equity. But during the last decade there has been an abrupt switch to market based governance styles and much influential advocacy to reduce the state role in health in order to enforce overall compression of public expenditure an reduce fiscal deficits. People have therefore been forced to switch between weak and efficient public services and expensive private provision or at the limit forego care entirely except in life threatening situations, in such cases sliding into indebtedness.

Health status of any population is not only the record of mortality and its morbidity profile but also a record of its resilience based on mutual solidarity and indigenous traditions of self-care—assets normally invisible to he planner and the professional. Such resilience can be enriched with the State retaining a strategic directional role for the good health of all its citizens in accordance with the constitutional mandate. Within such a framework alone can the private sector be engaged as an additional instrument or a partner for achieving shared public health outcomes. Similarly, in indigenous health systems must be promoted to the extent possible to become another credible delivery mechanism in which people have faith and away fond for the vat number of less than folly qualified doctors in rural areas to get skills upgraded. Public programs in rural and poor urban areas engaging indigenous practitioners and community volunteers can prevent much seasonal and communicable disease using low cost traditional knowledge and based on the balance between food, exercise medicine and moderate living. Such an overall vision of the public role of the heterogenous private sector must inform the course of future of state-led health care in the country.

KEY ACHIEVEMENTS IN HEALTH

Our overall achievement in regard to longevity and other key health indicators are impressive but in many respects uneven across States, The two Data Annexure at the end indicate selected health demographic and economic indicators and highlight the changes between 1951 and 2001. In the past five decades life expectancy has increased from 50 years to over 64 in 2000. IMR has come down from 147 to 70. Crude birth rates have dropped to 26.1 and death rates to 8.7.

At this stage, a process understanding of longevity and child health may be useful for understanding progress in future. Longevity, always a key national goal, is not merely the reduction of deaths as a result of better medical and rehabilitative care at old age. In fact without reasonable quality of life in the extended years marked by self-confidence and absence of undue dependency longevity may men only a display of technical skills. So quality of life requires as much external bio-medical interventions as culture-based acceptance of inevitable decline in faculties without officious start at sixty but run across life lived at all ages in reduction of mortality among infants through immunization and nutrition interventions and reduction of mortality among young and middle aged adults, including adolescents getting inform about sexuality reproduction and safe motherhood. At the same time, some segments will remain always more vulnerable—such as women due to patriarchy and traditions of infra-family denial), aged (whose survival but not always development will increase with immunization) and the disabled (constituting a tenth of the population).

Reduction in child mortality involves as much attention to protecting children from infection as in ensuring nutrition and calls for a holistic view of mother and child health services. The cluster of services consisting of antenatal services, delivery care and post-mortem attention and low birth weight, childhood diarrhoea and ARI management are linked priorities. Programme of immunization and childhood nutrition seen in better performing stats indicate sustained attention to routine and complex investments into growing children as a group to make them grow into persons capable of living long and well often interest fades in pursuing the unglamorous routine of supervised immunization and is substituted by pulse campaigns, etc. which in the long-run turn out counter-productive. Indeed. persistence with improved routines and care for quality in immunization would also be a path way to reduce the world's highest rate of maternal mortality.

In this context we may refer to the large ratio-based rural health infrastructure consisting of over 5 lakh trained doctors working under plural systems of medicine and a vast frontline force of over 7 lakh ANMs, MPWS and Anganwadi workers besides community volunteers. The creation of such public work force should be seen as a major achievement in a country short of resources and struggling with great disparities in health status. As part of rural Primary health care network lone, a total of 1.6 lakh sub-centers, (with 1.27 lakh ANMs in position) and 22975 PHCs and 2935 CHCs (with over 24000 doctors and over 3500 specialists to serve in them) have been set-up. To promote Indian systems of medicine and homeopathy there are over 22000 dispensaries, 2800 hospitals. Besides 6 lakh angawadis serve nutrition needs of nearly 20 million children and 4 million mothers. The total effort has cost the bulk of the health development outlay, which stood at over Rs. 62.500 crores or 3-64% of total plan spending during the last fifty years.

On any count these are extraordinary infrastructural capacities created with resources committed against odds to strengthen grass roots. There have been facility gaps, supply gaps and staffing gaps, which can be filled up only by allocating about 20% more funds and determined ill to ensure good administration and synergy from greater congruence of services, but given the sheer size of the endeavor there will always be some failure of commitment and in routine functioning. These get exacerbated by periodic campaign mode and vertical programme, which have only increased compartmentalized vision and over-medicalization of health problems. The initial key mistake arose from the needless bifurcation of health and family welfare and nutrition functions at all levels instead of promoting more holism. As a result of all this the structure has been precluded from reaching its optimal potential. It has got more firmly established at the periphery/sub-center level and dedicated to RCH services only. At PHC and CHC levels this has further been compounded by a weak referral system. There has not been enough convergence in "escorting" children through immunization coverage and nutrition education of mothers and ensuring better food to children, including cooked mid-day meals and health checks al schools. There has also been no constructive engagement between allopathic and indigenous systems to build synergies, which could have improved people's perceptions of benefits from the infrastructure in ways that made sense to them.

One key task in the coming decades is therefore to utilize fully that created potential by attending to well known organizational motivational and financial gaps. The gaps have arisen partly from the source and scale of funds and partly due to lack of persistence, both of which can be set right. PHCs and CHCs are funded by States several of whom are unable to match Central assistance offered and hence these centers remain inadequate and operate on minimum efficiency. On the other hand, over two-thirds cost of three-fourths of sub-centers are fully met by the Center due to their key role in family welfare services. But in equal part these gaps are due to many other non-monetary factors such as undue centralization and uniformity, fluctuating commitment to key routines at ground level, insufficient experimentation with alternatives such as getting public duties discharged through private professionals and ensuring greater local accountability to users.

Health Status Issues

The difference between rural and urban indiactors of health status and the wide interstate disparity in health status are well known. Clearly the urban rural differentials are substantial and range from childhood and go on increasing the gap as one grows up to 5 years. Sheer survival apart there is also the we known under provision in rural areas in practically all social sector services. For the children growing up in rural areas the disparities naturally tend to get even worse when compounded by the widely practiced discrimination against women, starting with foeticide of daughters.

In spite of overall achievement it is a mixed record of social development specially failing in involving people in imaginative ways. Even the averaged out good performance ideas wide variations by social class or gender or region or State. The classes in may States have had to suffer the most due to lack of access or denial of access or social exclusion or all of them. This is clear from the fact that compared to the riches quintile, the poorest had 2.5 times more IMR and child mortality, TFR at double the rates and nearly 75% malnutrition—particularly during the nineties.

Not only are the gaps between the better performing and other States-wide but in same cases have been increasing during the nineties. Large differences also exist between districts within the same better performing State urban areas appear to have better health outcomes than rural areas although the figures may not fully reflect the situation in urban and peri-urban slums with large in migration with conditions comparable to rural pockets. It is estimated that urban slum population will grow at double the rate of urban population growth in the next few decades. India may have by 2002 a total urban population of close to 600 million living in urban areas with an estimated 145 million living in slums in 2001. What should be a fair measure for assessing success in enhancing health status of population in any forecast on health care?

Disease Load in India and China

We need a basis for comparative scenario building. Among the nations of the world China alone rank in size and scale and in complexity comparable to India differences between an open and free society and a semi-controlled polity do matter. The remarkable success in China in combating disease is due to sustained attention on the health of the young in China, and of public policy backed by resources and social mobilization. While comparing China and India in selected aspects of disease load, demography and public expenditures on health, the record on India may seem mixed compared to the more all round progress made by China. But this should also be seen in the perspective of the larger burden of disease in India compared to China and of the transactional costs of an open and free democracy.

Though India and China recorded the same rate of growth till 70s, China initiated reforms a full decade earlier. This gave it a head stat for a higher growth rate and has resulted in an economic gap with India which has become wider over time. This is because domestic savings in China are 36% of GDP whereas in India it hovers at 23%, mostly in household savings. Again. China attracted $40 billion in foreign direct investment against $2 billion in India. Special economic zones and relaxed labour laws have helped. Public expenditure on health in China has been consistently higher underlining the regressive nature of financing of health are in India. Nevertheless, it is not too unrealistic to expect that India should be able to reach by 2010 at least three-fourth the current level of performance of China in all key health indices. India's current population is not a bit more than 75% that of China and India will of course be catching up even more with China into the 21st century. This would be offset by the handicap that Indian progress will be moderated by the fact that it is an open free and democratic society. A practical rule-of-thumb measure for an optimistic forecast of future progress in India could be—that between 2000 and 2010 India should do three-fourths as well as China did in 1990-2000 and, after 2010, India should try to catch up with the rate of performance of China and do just as well thereafter. This will translate into, for instance, a growth rate of about 8% for India till 2010 and as close to 10% as possible thereafter thus enabling doubling first in ten years and doubling twice over every seven years thereafter prior to 2025. Keeping this perspective in mind, we may now examine the profile of major disease control effort; the effectiveness of available instruments for delivery and financing public health action and assess factors relevant to the remaining event of vulnerability within jout emerging social pyramid over next two or three decades.

MAJOR DISEASE CONTROL EFFORTS

A careful analysis of the Global Burden of Disease (GBD) study focusing on age-specific morbidity during 2000 in ten most common diseases (excluding injuries) shows that sixty percent of morbidity is due to infectious diseases and common tropical diseases, a quarter due to life-style disorders and 13% due to potentially preventable peri-natal conditions. Further domestic R&D has been so far muted in its efforts against an estimated annual aggregate health expenditure in India of Rs. 80,000 crores R&D expenditure in India for public and private sector combined was Rs. 1150 crores only. India must play a larger part in its own efforts at indigenous R&D as very little world-wide expenditure on R&D is likely to be devoted to infectious diseases. For instance out of the 1233 new drugs that came into the market between 1975 and 1997 only 11 were indicated specifically for tropical country diseases.

We have already the distinction of elimination or control acceptable to public health standards of smallpox and guinea worm diseases in the draft National Health Policy-2010. It has now been proposed to eliminate or control the following diseases within limits acceptable to public health practice—A good deal of the effort would be feasible.

- Polio Yaws and leprosy by 2005 which seems distinctly feasible though the removal of social stigma and reconstructive surgery and other rehabilitation arrangements in regard to leprosy would remain inadequate for a decade or more.
- Kalaazar by 2010 and Filariasis by 2010 which also seems feasible due to its localized prevalence and the possibility of greater community based work involving PR institutions in the simple but time-limited tasks or public health programs.
- Blindness prevalence to 0.5% by 2010 sees less feasible due to a graying population. At present the programme is massively supported by foreign aid as there are many other legitimate demands on domestic health budgets.
- AIDS reaching zero growth by 2007 appears to be problematic as there are disputes even about base data on infected population. On most reckonings, affordable vaccines are not likely to be available soon nor anti-retro viral drugs appear likely at affordable prices in the near future. Further the prevalence curve of Aids in India is yet to show its shape. There is also larger unresolved question of where HIV/ATDS should be fitted in our priorities of public health, especially in this massively foreign aided programme what happen if aid does not become available at some point.

Unfinished Burden of Communicable Diseases

Apart from the above, there remains a vast unfinished burden in preventing controlling or eliminating other major communicable diseases and in bringing down the risk of deaths in maternal and peri-natal conditions. Endemic diseases arising from infection or lack of nutrition continue to account for almost two-thirds of morality and morbidity in India. Indeed eleven out of thirteen diseases recommended by the Bhore Committee were infectious diseases and at least three of them may well continue to be with us for the next two decades Baring Leprosy which is almost on the path to total control by 2005, the other key communicable diseases will be TB, Malaria and Aids—to which diarrhoea in children and complicated and high risk maternity should be added in view of their pervasive incidence and avoidable mortality among the poorer and under served sectors.

Tuberculosis

Tuberculosis has had a world wide resurgence including in India. It is estimated lhai about 14 million persons are infected, i.e. 1.55 of total population suffer from radio logically active Tuberculosis. About 1.5 million cases are identified and more than 300 000 deaths occur every year. Between NFHS 1 and NFHS 2 the prevalence has increased from 4678 per lakh population to 544. Unfortunately, prevalence among working age adults (15-59) is even higher as 675. All these may well be underestimates in so far as patients are traced only through hospital visit. Only about half reach the hospital. Often wrong diagnosis by insufficiently trained doctors or misunderstood protocols is another key problem both public and private sectors. TB is a widespread disease of poverty among women living and working in ill ventilated places and other undernourished persons in urban slums it is increasingly affecting the younger adults also in the economically productive segments. No universal screening is possible. Sputum positive test does not precede diagnosis but drugs are prescribed on the basis of fever and shadows as a result incomplete cure becomes common and delayed tests only prove the wrong diagnosis too late. Improved diagnosis through better training and clear protocols and elimination of drug resistance through incomplete cure should be priority. Treatment costs in case of drug resistance can soar close to ten times the normal level of Rs. 3000 to 4000 per person treated. Similarly even though the resistant strain may cover only 8% at present, it could suddenly rise and as it approaches 20% or so, there is a danger that TB may get out of control. The DOTS programme trying for full compliance after proper diagnosis is settling down but already has some claims of success. More than 3000 laboratories have been set-up for diagnosis and about 1.5 lakh workers trained and with total population coverage by 2007 cure rates (already claimed to have doubled) may rise substantially. There is reason to hope that DOTS programs would prove a greater success over time with increased community awareness aeneration. The key issue is how soon and how well can it be integrated into the PHC system and made subject to routines of local accountability, without which no low cost regime of total compliance is feasible in a country as large as India.

An optimistic assessment could be that with commitment and full use of infrastructure it will be possible to arrest further growth in absolute numbers of TB cases keeping it at below 1.5 million till 2010 even though the population will be growing. Once that is done TB can be brought down to less than a million lie within internationally accepted limits and disappears as a major communicable disease in India by 2020.

Malaria

As regards malaria, we have had a long record of success and failure and each intervention has been thwarted by new problems and plagued by recrudescence. At present India has a large manpower fully aware of all aspects of malaria about often low in motivation. It can be transformed into a large-scale work force for awareness generation, tests and distribution of medicine. In spite of past successes, there is evidence of reemergence with focal attacks of malaria with the virulent falciparum variety especially in tribal areas. In priority tribal area malaria stands fully funded by the center. About 2 million cases of malaria are recorded allover India every year with seasonal high incidence local failures of control. Drug resistance in humans and insecticide resistant strains of mosquitoes present a significant problem. But there is a window of opportunity in respect of DDT sensitive areas in eastern India where even now malaria incidence can be brought down by about 50% within a decade and be beneficial for control of kalazaar and JE. There is growing interest and community awareness of biological methods of control of mosquito growth. Unfortunately diligent ground level public health work is in grave disarray in these areas but can be improved by better supervision greater use of panchayatraj institutions and buildings on modest demonstrated successes. As regards a vaccine, there seems to be no sufficient incentive for international R&D to focus on a relatively lower priority or research. Rollback malaria programmes of the WHO are more likely to concentrate on Africa whose profile of malaria is not similar to ours. The search for a vaccine continues but has little likelihood of immediate success.

In spite of various difficulties, if the restructuring of the malaria workforce and the strengthening of health infrastructure takes place, one can expect that the incidence can be reduce by a third or even upto half in the next decade or so. For this it is necessary that routine tasks like timely spraying and logistics for taking blood slides testing and their analysis and organic methods of reducing mosquito spread, etc. are down staged to community level and performed under supervision through panchayats with commonality participation public education and local monitoring. Malaria can certainly be reduced by a third even upto a half in ten years, and there is a prospect of near freedom from malaria for most of the country by 2020.

The Case of AIDS

There is finally the case of HIV/AID. The magnitude in the numbers of HIV infected and of AIDS patients by 2025 can be known only as trends emerge over a decade from now. When better epidemiological estimates are available but at present these figures are hotly contested. We cant start with the number infected with HIV as per NACO sentinel surveillance in 2000 a cumulative total 3.86 million, a figure disputed in recent public health debate. We can then assume that about 10% will turn into full-blow cases of severe and intractable stage of Aids. There is as yet no basis to know how many of those infected will become AIDS patients, preventive efforts focused on behaviour change will show up firmly only after a decade or so. During this period one can assume an additional 10% growth to account for new cases every year. The Draft NHP 2001 seeks to stop further infection by educating and counseling and condom supplies to level it off around 2007, which seems somewhat ambitious. We have yet to make a decisive dent into the problem of awareness with the broader population and so far we have been at work only on high risk groups. NFHS 2 shows only a third of women reporting that they even knew about the HIV/AIDS. Further such awareness efforts must be followed by multi-pronged and culturally compatible techniques of public education that go beyond segments easier to be convinced or behaviour changed. There are voices already raised about the appropriateness of IEC mass media content and of the under emphasis of face to face counseling, calling for innovative mobilization strategies rooted in indigenous belief systems.

What it implies is that we may be carrying by 2015 close to 5 million infected and upto a tenth of them could turn into full blown cases. We may not be able to level off infection by 2007. Further these magnitudes may turn out in actual fact to be wildly off the mark. On any account it is clear that AIDS can lead to high mortality among the productive groups in society affecting economic functioning as also public health. Even if 10% of them say 50 to 60000 cases becomes full blown cases the state has the onerous and grim choice to look at competing equities and decide on a policy for free treatment of AIDS patients with expensive anti-retroviral drugs. And if it decides not to the issue remains as to how to evolve humane balanced and affordable policies that do not lead to a social breakdown. In about a decade vaccine development may possibly be successful and drugs may be more effective but they may not always be affordable nor can be given free.

There would hopefully be wider consultation with persons with caring sensibilities including AIDS patients on how to counsel in different eventualities and to get the balance right between hospital and home care and how to develop a humane affordable policy for anti-retroviral drugs for AIDS patients. Is there a case for providing them with drug free of cost merely to extend their lives for few years? The matter involves a true dilemma, for public health priorities themselves certainly argue for more funds should address diseases constituting bigger population-based hazards. Investments made in such expensive interventions can instead be made in supporting hospice efforts in the voluntary and private sectors.

Whatever position may emerge in research or spread of infection of case fatalities, a multi-pronged attempt for awareness, must continue and tough choices must get discussed openly without articulate special, often urban middle class interests denying other views and especially public health priorities of the poor. The promotion of barrier protection must increase but has to related to a system of values, which would be acceptable to the people's beliefs. We need to strengthen sentinel surveillance systems and awareness effort. We also need sensitive feedback on the effects they leave on younger minds for a balanced culturally acceptable strategy. All this is feasible and can be accomplished if we are not swept away by the power of funding and advocacy and fear of being accused to be out of line with dominant world opinion.

In any case many of the ill cannot afford the high prices or have access to it from public agencies. The strict patent regimen under TRIPS is bound to prevail, notwithstanding the ambivalently worded Doha decision of WTO that public health emergencies provide sufficient cause of countries to use the flexibility available from various provisions of TRIPS. A recent analysis reveals that the three drug regimen recommended will cost $10000 per person per year from Western companies and the treatment will be lifelong. Three Indian companies are offering to Central Government anti-retro viral drugs at $600/Rs. 30,000/per person per year and to an international charity at an even lower price $ 350/Rs. 13,000/per year provided it was distributed for humanitarian relief free in S. Africa. It has been public policy in Brazil that the drug is supplied free to all AIDS should be no exception. If drugs are supplied acting on a public health emergency basis and prices can stabilize at Rs. 1000 or so per year the public health budget should be able to accommodate the cost weighed against true public criteria. But the aim of leveling off infection of 2007 still seems unlikely.

Maternal and Parental Deaths

Maternal and parental deaths are sizeable but the advantage here is that they can be prevented merely by more intensive utilization of existing rural health infrastructure. Policy and implementation must keep steady focus on key items such as improved institutional deliveries, better trained birth attendants and timely antenatal screening to eliminate anaemia and at the same time isolate cases needing referral or other targeted attention. After all Tamil Nadu has by such methods ensured closed to 90% institutional deliveries backed by a functional referral. Firm administrative will and concurrent supervision of specified screening tasks included in MCH services can give us a window of opportunity to dramatically bring down within a few years alarming maternal mortality currently one of the highest in the world. From NFHS I data, it was estimated at 424 per lac births, it has risen to 540 per lac births in NFHS II, but the WHO estimate puts it higher at 570. There can be a systematic campaign over five years to increase institutional deliveries as near as possible to the Tamil Nadu level, also taking into account assisted, home deliveries by trained staff with doctors at call. For the interim TBAs should be relied on through a mass awareness campaign involving Gram Panchayats too. Over a period of time there is no reason why ANMs entitled benefits of children to help in their growth and not remain as welfare measure. Using the infrastructures fully and with community participation and extensive social mobilization many tasks in nutrition are feasible and can be in position to make impact by 2010.

Child Health and Nutrition

Associated with this is the issue of infant and child mortality, (70 out of 1000 dying in the first year and 98 before vide years) and low birth weight (22% UW at birth ands 47% EJW at below 3 years) most mortality occurs from diarrhoea and the stagnation in IMR in the last few year is bound to have a negative effect on population stabilization goals. A recent review of the Ninth plan indicated that even with accelerated efforts we may reach at best IMR/50 by 3002, but more like IMR/56, since the easier part of the problem is taking child mortality is over every pomt gain hereafter will deal with districts at greater risk and needing better organizational efficiencies in immunization. At the same time, more streamlined RCH services are getting established as part of public systems and through private partnerships Therefore, there is every reason to hope that the NPP 2000 target of 30 per thousand live births by 2010 will be met barring a few pockets of inaccessible and resource lean areas with stubborn persistence of poverty and dominantly composed of weaker sections (e.g. in part of Orissa as seen from NFHS II).

As regards childhood diarrhoea, deaths are totally preventable simple community action and public education by targeting children of low birth weights and detecting early those children at risk from malnutrition through proper low cost screening procedure, the present arrangement has got too burdened with attempting total population coverage getting all children weighed even once in three months and making ANMs depots for ORS and for simple drugs for fever and motivating the community to take pride in healthy children are the lessons of the success of the Tamil Nadu Nutrition Project. If this is done there is a reasonable chance of two-thirds decline in moderate malnutrition and abolition of serious grades completely by 2015. The success can be built upon till 2025 for reaching levels comparable to China.

Concentration on preventive measures of maternal and child health and in particular improved nutrition services will be particularly useful because it will help that generation to have a head start in good health who are going to be a part of the demographic bonus. The bonus is a young adult bulge of about 340 million (with not less than 250 million from rural population and about 100 million born in this century). The bonus will appear in a sequence with South Indian States completing the transition before North Indian States spread it over the next three decades to ensure best results at this stage the present nutritional services must be converted into targeted (and entitled) benefits of children to help in their growth and not remain as welfare measure. Using the infrastructures fully and with community participation and extensive social mobilization many tasks in nutrition are feasible and can be in position to make impact by 2010.

Mild and moderate malnutrition still prevalent in over half of our young populaaon can be halved if food as the supplemental pathway to better nutrition becomes a priority both for self-reliance and lower costs. There has been a tendency for micro-nutrient supplementation to overwhelm food derived nourishment. This trend is assisted by foreign aid but over a long-run may prove unsustainable. By engaging the adolescents into proper nutrition education and reproductive health awareness we can seamlessly weave into the nutritional security system of our country a corps of informed interconnected and imaginative ideas can be tried out. Such social mobilization at low cost can be the best preventive strategy as has been advocated for long by the Nutrition Foundation of India (< Gopalan 2001) and can be a priority in this decade over the next two plan periods.

Unfinished Agenda—Non-communicable Diseases and Injuries

Three major such diseases viz., cancer cardiovascular diseases and renal conditions—and neglect in regard to mental health conditions - have of late shown worrisome trends. Cures for cancer are still elusive in spite of palliatives and expensive and long drawn chemo—or radio-therapy which often inflict catastrophic costs. In the case of CVD and renal conditions known and tried procedures are available for relief. There is evidence of greater prevalence of cancer even among young adults due to the stress of modern livmg. In India cancer is a leading cause of death with about 1.5 to 2 million cases at anytime to which 7 lac new cases are added every year with 3 lakh deaths. Over 15 lakh patients require facilities for diagnosis and treatment. Studies by WHO show that by 2026 with the expected increase in fife expectancy, cancer burden in India will increase to about 14 lac cases. CVD cases and Diabetes cases are also increasing with an 8 to 11% prevalence of the latter due to fast lifestyles and lack of exercise. Traumas and accidents leading to injuries—are offshoots of the same competitive living conditions and urban traffic conditions Data show one death every minute due to accidents or more than 1800 deaths every day—in Delhi alone about 150 cases are reported every day from accidents on the road and for every death 8 living patients are added to hospitals due to injuries. There is finally the emerging aftermath of insurgencies and militant violence leading to mental illnesses of various types. It is estimated that 10 to 20 persons out of 1000 population suffer from severe mental illness and 3 to 5 times more have emotional disorder. While there are some facilities for diagnosis and treatment exist in major cities there is no access whatever in rural areas. It is acknowledged that the only way of handling mental health problems is through including it into the primary health care arrangements implying trained screening and counseling at primary levels for early detection.

All these are eminently feasible preventive steps and can be put into practice by 2005 and we should be doing as well or better than China by 2020 considering the greater load of non-communicable diseases they bear now. The burden of non-communicable diseases will be met more and more by private sector specialized hospitals which spring up in urban centers. Facilities in prestigious public centers will also be under strain and they should be redesigned to take advantage of community-based approach of awareness, early detection and referral system as in the mode) developed successfully in the Regional Cancer Center, Keraia. Public sector institutions are also needed to provide a comparator basis for costs and evaluating technology benefits. For the less affluent sections prolonged high tech cure will be unaffordable. Therefore, public funds should go to promote a routine of proper screening health education and self-care and timely investigations to see that interventions are started in stages I and II.

HEALTH INFRASTRUCTURE IN THE PUBLIC SECTOR

Issues in regard to public and private health infrastructure are different and both of them need attention but in different ways. Rural public infrastructure must remain in mainstay for wider access to health care for all without imposing undue burden on them. Side by side the existing set of public hospitals at district and sub-district levels must be supported by good management and with adequate funding and user fees and out contracting services, all as part of a functioning referral net work. This demands better routines more accountable staff and attention to promote quality. Many reputed public hospitals have suffered from lack of autonomy inadequate budgets for non-wage O&M leading to faltering and poorly motivated care. All these are being tackled in several states are part health sector reform, and will reduce the waste involved in simpler cases needlessly reaching tertiary hospitals direct. These attempts must persist without any wavering or policy changes or periodic denigration of their past working. More autonomy to large hospitals and district public health authorities will enable them to plan and implement decentralized and flexible and locally controlled services and remove the dichotomy between hospital and primary care services. Further, most preventive services can be delivered by down staging to a public health nurse much of what a doctor alone does now. Such long term commitment for demystification of medicine and down staging of professional help has been lost among the politicians bureaucracy and technocracy after the decline of the PHC movement. One consequence is the huge regional disparities between states which are getting stagnated in the transition at different stages and sometimes, polarized in the transition. Some feasible steps in revitalizing existing infrastructure are examined below drawn from successful experiences and therefore feasible elsewhere.

Feasible Steps for Better Performance

The adoption of a ratio based approach tor creating facilities and other mpuls has led to shortfalls estimated upto twenty percent. It functions well whereever there is diligent attention to supervised administrative routines such as orderly drugs procurement, adequate, O&M budgets and supplies and credible procedures for redressal of complaints. Current PHC· CHC budgets may have to be increased by 10% per year for five years to draw level. The proposal in the Draft NHP 2001 is timely that State health expenditures be raised to 7% by 2015 and to 8% of State budgets thereafter. Indeed the target could be stepped up progressively to 10% by 2025. it also suggests that Central funding should constitute 25% of total public expenditure in health against the present 15%. The peripheral level at the sub center has not been (and may not now ever be) integrated with the rest of the health system having become dedicated solely to reproduction goals. The immediate task would be to look deepening the range of work done at all levels of existing centers and in particular strengthen the referral links and fuller and flexible utilization ofPHC/CHCs. Tamil Nadu is an instance where a review showed that out of 1400 PHCs 94% functioned in their own buildings and had electricity, 98% of ANMs and 95% of pharmacists were in position. On an average every PHC treated about 100 patients 224 out of the 250 open 24 hour PHCs had ambulances. What this illustrates is that every State must look for imaginative uses to which existing structures can be put to fuller use such as making 24 hours services open or trauma facilities in PHCs on highway locations, etc.

The persistent under funding of recurring costs had led to the collapse of primary care in many states, some spectacular failures occurring in malaria and kalazar control. This has to do with adequacy of devolution of resources and with lack of administrative will probity and competence in ensuring that determined priorities in public health tasks and routines are carried out timely and in full. Only genuine devolution or simpler tasks and resources to panchayats, where there will be a third women members—can be the answer as seen in Kerala or M.P. where panchayats are made into fully competent local governments with assigned resources and control over institutions in health care. Many innovative cost containment initiatives are also possible through focused management—as for instance in the streamlining of drug purchase stocking distribution arrangements in Tamil Nadu leading to 30% more value with same budgets.

The PHC approach as implemented seems to have strayed away from its key thrust in preventive and public health action. No system exists for purposeful community focused public information or seasonal alerts or advisories or community health information to be circulated among doctors in both private practice and in public sector. PHCs were meant to be local epidemiological information centers which could develop simple community.

Tertiary hospitals had been given concessional land, customs exemption and liberal tax breaks against a commitment to reserve beds for poor patients for free treatments. No procedures exist to monitor this and the disclosure systems are far from transparent, redressal of patient grievances is poor and allegations of cuts and commissions to promote needless procedure are common.

The bulk of non-corporate private entities such as nursing homes are run by doctors and doctors-entrepreneurs and remain unregulated either in terms of facility of competence standards or quality and accountability of practice and sometimes operate without systematic medical records and audits. Medical education has become more expensive and with rapid technological advances in medicine, specialization has more attractive rewards. Indeed the reward expectations of private practice formerly spread out over career long earnings are squeezed into a few years, which becomes possible only by working in hi-tech hospital some times run as businesses. The responsibilities or private sector in clinical and preventive public health services were not specified though under the NHP 1983 nor during the last decade of reforms followed up either by government of profession by any strategy to engage allocate, monitor and regulate such private provision nor assess the costs and benefits or subsidization of private hospitals. There has been talk of public private partnerships, but this has yet to take concrete shape by imposing pubic duties on private professionals, wherever there is agreement on explicitly public health outcomes. In fact, it has required the Supreme Court to lay down the professional obligations of private doctors in accidents and injuries who used to be refused treatment in case of potential becoming part of a criminal offence.

The respective roles of the public and private sectors in health care has been a key issue in debate over a long time. With the overall swing to the right after the 1980s, it is broadly accepted that private provision of care should take care of the needs of all but the poor, doing so, risk pooling arrangements should be made to lighten the financial burden on theirs who pay for health care. As regards the poor with priced services. Taking into account the size of the burden, the clinical and public health services cannot be shouldered for all by government alone. To a large extent this health sector reform in India at the state level confirms this trend. The distribution of the burden, between the two sectors would depend on the shape and size of the social pyramid in each society. There is no objection to introduce user fees, contractual arrangements, risk pooling, etc. for mobilization of resources for health care. But, the line should be drawn not so much between public and private roles, but between institutions and health care run as businesses or run in a wider public interest as a social enterprise with an economic dimensions. In a market economy, health care is subject to three links, none of which should become out of balance with the other—the link between state and citizens' entitlement for health, the link between the consumer and provider of health services and the link between the physician and patient.

HEALTH FINANCING ISSUES

Public Expenditure Levels

Fair financing of the costs of health care is an issue in equity and it has two aspects how much is spent by Government on publicly funded health care and on what aspects? And secondly, how huge does the burden of treatment fall on the poor seeking health care? Health spending in India at 6% of GDP is among the highest levels estimated for developing countries. In per capita terms it is higher than in China Indonesia and most African countries but lower than in Thailand. Even on PPP $ terms India has been a relatively high spender information sheets based on reporting from a network associating private doctors also as has been done successfully at CMC Vellore in their rural health projects or by the Khoj projects of the Voluntary Health Association of India. It is only through such community-based approach that revitalization of indigenous medicines can be done and people trained in self-care and accept responsibility for their own health.

PHC approach was also intended to test the extent to which non-doctor based health care was feasible through effective down staging of the delivery of simpler aspects of a care as is done in several countries through nurse practitioners and physician assistants, ANMs; physician assistants, etc. can each get trained and recognized to work in allotted areas under referral/supervision of doctors. This may indeed be more acceptable to the medical profession than the draft NHP proposal to restart licentiates in medicine as in the thirties and give them shorter periods of training to serve rural areas. Such a licentiate system cannot now be recalled against the profession's opposition nor would people accept two level services.

Finally, it is important 10 noie some dangers inherem m arrangemenis itiai promote delivery systems substantially outside government channel either through NGOs or through registered societies at State and district levels. Clearly this may by a better approach than leaving it to the market and welcome as path breaking of innovative efforts as a precursor to launching a public program. But as a long-run delivery mechanism it is neither practical nor sustainable as such arrangements tend to bypass government under our constitutional scheme of parliamentary responsibility and would also cut into the potential of panchayatraj institutions. Each major disease control program has now got a separate society at state and district levels often as part of access to foreign aid. What is lost is the principle of parliamentary accountability over the flow of funds that arise out of voted budgets and international agreements to which Government is a party and answerable to parliament. Like campaign modes and vertical interventions, the registered society approach would weaken the long-term commitment and integrity of public health care systems.

SHAPE OF THE PRIVATE SECTOR IN MEDICINE

The key features of the private sector in medical practice and health care are well known. Two questions are relevant. What role should be assigned to it? How far and how closely should it be regulated? Over the last several decades, independent private medical practice has become widespread but has remained stubbornly urban with polyclinics, nursing homes and hospitals proliferating often through doctor entrepreneurs. At our level tertiary hospitals in major cities are in may cases run by business houses and use corporate business strategies and hi-tech specialization to create demand and attract those with effective demand or the critically vulnerable at increasing costs. Standards in some of them are truly world class and some who work there are outstanding leaders in their areas. But given the commodification of medical care as part of a business plan it has not been possible to regulate the quality, accountability and fairness in care through criteria for accreditation, transparency in fees, medical audit, accountable record keeping, credible grievance procedures, etc., such accreditation, standard setting and licensure systems are best done under self-regulation, but self-regulation systems in India medical practice have been deficient in many respects creating problem in credibility. Acute care has become the key priority and continues to attract manpower and investment into related specialty education and facilities for technological improvement. Common treatments, inexpensive diagnostic procedures and family medicine are replaced and priced out of the reach of most citizens in urban areas.

Public health spending accounts for 25% of aggregate expenditure the balance being out of pocket expenditure incurred by patients to private practitioners of various hues. Public spending on health in India has itself declined after liberalization from 1.3% of GDP in 1990 to 0.9% in 1999. Central budg*et al*locations for health have stagnated at 1.3% to total Central budget. In the States it has declined from 7.0% to 5.5.% of State health budget. Consider the contrast with the Bhore Committee recommendation of 15% committed to health from the revenue expenditure budget. Indeed WHO had recommended 55 of GDP for health. The current annual per capita public health expenditure is no more than Rs. 160 and a recent World Bank review showed that over all primary health services account for 58% of public expenditure mostly but on salaries, and the secondary/ tertiary sector for about 38%, perhaps the greater part going to tertiary sector, including government funded medical education. Out of the total primary care spending, as much as 85% was spent on or curative services and only 15% for preventive service. <World Bank 1995> about 47% of total Central and State budget is spent on curative care and health facilities. This may seem excessive at first sight but in face the figure is over 60% in comparable countries, with the bulk of the expenditure devoted publicly funded care or on mandated or voluntary risk pooling methods, in India close to 75% of all household expenditure on health is spend from private funds and the consequent regressive effects on the poor is not surprising.

In this connection. The proposals in the draft NHP 2000 are welcome seeking to restore the key balance towards primary care, and bring it to internationally accepted proportions in the course of this decade.

Private Expenditure Trends

Many surveys confirm that when services are provided by private sector it is largely for ambulatory care and less for inpatient carte. There are variations in levels of cost, pricing, transactional conveniences and quality of services. There is evidence to suggest that disparities in income as such do not make a difference in meeting health care costs, except for catastrophic or life threatening situations. Finally, it has been established that between 2/3rds to 3/4ths of all medical expenditure is spend on privately provided care every household on the average spends up to 10% of annual household consumption in meeting health care needs. This regressive burden shows up vividly in the cycle of incomplete cure followed by recurrence of illness and drug resistance that the poor face in diseases like TB or Kalazar or Malaria especially for daily wage earners who cannot afford to be out of work.

Privatization has to be distinguished from private medical practice which has always been substantial within our mixed economy. What is critical however is the rapid commercialization of private medical practice in particular uneven quality of care. There are complex reasons for this trend. First is the high scarcity cost of good medical education, and second the reward differential between public and corporate tertiary hospitals leading to the reluctance of the young professional to be lured away from the market to public service in rural areas and finally there is the compulsion of returns on investment whenever expensive equipment is installed as part of practice. Increasingly, this has shifted the balance from individual practice to institutionalizes practice, in hospitals, polyclinics, etc. this conjunction explodes into unbearable cost escalation when backed by a third party payer system. This in turn induces increases in insurance premiums making such cover beyond the capacity to pay. There is a distinct possibility of such cycles of cost escalation periodically occurring in the future, promoted further by global transfer of knowledge and software, tele-medicine, etc. especially after the advent of predictive medicine and gene manipulation.

Doctors practicing in the private sector are sometimes accused of prescribing excessive, expensive and risky medicines and with using rampant and less than justified use of technology for diagnosis and treatment. Some method of accreditation of hospitals and facilities and better licensure systems of doctors is likely within a decade. This will enables some moderation in levels of charges in using new technology. High cost of care is sometimes sought to be justified as necessary due to defensive medicine practiced in order to meet risks under the Consumer Protection Act. There is little evidence from decisions of Consumer Courts to justify such fears. While the line between mistaken diagnosis and negligent behaviour will always remain thin, case law has already begun to settle around the doctor's ability to apply reasonable skills and not the highest degree of skill. What has been established is the right of the patient to question the treatment and procedures if there is failure to treat according to standard medical practice or if less than adequate care was taken. As health insurance gets established it may impost more stringent criteria and restrictions on physician performance which may tempt them into defensive medicine. There may also be attempt to collusive capture and (indirect ownership) of insurance companies by corporate hospitals as in other countries. Advances in medical technology are rapid and dominant and easily travel world wide and often seen as good investment and brand equity in the private sector. Private independent practices—and to smaller extent hospitals, dispensaries, nursing homes tele—are seen as markets for medical services with each segment seeking to maximize gains and build mutually supporting links with other segments. More than one study on the quality of care indicates that sometimes more services are performed to maximize revenue, and services/medicines are prescribed which ffl-e not always necessary. Allegations are also widely made of collusive deals between doctors and hospitals with commissions and cuts exchanged to promote needless referral, drugs or procedures <World Bank A 1995> Appropriate regulation is likely in the next decade for minimum standards and accountability and that should consist of a balanced mix of self-regulation external regulation by standard setting and accreditation agencies including private voluntary health insurance.

How far can Health Insurance Help?

What constitutes a fair distribution of the costs of care among different social groups will always be a normative decision emerging out of political debate. It includes risk pooling initiatives for sharing costs among the healthy and the sick leading to insurance schemes as a substitute for or as supplementary to State provision for minimum uniform services. It also covers risk sharing initiatives across wealth and income involving public policy decisions on progressive taxation, merit subsidy and cross-subsidization by dual pricing. Both will continue to be necessary in our conditions with more emphasis on risk sharing as growth picks up. Risk pooling within private voluntary and mandated insurance schemes has become inevitable in all countries because of the double burden of sickness and to ensure that financial costs of treatment do not become an excessive burden relative to incomes. It is difficult but necessary to embed these notions of fair financing into legislation, regulations and schemes and programs equity is aimed at in health care.

With the recent opening up of the general Insurance sector to foreign companies, there is the prospect of two trends. New insurance product will be putout so expand business more be deepening than widening risk covered. The second trend would be to concentrate on urban middle and upper classes and settled jobholders with capacity to pay and with a perceived interest in good health of the family. Both trends make sound business sense in a vast growth market and would increase extensive hospital use and protection against huge hospitalization expenses, and promoted by urban private hospitals since their clientele will increase.

Insurance is a welcome necessary step and must doubtless expand to help in facilitating equitable health care to shift to sections for which government is responsible. Indeed for those not able to access insurance it is government that will have to continue to provide the minimum services, and intervene against market failures including denial through adverse selection or moral hazard. Indeed in the long-run the degree of inequity in health care after insurance systems are set-up will depend ironically on the strength and delivery of the public system as a counterpoise in holding costs and relevance in technology.

The insurable population in India has been assessed at 250 million and at an average of Rs. 1000 per person the premium amount per year would be Rs. 25,000 crores and is expected to treble in ten years. While the insurance product will dutifully reflect the demands of this colossal market and related technological developments in medicine, it should be required to extend beyond hospitalization and cover domiciliary treatment too in a big way; for instance, extending cover to ambulatory maternal and selected chronic conditions like Asthma more prevalent among the poor. The insurance regulatory authority has announced priority in licensing to companies set-up with health insurance as key business and has emphasized the need for developing new products on fair terms to those at risk among the poor and in rural areas. Much will turn on what progress takes place through sound regulation covering aspects indicated below. In order to be socially relevant and cominercially viable the scheme must aim at a proper mix of health hazards and cover many broad social classes and income groups. This is possible in poor locations or communities only if a group view is taken and on chat basis a population-based risk is assessed and community rated premiums determined covering families for all common illnesses and based on epidemiological determined risk. In order that exclusions, co-payments deductibles, etc. remain minimum and relevant to our social situation, some well judged government merit subsidy can be incorporated into anti-poverty family welfare or primary education or welfare pension schemes meant for old age. Innovative community-based new products can be developed by using the scattered experience of such products for instance in SEWA, so that a minimum core cover can be developed as a model for innovative insurance by panchayats with reinsurance backup by companies and government bearing part of promotional costs. The bulk of the formal sector maybe covered by an expanded mandatory insurance with affordable cover and convenient modes of premium payment. Outside the formal manufacturing sector innovate schemes can be designed around specific occupation groups in the informal sector which are steadily becoming a base for old age pension entitlements, as in Kerala and Tamil Nadu—and brought under common risk rating. Finally, as in the West health insurance should develop influence and capacity as bulk purchaser or medical and hospital services to impact on quality and cost and provide greater understanding about Indian health and illness behaviours, patterns of utilization of care and intra-family priorities for accessing medical care. Health insurance should be welcomed as a force for a fairer health care system. But its success should be judged on how well new products are developed with a cover beyond hospitalization, how fairly and inclusively the cover is offered and how far community rated premiums are established. The IRDA has an immense responsibility and with its leadership one can optimistically expect about 30% coverage by 2015 relieving the burden on the public systems.

HEALTH PERCEPTIONS AND PLURAL SYSTEMS

Health perceptions play an important part in ensuring sound health outcomes. To a large extent they are culturally determined but also subject to change with economic growth and social development. People intuitively develop capacity to make choices tor being treated under the western of indigenous systems of medicines, keep a balance between good habits traditionally developed for healthy living and modern lifestyles, decide on where to go for chrome and acute care and how to apportion intra-family utilization of health care resources. The professional is generally bound by his discipline and its inherent logic of causation and effect and tends to discount even what work as successful practice, I fit does not fall within the accepted understanding of his profession. Some movement is occurring among eminent allopathic doctors trying, for instance, to rework Ayurveda theory in a modern idiom starting from respectful reverse analysis for actual successful contemporary practice of Ayurveda and provide a theoretical frame linking it to contemporary needs. There is evidence from public health campaigns in Tamil Nadu where every seventh person spontaneously expressed a preference for Sidda Medicine. Homeopathy for chronic ailment is widely accepted. The herbal base for Ayurvda medicine widely practiced in the Himalayan belt has down world attention a huge export market remains to be tapped according to the knowledgeable trade sources but the danger of bio-privacy remains and legal enablements should be put in place soon that would fully expand on our rights under the WTO agreements. The draft national policy on ISI *v.* IH has attempted to place these plural systems in a modem service delivery and research and education context, it has covered its natural resource base, traditional knowledge base and development of institutions to carry a national heritage forward. There is hope for the survival and growth of the sector only if it becomes an example of convergence between people's and planner's perceptions and ensure its relevance, accountability and affordability to contemporary illnesses and conditions. At the same time it is undeniable that there is much cross practice by ISM practitioners which usually include prescriptions we western medicine as part of indigenous treatment.

Appropriate regulation is needed to protect people from fraud and other dangers but the larger question is how to make the perceptions of the professionals and planners regarding indigenous system of medicine less ambivalent. The separate department for ISM&H should be able to bring about functional integration of ISM and western medicine in service delivery at PHC levels by 2005 whereby it will usher in an uniquely Indian system of care.

EMERGING SCENARIO

What then can we conclude about the prospects of health care in India in 2020? An optimistic scenario will be premised on an average 8% rate of economic growth during this decade and 10% per annum thereafter. If so, what would be the major fall out in terms of results on the health scene? In the first place, longevity estimates can be considered along the following lines. China in 2000 had a life-expectancy at birth of 69 years (M) and 73 years (F) whereas India had respectively 60 (M) and 63 (F). More importantly, healthy life expectancy at birth in China was estimated in the World Health Report 2001 at 61 (M) and 63.3 (F) whereas in India figures were 53 (M) and 51.7 (F). If we look at the percentage of life expectancy years lost as a result of the disease burden and effectiveness of health care systems, Chinese men would have lost 11.6 years against Indian men losing 12.7 years. The corresponding figures are 13.2 for Chinese women and 17.5 for Indian women. Clearly, an integrated approach is necessary to deal with avoidable mortality and morbidity and preventive steps in public health are needed to bridge the gaps, especially in regard to the Indian women. Taking all the factors into consideration, longevity estimates around 20-25 could be around 70 years, perhaps, without any distinction between men and women.

This leads us to the second question of the remaining disease burden in communicable and non-communicable diseases, the effective of interventions, such as, immunization and maternal care and the extent of vulnerability among some groups. These issues have been death with in detail earlier. Clearly an optimistic forecast would envisage success in polio, yaws, leprosy, kalazar, filaria and blindness. As regards TB it is possible to arrest further growth in absolute numbers by 2010 and thereafter to bring it to less than a million within internationally accepted limits by 2020. With regard to Malaria, the incidence can be reduced by a third or even upto half within a decade. In that case, one can expect near freedom from Malaria from most of the countries by 2020. As regards AIDS, it looks unlikely that infection can be leveled of by 2007. The prognosis in regard to the future shape of HIV/AIDS is uncertain. However, it can be a feasible aim to reduce maternal mortality from the present 400 to 100 per lakh population by 2010 and achieve world standards by 2020. As regards child health and nutrition, it is possible to reach IMRV30 per thousand live births by 2010 in most parts of the country though in some areas, it may take a few years more. What is important is the chance of two-thirds decline in moderate malnutrition, and abolition of serious malnutrition completely by 2015 in the case of Cancer, it is feasible to set-up an integrated system for proper screening, early detection, self-care and timely investigation and referral. In the matter of disease burden as a whole, it is feasible to attempt to reach standards comparable to China from 2010 onwards.

Taking the third aspect viz. fairness in financing of health care and reformed structure of health services, an optimistic forecast would be based on the fact that the full potential of the vast public health infrastructure would be fully realized by 2010. its extension to urban areas would be moderated to the extent substantial private provision of health care is available in urban areas, concentrating on its sensible and effective regulation. A reasonably wide network of private voluntary health insurance cover would be available for the bulk of the employed population and there would be models of replicable community-based health insurance available for the unorganized sector. As regards the private sector in medicine, it should be possible in the course of this decade to settle the public role of private medical practice—independent or institutional. For this purpose, more experiments are to be done for promoting public private partnerships, focusing on the issue of how to erect on the basis of shared public health outcome as the key basis for the partnership. A sensible mixture of external regulation and professional self-regulation can be device in the consultation with the profession to ensure competence, quality and accountability. The future of plural systems in medical understanding and evaluation of comparative levels of competence and reliability in different systems—a task in which, the separate department for Indian systems of medicine and homeopathy will play a leading role in inducting quality into the indigenous medical practices.

The next issue relates to the desirable level of public expenditure towards health services. China devotes 4.5% to its G-DP as against India devoting 5.1%. but this hides the fact that in China, public expenditure constitutes 38% whereas in India, it is only 15% of total health expenditure. An optimistic forecast would be that the level of public expenditure will be raised progressively such that about 30% of total health expenditure would be met out of public funds by progressively increasing the health budget in states and the central and charging user fees in appropriate cases. The figure mentioned would perhaps correspond to the proportion of the population which may still need assistance is social development.

Finally it is proper to remember that health is at bottom an issue in justice. It is in this context that we should ask the question as to how far and in what way has politics been engaged m health care? The record is disappointing. Most health sector issues figuring in political debate are those that affect interest groups and seldom central to choices in health care policy. For instance conditions of service and reward systems for Government doctors have drawn much attention often based on inter-service comparison of no wider interest. Inter-system problems of our plural medical care have drawn more attention from courts than from politics.

Hospital management and strikes, poor working of the MCI and corruption in recognition of colleges, dramatic cases of spurious drug supply, etc. have been debated but there has been no sustained attention on such issues as why malaria recrudescence is so common in some parts of India or why complaints about absence of informed consent or frequent in testing on women, or on the variations in prices and availability of essential drugs or for combating epidemic attacks in deprived areas seldom draw attention. The far reaching recommendations made by the Hathi Committee report and or the Lentin Commission report, have been implemented patchily. The role to be assigned to private sector in medicine, the need for a good referral system or the irrationality in drug prescriptions have seldom been the point of political debate. Indeed the lack luster progress of MNP over the Plans shows political disinterest and the only way for politics to become more salient to the health of the poor and the reduction of health inequalities is for a much greater transfer of public resources for provision and financing—as has happened in the West, not only in UK or Canada but in the US itself with a sizable outlay on Medicaid and Medicare.

Index